ADVANCES IN ABDOMINAL SURGERY

ADVANCES IN ABDOMINAL SURGERY

Edited by

Everardo Zanella

Professor of Surgery and Chairman,
Department of Surgery,
University of Rome "Tor Vergata",
Rome, Italy

A survey of researches funded by the Italian Ministry of the University and of Scientific and Technological Research

KLUWER ACADEMIC PUBLISHERS
DORDRECHT / BOSTON / LONDON

A C.I.P. Catalogue record for this book is available from the Library of Congress.

ISBN 0-7923-5988-7

Published by Kluwer Academic Publishers,
P.O. Box 17, 3300 AA Dordrecht, The Netherlands.

Sold and distributed in North, Central and South America
by Kluwer Academic Publishers,
101 Philip Drive, Norwell, MA 02061, U.S.A.

In all other countries, sold and distributed
by Kluwer Academic Publishers,
P.O. Box 322, 3300 AH Dordrecht, The Netherlands.

Printed on acid-free paper

Printed in the Netherlands.

Contents

List of Contributors

D. Altomare
Institute of Surgical Clinics, University of Bari, Bari, Italy
M. Bacosi
Department of Gastroenterology, University of Rome "La Sapienza", Rome, Italy
L. Baldassarri
Laboratory of Ultrastructure, ISS, Rome, Italy
C. Baldi
Institute of Surgical Clinics, University of Siena, Siena, Italy
A. Basoli
2nd Department of Surgery, University of Rome "La Sapienza", Rome, Italy
G. Batignani
Department of Clinical Pathophysiology, Surgical Unit, University of Florence, Florence, Italy
A. Benevento
Department of Surgery, University of Pavia in Varese, Varese, Italy
A. Bertolotti
4th Chair of Surgical Methodology, University of Rome "La Sapienza", Rome, Italy
P. Boccasanta
Department of General Surgery and Surgical Oncology, University of Milan, Milan, Italy
G. Branca
Institute of Microbiology, Catholic University of the Sacred Heart, Rome, Italy
O. Buonomo
Department of Surgery, University of Rome "Tor Vergata", Rome, Italy
G. Carcano
Department of Surgery, University of Pavia in Varese, Varese, Italy
C.U. Casciani
Department of Surgery, University of Rome "Tor Vergata", Rome, Italy
F. Cetta
Institute of Surgical Clinics, University of Siena, Siena, Italy
A. Conti
Department of Surgery and Anesthesiology, 1st Surgical Clinics, University of Bologna, Bologna, Italy
M. Delle Monache
Department of Gastroenterology, University of Rome "La Sapienza", Rome, Italy

M. Di Paola
4th Chair of Surgical Methodology, University of Rome "La Sapienza", Rome, Italy
R. Di Rosa
Department of Clinical Medicine, University of Rome "La Sapienza", Rome, Italy
R. Dionigi
Department of Surgery, University of Pavia in Varese, Varese, Italy
L. Dominioni
Department of Surgery, University of Pavia in Varese, Varese, Italy
GF. Donelli
Laboratory of Ultrastructure, ISS, Rome, Italy
G. Fadda
Institute of Microbiology, Catholic University of the Sacred Heart, Rome, Italy
A.M. Farinon
Department of Surgery, University of Rome "Tor Vergata" , Rome, Italy
F. Fiocca
2nd Department of Surgery, University of Rome "La Sapienza", Rome, Italy
E. Giarnieri
Department of Experimental Medicine, University of Rome "La Sapienza", Rome, Italy
M.R. Giovagnoli
Department of Experimental Medicine, University of Rome "La Sapienza", Rome, Italy
S. Gobbi
Institute of Surgical Clinics, University of Parma, Parma, Italy
V.M. Greco
Department of Surgery and Anesthesiology, 1st Surgical Clinics, University of Bologna, Bologna, Italy
F. Leone
Institute of Microbiology, Catholic University of the Sacred Heart, Rome, Italy
M. Lise
Department of Surgery and Oncology, 2nd Surgical Clinics, University of Padua, Padua, Italy
A. Lombardi
4th Chair of Surgical Methodology, University of Rome "La Sapienza", Rome, Italy
L. Lupo
Institute of Surgical Clinics, University of Bari, Bari, Italy
A. Marchet
Department of Surgery and Oncology, 2nd Surgical Clinics, University of Padua, Padua, Italy

D. Marrano
Department of Surgery and Anesthesiology, 1st Surgical Clinics, University of Bologna, Bologna, Italy
E. Martinelli
Institute of Surgical Clinics, University of Bari, Bari, Italy
V. Mazzarella
Department of Surgery, University of Rome "Tor Vergata", Rome, Italy
P. Mazzella
Institute of Microbiology, Catholic University of the Sacred Heart, Rome, Italy
G. Midiri
4th Chair of Surgical Methodology, University of Rome "La Sapienza", Rome, Italy
G. Montalto
Institute of Surgical Clinics, University of Siena, Siena, Italy
D. Nitti
Department of Surgery and Oncology, 2nd Surgical Clinics, University of Padua, Padua, Italy
G. Nuzzo
Institute of Surgical Pathology, Catholic University of the Sacred Heart, Rome, Italy
O.C. Pannarale
Institute of Surgical Clinics, University of Bari, Bari, Italy
S. Passini
Department of Clinical Pathophysiology, Surgical Unit, University of Florence, Florence, Italy
G. Peloni
Department of Surgery, University of Pavia in Varese, Varese, Italy
Al. Peracchia
Department of General Surgery and Surgical Oncology, University of Milan, Milan, Italy
An. Peracchia
Institute of Surgical Clinics, University of Parma, Parma, Italy
N. Pietra
Institute of Surgical Clinics, University of Parma, Parma, Italy
F. Pisani
Department of Surgery, University of Rome "Tor Vergata", Rome, Italy
F. Puglisi
Institute of Surgical Clinics, University of Bari, Bari, Italy
G.L. Ricci
Department of Gastroenterology, University of Rome "La Sapienza", Rome, Italy
R. Rosati
Department of General and Minimally Invasive Surgery, Hospital "Humanitas", Rozzano (Milan), Italy

M. Roselli
Department of Surgery, University of Rome "Tor Vergata", Rome, Italy
F.A. Rovera
Department of Surgery, University of Pavia in Varese, Varese, Italy
M. Rubino
Institute of Surgical Clinics, University of Bari, Bari, Italy
F. Rulli
Department of Surgery, University of Rome "Tor Vergata" , Rome, Italy
F. Russo
Department of Gastroenterology, *University of Rome "La Sapienza", Rome, Italy*
L. Sarli
Institute of Surgical Clinics, University of Parma, Parma, Italy
G. Serio
Institute of Hygene, University of Bari, Bari, Italy
M. Sianesi
Chair of Surgical Pathology, University of Parma, Parma, Italy
T. Spanu
Institute of Microbiology, Catholic University of the Sacred Heart, Rome, Italy
G. Splendiani
Department of Surgery, University of Rome "Tor Vergata" , Rome, Italy
A. Tesoriere
4th Chair of Surgical Methodology, University of Rome "La Sapienza", Rome, Italy
G. Tisone
CNR, Rome, Italy
F. Tonelli
Department of Clinical Pathophysiology, Surgical Unit, University of Florence, Florence, Italy
C. Tozzo
Department of Surgery, University of Rome "Tor Vergata" , Rome, Italy
A. Vecchione
Department of Experimental Medicine, University of Rome "La Sapienza", Rome, Italy
G. Velardi
Institute of Microbiology, Catholic University of the Sacred Heart, Rome, Italy
G. Vieceli
Department of Surgery and Oncology, 2nd Surgical Clinics, University of Padua, Padua, Italy
E. Zanella
Department of Surgery, University of Rome "Tor Vergata" , Rome, Italy
M. Zuckermann
Institute of Surgical Clinics, University of Siena, Siena, Italy

Foreword

General surgery consists of a main *corpus* of propaedeutic elements and clinical problems, which has been modified over the years by the separate development of numerous sub-specialistic branches.

Although a common basis on the physiopathology of surgical trauma and post-operative complications persists, as a result of general knowledge of surgical diseases, there is no doubt that in the spheres of doctrine and application, both research and clinical medicine have distinguished themselves autonomously in many surgical fields (orthopedics, neurosurgery, cardiovascular surgery, thoracic surgery, urology, etc.).

It is therefore difficult to define the present configuration of general surgery, but without question abdominal surgery occupies a position of pre-eminent importance within the general framework. We are dealing, in fact, with pathological pictures which occur in a section of the body of vast proportions, in which structures, organs, and morphologically complex spaces are arranged to carry out important functions. They are, therefore, subject to considerably complex pathological alterations, such as to establish an interesting field of diagnostic discussion and an exciting training-ground for surgical activity. It can be affirmed that the diagnosis and cures of abdominal surgical diseases constitute a test of the surgeon's experience.

Diagnosis is often entrusted to a differential process, the results of which may be confirmed today by complementary diagnostics . This, however, must be guided by predominating clinical considerations, the exaggerated use of diagnostic techniques, detached from clinical examination, being the cause of very serious errors, which can mislead decision making and human contact, which is the basis of correct medical practice.

It must not be forgotten that the peritoneal cavity and retroperitoneal spaces, with such interesting morpho-functional characteristics, as yet not completely known, are cause of great theoretical and applicational conjecture concerning abdominal surgical diseases; therefore there is still ample space for scientific research in abdominal surgery.

With these objectives, for some years a research programme on national scale has been financed with funds specifically provided by the Italian Ministry of University and of Scientific and Technological Research. The co-ordination of many proposed and partly financed fields of research has been a particularly

demanding task, mainly due to the difficulties of selection, an aspect well known to whoever is involved in promotion of research and evaluation of the results.
Over the years, a number of studies have been abandoned for various reasons, so a selection of research studies originally begun, has been collected in this volume. Frequently it has been a question of auto-selection because the critical process of testing research hypotheses, and analysing procedures and results of the research itself, has permitted many good researchers to reach a conclusion and bring it to the readers attention, only if the production was of quality methodology and had provided tested results, even if they were not always conclusive. The published articles are grouped in Sections, and as from now I can affirm that this is a first part, to be followed by a naturally indispensable sequence, with the results of further studies which are in the process of being completed.
The grouping together of these items of research renders valid the method of co-ordinating subject-matter dealing with a significant section of the human body; if nothing else, because of the clear inter-relations to be found in the clinical courses of diseases of different nature and origin. Is not this the reason for elaborating hypotheses , especially in experimental research, which then meet with positive responses in the clinical field?
For example, I believe that the subject of infections never loses interest, due to a constant renewal of problems of pathogenesis , epidemiology and evolution as they occur, above all, in specific topographical areas such as in peritoneal cavities or in retroperitoneal spaces, in parenchymatous organs like the pancreas or hollow viscus like the gallbladder. As a natural consequence, the branch of surgery dealing with the liver and pancreas earnestly proposes further physiopathological studies of the great important syndromes, which are characteristic of parenchymatous and hollow viscus, both in inflammatory and degenerative or neoplastic pathology.
Colorectal surgery is rich in subject-matter to be studied, conveniently coinciding with advances in the field of immunology, which serve both diagnostic and therapeutic ends, also with suggestions for new surgical approaches.
Surgical techniques must necessarily be valued also in the sphere of their application, and for results achieved, in minimally invasive surgery: an intentionally critical contribution can only show how valid this particular trend may be, above all as applied to abdominal surgery.
Concerning transplants of abdominal organs, we cannot ignore the need for professional preparation that should be not exaggeratedly specialistic, but sufficiently extensive to comply with general surgery education, which is beneficiary in organ transplantation.
Though as yet an uncompleted mosaic, I believe that the programme of research in abdominal surgery has provided good quality first results, such as to justify the choice of the theme, and to motivate good researchers to continue carrying out

scientific and technological research in accordance with the intentions of the Ministry of the University.
The satisfaction accorded me by this collection will be completed with future contributions, but above all by the opinions of surgeons involved in research, who read these chapters.

EVERARDO ZANELLA
Professor of General Surgery
University of Rome "Tor Vergata"

Scientific Secretariat

A.M.FARINON
F.RULLI
M.LAZZARI

Department of Surgery
University of Rome "Tor Vergata"
Rome, Italy

Acknowledgments
We are indebted with Mrs. W Rubertelli for secretarial assistance, and with Mrs. M. A. Smith for english revision.

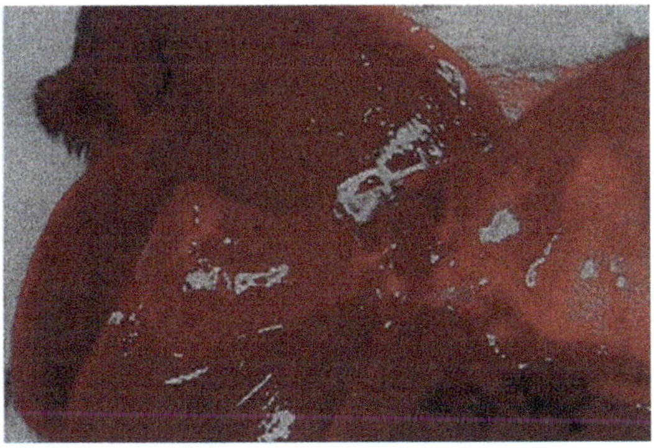

Figure 1. Acute cholecystitis in the Guinea pig. Note the intense redness of the viscus post mortem specimen. (From p. 35)

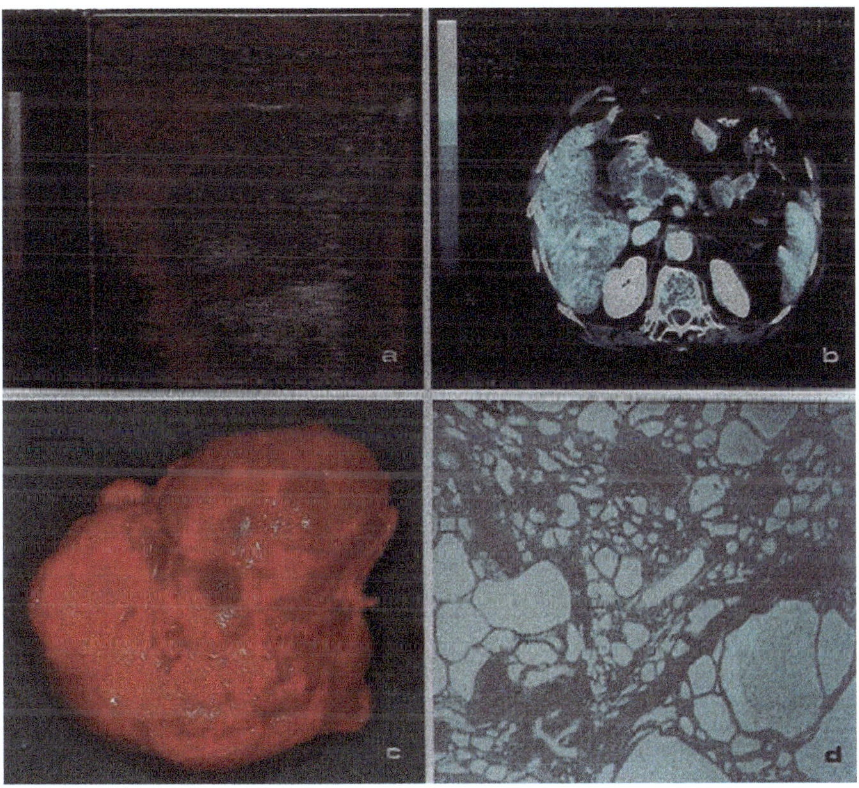

Figure 1. Case n.8 : M.I. , 65 year old female. Ultrasound (a) and C.T. scan (b) show a serous cystadenoma located in the neck and body of the pancreas; the gross appearance of the surgical specimen (c), obtained by middle pancreatic resection, is characterized by numerous small cysts; histological features (d) display cysts containing flocculent material. (From p. 83)

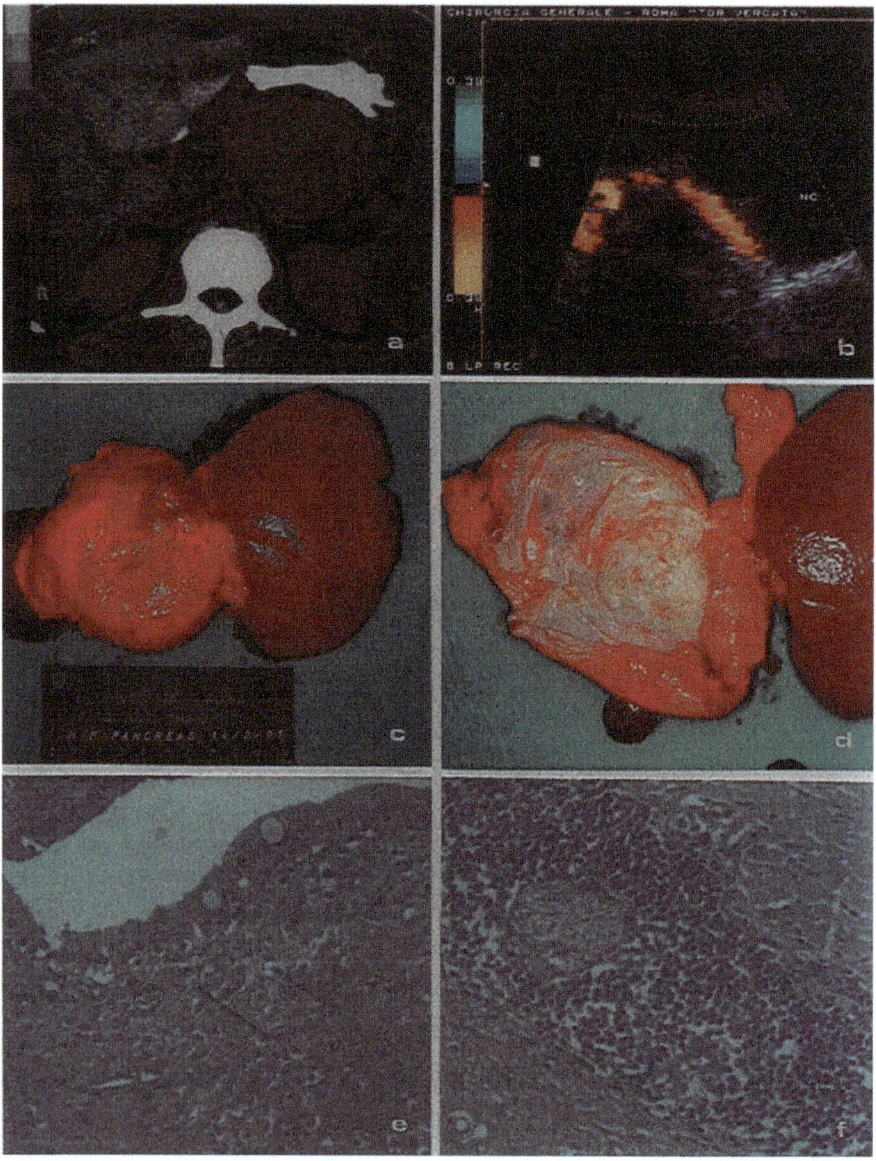

Figure 2. Case n.7 :P.N. **32** year-old female.C.T.scan (a) and echo-color-doppler (b) show a cystic biloculated mass of the pancreatic tail; grown features of the outer (c) and cut (d) surface of the surgical specimen are detailed, as well as histological appearances demonstrating a mucinous cystic neoplasm of the pancreas with ovarian-like stroma (e) and with adjacent fibrotic tissue exhibiting focal perineural pseudoinvasion (f) (From p. 85)

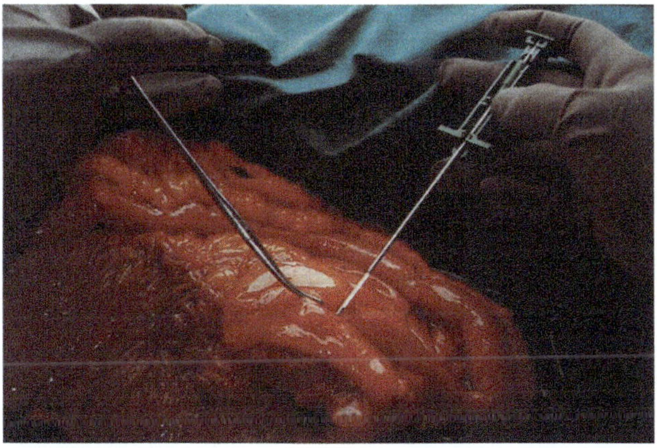

Figure 1. Therefore the eleven T3 colo-rectal cancer patients of this study were also evaluated by means of multiple full thickness sampling performed by inserting a 14 gauge trucut from the outside of the sierosa through the tumour as far as the lumen. (From p. 170)

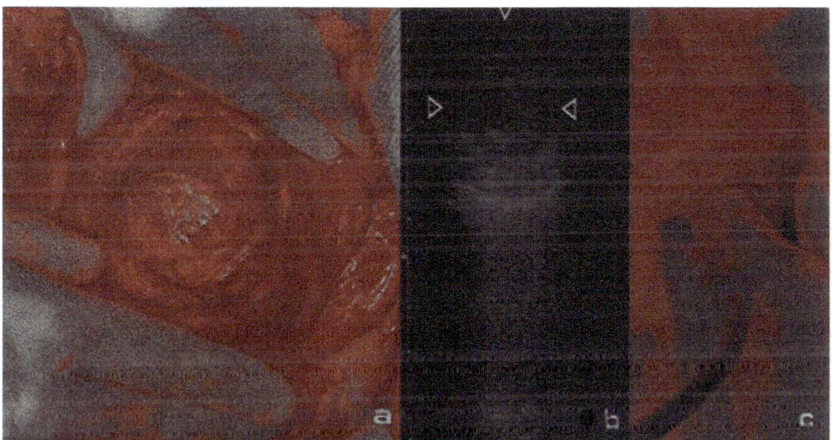

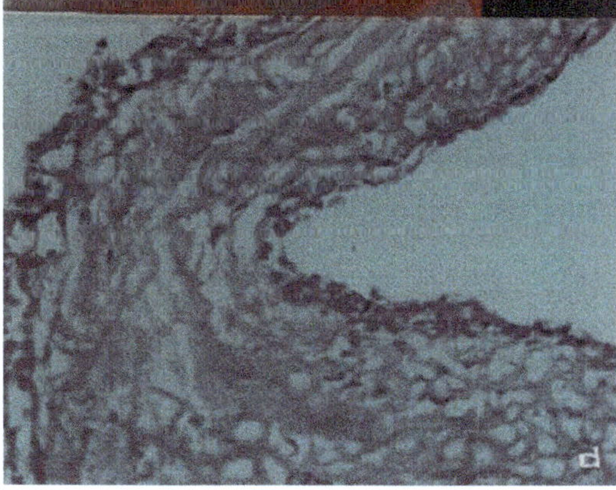

Figure 3. Case n. 9: A.I. ,73 year old female.Intra-operative findings (a) of a mass in the pancreatic head, which revealed microcystic features at intra-operative ultrasonography (b,c), with a cytologically benign appearance (d).
(From p. 91)

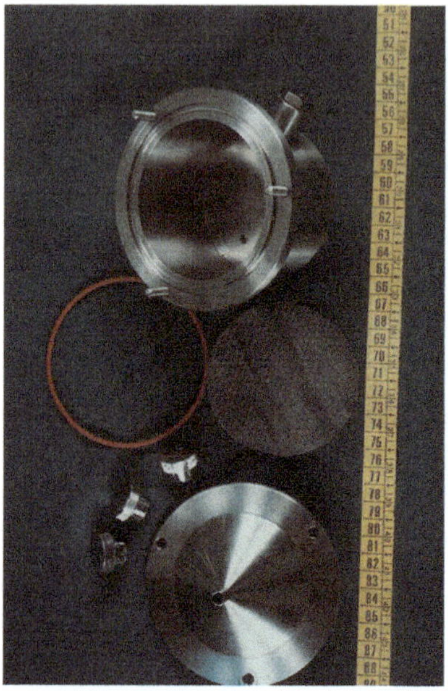

Figure 4a

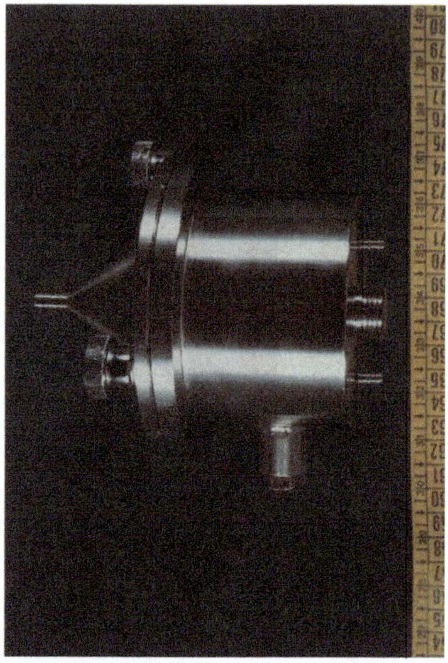

Figure 4b

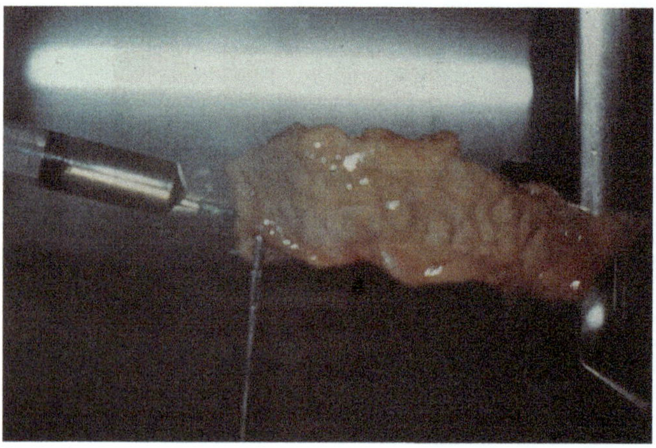

Figure 3

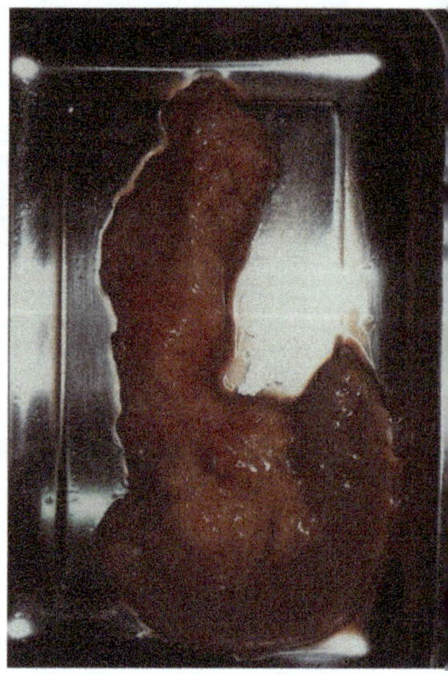

Figure 1

Figure 4. Upper and lower components of stainless steel isolation chamber, separated by a micropore screen allowing passage of particles below 400 micron in size (a). Assembled chamber (b). (From p. 228)

Figure 3. Marked gland distension induced by intraductal collagenase injection. (From p. 227)

Figure 1. Duodeno-pancreatic bloc without vascular pedicles, at the end of the harvesting phase. (From p. 225)

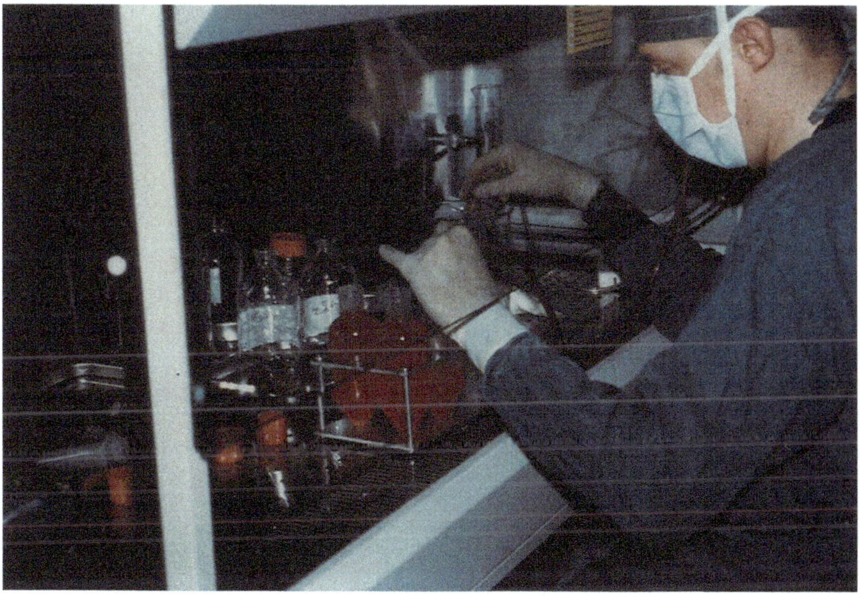

Figure 12. Preparation of the solutions necessary for pancreas digestion in a laminar flow room. (From p. 236)

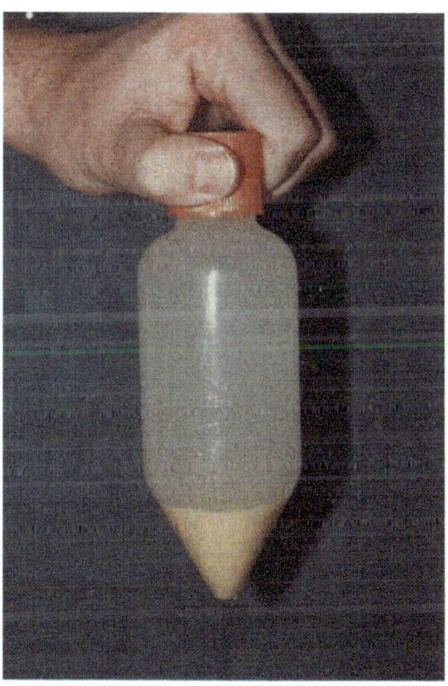

Figure 6. Post-centrifugation Corning tube containing mixed pancreatic material pelleted at the bottom (From p. 230)

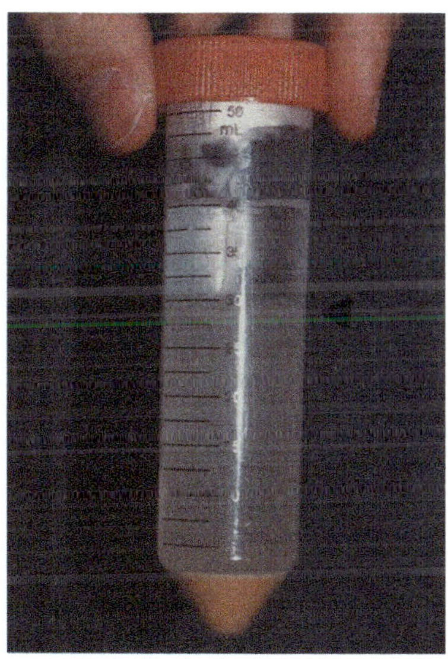

Figure 7. At the end of the purification phase, islets are pelleted at the interface between Ficoll solutions 1096 and 1037. Non-islet material is deposited at the bottom. (From p. 231)

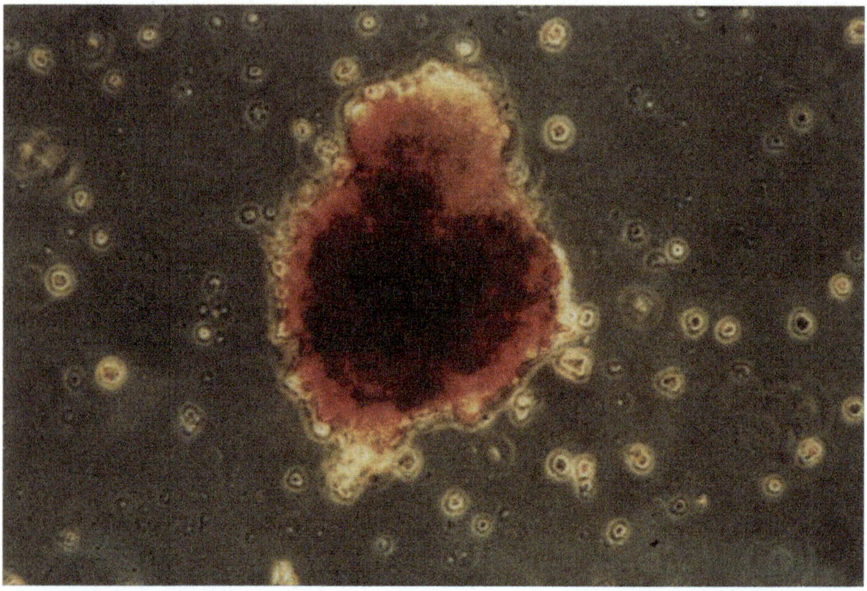

Figure 5. Dithizone stained pancreatic islet observed with inverted light microscopy at the end of digestion. (From p. 229)

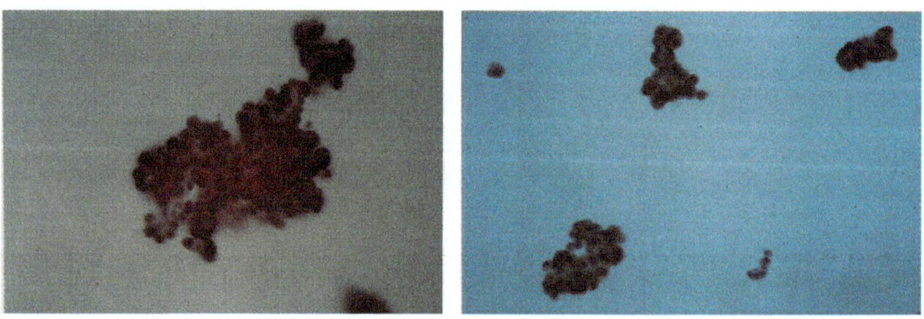

a b

Figure 13 . Identification of intact islets: normal nucleus/cytoplasm ratio, normal nucleus and intercellular contacts. No pyknosis and/or intracellular necrosis and no cytoplasmatic degeneration (40x magnification) (a). By immmunohistochemical analysis with antichromogranin A antibody, islet cells are identified that are rich intracytoplasmic granules (25x magnification) (b). (From p. 237)

CHAPTER 1

INFECTED PANCREATIC NECROSIS COMPLICATED BY MULTIPLE ORGAN FAILURE.

LORENZO DOMINIONI, ANGELO BENEVENTO, GIULIO CARCANO, GIUSEPPE PELONI, and RENZO DIONIGI

Department of Surgery, University of Pavia in Varese, Varese, Italy

Summary

Sixteen patients with severe bacteriologically proven infected pancreatic necrosis (IPN) undergoing sequential surgical treatment were studied in prospective. The severity of IPN was documented prior to operation with the following scores: 1) degree of necrosis by CT scan [< 30% in three patients (19%); 30 - 50% in nine patients (56%); > 50% in four patients (25%)]; 2) Elebute and Stoner's sepsis score (16±4 points); 3) Goris'score of multiple organ failure (MOF) (5±2 points).

Sequential surgical treatment was carried out by the same surgical team, as follows: 1) abdominal laparotomy second look through a zipper for the first 7-10 days; 2) open abdomen and repeated peritoneal debridements for the following 7-10 days; 3) continuous closed peritoneal lavage with multiple drainage, until eradication of infection (range: 15-85 days).

No patient required further re-exploration. Mortality occurred in 3/16 patients (19%), due to MOF in all 3 cases. The 13 survivors (81%) were discharged convalescent with closed abdominal wound, feeding orally, after 73±33 days, without fistulae.

These results indicate that by treating severe IPN with the technique of sequential abdominal laparatomy second look, open drainage and continuous closed lavage, a low 19% mortality can be achieved. This study also provides an assessment of the pre-operative severity of sepsis and of MOF in every patient with IPN; these data could facilitate future comparison with results obtained with other treatment modalities.

Key Words: Infected pancreatic necrosis; sequential surgical treatment; sepsis score, MOF, APACHE II.

Introduction

Severe forms of acute pancreatitis, characterized by infected necrosis and haemorrhage, are relatively uncommon, occurring in approximately 3-15% of patients with acute pancreatic inflammation [1,2]. Aggressive multimodal therapy in the early stage of severe necrotizing pancreatitis improves survival, patients with septic complications, however, tend to die from multiple organ failure (MOF) at a later stage [3,4]. The site of necrosis, especially if located in the head of the pancreas, was recently confirmed as correlating with disease severity, by

E. Zanella (ed.), Advances in Abdominal Surgery, 1–11.

Kemppainen et al. [5].
The reported mortality rates of infected pancreatic necrosis (IPN) range widely, from 20 to 70% [6]; such difference in outcome obviously relates to the variable severity of pancreatic disease, and possibly also to differences in modalities of surgical treatment. In recent years acute pancreatitis complicated by infection has been classified into 3 categories, according to clinical, morphological, and laboratory criteria: 1) infected pancreatic necrosis (IPN); 2) pancreatic abscess (PA); 3) infected pseudocyst [9]. Such classification is of prognostic relevance; in fact the mortality rate of IPN is much higher than that of pancreatic abscess and of infected pseudocyst [7,8].
Three main patterns of surgical treatment of IPN are currently widely used: 1) "conventional treatment" , consisting of pancreatic necrosectomy and multiple drainage; 2) necrosectomy followed by "continuous lavage" of the peritoneum and of the involved retroperitoneal area; 3) "open abdominal handling", consisting of pancreatic necrosectomy, followed by various combinations of planned or staged re-operation for peritoneal debridement. The results of these strategies were reviewd by D'Egidio and Schein [2] in 1991: mortality rates of documented IPN after "conventional treatment", "continuous lavage" and "open abdominal management" were 42% (range, 24-48), 18% (range, 14-27) and 21% (range, 11-55) respectively. The results of these treatments, however, cannot be compared objectively; in fact in most previous reports the severity of IPN, which obviously affects survival, had not been assessed with adequate indices prior to operation [2,4,9].The purpose of the present prospective study is to describe the results of our modality of sequential surgical treatment of IPN complicated by MOF, in 16 patients for whom specific scoring systems were used for the prior to operation assessment of the severity of sepsis and of MOF.

Material and methods

Patients
From 1988 to 1996, 16 consecutive patients [12 M, 4 F; mean age: 54±10 years (range, 34 - 70 years)] with infected (peri)pancreatic necrosis (IPN) complicated by MOF were treated prospectively at the Department of Surgery of the University of Pavia in Varese, by the same surgical team (R.Dionigi as operator or supervisor), with the sequential technique of necrosectomy, abdominal re-laparotomy, open abdomen and continuous closed lavage, as described in detail below.
The patients were referred to our Department, after initial medical treatment carried out in other hospitals had failed to control the progression of pancreatic inflammation. The cause of pancreatitis was gallstones in seven patients (44%), post-surgical or post-ERCP in four patients (25%) and idiopathic in five cases (31%) (Table 1).

TABLE 1. CLINICAL DATA AND OUTCOME OF 16 PATIENTS WITH INFECTED PANCREATIC NECROSIS.

Patient No./Sex	Age (Years)	Aetiology of Pancreatitis	Organ Failures	No. of Re-explorations in Theatre	Outcome	Intensive Care Unit Stay (Days)	Postop. Day of Discharge
P.P. 1/M	34	Idiopathic	Respiratory, renal, cardiovasc.	6	Survived	42	135
L.G. 2/M	44	Biliary	Respiratory, renal, hepatic	5	Survived	8	37
S.A. 3/M	55	Post-surgery	Hepatic, renal, centr. nerv. syst.	9	Survived	12	95
M.G. 4/F	59	Post-surgery	Respiratory, renal	6	Died (MOF)	11(11)*	/
C.S. 5/M	45	Post-surgery	Respiratory, renal, hepatic	9	Survived	14	33
C.G. 6/M	56	Biliary	Respiratory, renal, cardiovasc., centr. nerv. syst.	8	Died (MOF)	17(32)*	/
C.A. 7/M	59	Biliary	Respiratory, renal, cardiovasc.	12	Survived	20	31
B.F. 8/M	50	Biliary	Respiratory, hepatic, haematologic	7	Survived	10	101
B.D. 9/F	70	Idiopathic	Respiratory, cardiovasc., haematologic	20	Survived	31	71
N.F. 10/M	59	Biliary	Respiratory, renal, cardiovasc., hepatic	10	Died (MOF)	72(122)*	/
L.A. 11/F	58	Post-ERCP	Respiratory, renal	10	Survived	57	94
S.D. 12/F	37	Biliary	Respiratory, centr. nerv. syst., haematologic	7	Survived	39	82
F.D. 13/M	63	Idiopathic	Respiratory, renal, hepatic, centr. nerv. syst.	9	Survived	64	113
C.C. 14/M	52	Biliary	Respiratory, cardiovasc., haematologic	4	Survived	28	74
P.A. 15/M	55	Idiopathic	Respiratory, hepatic, cardiovasc., haematologic	7	Survived	24	45
G.L. 16/M	47	Idiopathic	Cardiovasc., haematologic	3	Survived	16	39
Mean±SD	54±10	//	//	8±4	//	29±20(°)	73±33

( )* Postoperative day of death
(°) Mean value for survivors

Clinical management

After the initial diagnosis of acute pancreatitis, all patients had previously undergone intensive medical treatment in primary referral hospitals, with fluid-electrolyte resuscitation, nasogastric aspiration, parenteral nutrition, wide spectrum antibiotics and somatostatin. The clinical course of the disease had been monitored by ultrasonography and by CT scans repeated at short intervals.

Infection of pancreatic necrosis, that complicated the course of acute pancreatitis, was initially suspected on the basis of clinical and laboratory signs of sepsis. Lack of contrast enhancement in computerized tomography (CTCE) reinforced the clinical suspect of IPN, and this was the finding that usually prompted surgical treatment. The decision to operate and to carry out the sequential procedure of surgical treatment of the abdomen, was made when all of the following three criteria were met with: 1) persistent physical signs of peritonitis; 2) deterioration of laboratory indices of pancreatitis (elevated CRP, leukocytosis); 3) worsened CTCE of the pancreas, with contrast enhancement documenting peripancreatic inflammation and/or fluid collections. Due to the severity of the illness, treatment with abdominal re-exploration began shortly after admission (1 - 3 days) to our Department; at the onset of our surgical treatment the patients presented the organ failures indicated in Table 1.The interval between clinical onset of pancreatitis and beginning of sequential surgical treatment of IPN in our Department ranged from 1 to 11 weeks (an average of: 4 weeks). At laparotomy, all patients presented multiple foci of necrotic pancreatic and peripancreatic tissue, diffused signs of pancreatic inflammation and turbid or purulent exudate, not walled-off by granulation tissue. The diagnosis of IPN was confirmed by bacterial culture of necrotic pancreatic tissue, following the criteria proposed by Frey et al. [10].

Microbiological culture of (peri)pancreatic necrotic tissue revealed multiple bacterial flora in 12 patients (75%) and a single pathogen in 4 patients; in three patients (19%) C. albicans was isolated with other pathogens (Table 2).

Grading of IPN severity

The severity of IPN was assessed prior to operation by using multiple scoring methods. According to the CT grading of Balthazar et al. [11], grade C (diffused pancreatic and peripancreatic inflammation) was seen in four patients; grades D and E (one or more peripancreatic fluid collections) were observed in the other twelve patients.

Furthermore, the percentage of pancreatic necrosis was estimated by CTCE, by the ratio of decreased contrast enhancement in the area of normally perfused pancreas, as described by Ranson et al. [12]: in 3 patients (19%) the pancreatic necrosis was less than 30%; in 9 patients (56%) it ranged from 30 to 50% and in four patients (25%) it was more than 50%. In order to quantify the overall severity of the disease due to systemic complications of IPN, each patient was further assessed with a Sepsis Score [13], a MOF score [14] and with an APACHE II score [15], just before the beginning of open surgical treatment

TABLE 2. BACTERIAL AND FUNGAL ISOLATES IN THE 16 PATIENTS WITH IPN.

Isolate	Patient with Isolated Pathogens
Staphylococcus aureus	9
Pseudomonas aeruginosa	5
Candida albicans	3
Enterococcus faecalis	3
Escherichia coli	3
Klebsiella pneumoniae	2
Acinetobacter	2
Staphylococcus haemoliticus	2
Streptococcus cohni	1
Pseudomonas maltophylia	1
Bacteroides	1
Serratia spp.	1
Hafnia alvei	1
Enterococcus faecium	1
Morganella morganii	1
Tularensis glabrata	1
Enterobacter	1

(baseline measurements). The mean baseline scores were high (Sepsis Score: 16±4; MOF score: 5±2; APACHE II score: 11±3) (Table 3), indicating a high risk of mortality [14,16].

TABLE 3. ASSESSMENT OF SEVERITY OF INFECTED PANCREATIC NECROSIS BY SCORING SYSTEMS AT ONSET OF SURGICAL TREATMENT.

Patient No. / Sex	Age (Years)	Aetiology of Pancreatitis	Balthazar CT Grade	Pancreatic Necrosis % (CT Evaluation)	APACHE II Score	Sepsis Score	MOF Score
P.P. 1 / M	34	Idiopathic	E	30-50	14(°)	21	6
L.G. 2 / M	44	Biliary	D	30-50	8(°)	9	5
S.A. 3 / M	55	Post-surgery	D	<30	12(°)	15	5
M.G. 4 / F	59	Post-surgery	D	30-50	12(*)	15	4
C.S. 5 / M	45	Post-surgery	C	<30	10(°)	17	4
C.G. 6 / M	56	Biliary	C	30-50	15(*)	14	8
C.A. 7 / M	59	Biliary	C	30-50	10(°)	9	5
B.F. 8 / M	50	Biliary	C	<30	11(°)	8	5
B.D. 9 / F	70	Idiopathic	E	30-50	14(°)	18	6
N.F. 10 / M	59	Biliary	E	>50	14(*)	22	6
L.A. 11 / F	58	Post-ERCP	E	30-50	12(°)	20	2
S.D. 12 / F	37	Biliary	E	>50	12(°)	17	6
F.D. 13 / M	68	Idiopathic	E	30-50	16(°)	22	6
C.C. 14 / M	62	Biliary	D	>50	8(°)	20	5
P.A. 15 / M	55	Idiopathic	E	>50	4(°)	18	3
G.L. 16 / M	47	Idiopathic	D	30-50	6(°)	17	2
Mean±SD	54±10	//	//	//	11±3(°)	16±4	5±2

Mean APACHE II score of *survivors* (°) vs. *non survivors* (*): 11±3 vs. 14±1; P>0.05; difference not significant.

Sequential surgical treatment

Access to the pancreatic area was obtained through a bilateral subcostal or midline laparotomy, depending on the topographic area involved by necrosis, as documented by CTCE. The lesser sac was exposed by dividing the gastrocolic omentum, by entering the peripancreatic retroperitoneal space through the root of the transverse mesocolon, and by mobilizing the duodenum with the Kocher manoeuvre. The diagnosis of IPN was confirmed on finding foul-smelling necrotic pancreatic and peripancreatic tissue, associated with turbid or purulent fluid collections, and by microbiological culture. The head, body and tail of the pancreas were exposed and necrosectomy was performed. Debridement of portions of necrotic pancreatic and peripancreatic tissue was carried out whenever possible along a demarcation cleavage between viable and necrotic tissue,by digitoclasia, and by using the cannula of the aspirator as a dissector. The use of sharp instruments was spared, to avoid injury to the surrounding structures and to limit bleeding. The lesser sac, the pancreatic bed and the peritoneal recesses were thoroughly lavaged with several liters of saline, until a clear lavage solution was aspirated. Multiple abdominal drains with side holes were placed respectively: in the lesser sac through the transverse mesocolon, and through the divided gastrocolic omentum; in the inframesocolic space; in the right and left para-colic gutters. In addition, several long gauze packs were placed in the pancreatic bed after necrosectomy, and were brought out of the abdominal cavity at the corners of laparotomy.

At the end of the surgical procedure an abdominal wound zipper (Ethizip™) was sutured to the fascial margins of the laparotomy, to facilitate planned reopening of the abdominal cavity. Planned abdominal re-explorations, debridement and lavage of the lesser sac and of peripancreatic tissues were carried out every 24-48 hours during the first week of treatment; and subsequently every 72 hours, or at longer intervals, depending on the clinical course of each patient. During peritoneal debridement great care was taken to avoid injury to the jejunum and colon, using only the fingers to separate the intestinal loops and to find the cleavage planes leading to the pancreatic bed. At the time of each abdominal re-exploration the gauze packs were removed (and replaced, if necessary, to control bleeding); the peritoneum, the pancreatic and peripancreatic tissues were debrided of all necrotic tissue which could be separated without causing excessive bleeding; lavage of the peritoneum and retroperitoneal space was carried out; the patency of drainage tubes was controlled. After the initial 7-10 days of abdominal explorations, the zipper was removed, the wound was left open, and repeated peritoneal debridements were carried out for another 7-10 days. Subsequently, when two consecutive explorations failed to demonstrate significant residual necrotic tissue, and granulation tissue began to appear in the pancreatic bed, the wound was closed; if this was not feasible, the wound edges were approximated by sutures at the corners of the incision. Aseptic dressings with plastic drapes and gauzes were placed; the drainage tubes were left in place and were used to carry out continuous closed peritoneal and retroperitoneal lavage. with 5 - 15 liters of saline solution daily, until turbid fluid flowed out.

During sequential surgical treatment all patients underwent conventional multimodal medical therapy of septic pancreatitis, including total parenteral nutrition, wide spectrum antibiotics and somatostatin; supportive treatment of organ failures was carried out.

Results

The demographic and clinical data and the outcome of the 16 patients with IPN are presented in Tables 1, 3 and 4.

TABLE 4. MAJOR COMPLICATIONS AND OUTCOME.

Patient No. / Sex	Major Complications	Outcome
P.P. 1 / M	Diabetes, pancreatic fistula	Survived
L.G. 2 / M	None	Survived
S.A. 3 / M	Pancreatic fistula, severe bleeding	Survived
M.G. 4 / F	Septicemia, septic shock	Died (MOF)
C.S. 5 / M	None	Survived
C.G. 6 / M	Septicemia, septic shock	Died (MOF)
C.A. 7 / M	Pseudocyst	Survived
B.F. 8 / M	Pseudocyst	Survived
B.D. 9 / F	Pneumonia	Survived
N.F. 10 / M	Septicemia. septic shock	Died (MOF)
L.A. 11 / F	None	Survived
S.D. 12 / F	Severe bleeding, enteric fistula	Survived
F.D. 13 / M	None	Survived
C.C. 14 / M	Septicemia, pneumonia	Survived
P.A. 15 / M	Septicemia, severe bleeding, enteric fistula	Survived
G.L. 16 / M	Septicemia	Survived

The mean number of abdominal explorations per patient was 8+4 The duration of subsequent continuous lavage ranged from 15-85 days. The major complications observed during sequential surgical treatment were: septicemia (positive blood culture) in 6 patients (38%); severe bleeding in 3 patients (19%); pneumonia in 3 patients (19%); pancreatic fistula in 2 patients (13%); enteric fistula in 2 patients (13%); pseudocyst in 2 patients (13%); severe diabetes in 1 patient (6%).

The three patients with life-threatening bleeding required massive blood transfusion and emergency re-operation to control haemorrhage; all three patients survived. The four fistulae observed (2 pancreatic, 2 enteric) healed spontaneously before hospital discharge, with prolonged total parenteral nutrition.

Mortality was 3/16 patients (19%), due to MOF in all three cases. The mean duration of Intensive Care Unit (ICU) stay of survivors was 29±20 days.The 13 survivors (81%) were discharged with closed abdominal wound, feeding orally, after 73±33 days (Table 1).

Discussion

Trends in the treatment of septic complications of necrotizing pancreatitis have evolved in the last decade, as progress has been made in the evaluation of pathological changes occurring in the pancreas and in the peripancreatic tissues. Computerized tomography with contrast enhancement (CTCE) [12] and bacteriology by percutaneous aspiration of peripancreatic fluid collections [17,18] are especially important in order to obtain a precise diagnosis and assessment of the severity of pancreatic necrosis.

The important differential diagnosis between IPN and pancreatic abscess can be made on the basis of CTCE findings, although these two types of infections are practically indistinguishable in clinical and laboratory findings. IPN usually runs a much more severe clinical course than pancreatic abscess, and is associated with a greater risk of mortality [7,8].

The pancreatitis score described by Ranson in 1976 [19] is not useful in assessing the severity of established IPN. Indeed that score refers to the pathophysiological alterations detected during the first 48 hours from the clinical onset of pancreatitis, whereas surgical treatment of IPN is usually carried out from one to several weeks later.

We used several scoring systems for the grading of IPN severity, including radiological scores, the sepsis score and the MOF score. The criteria established in recent years for diagnosing the severity of IPN include also determination of the APACHE II score [4,15,22].

In our experience, however, the APACHE II score was not a reliable index of severity of IPN, when measured just before starting surgical treatment. In fact, at that time point of the clinical evolution of IPN, when MOF has already developed, the APACHE II score of non-survivors is not significantly different from the score of survivors (Table 3).

Moreover, a review of literature on APACHE II scores in patients with IPN, clearly shows that there is no correlation between scores and mortalities (Table 5). Furthermore, it is difficult to explain the large variability of the mean pre-operative APACHE II score of non-surviving patients in different studies (Table 5).

Therefore, the real value of using the APACHE II score for the grading of IPN is questionable; the structure of that scoring system in fact includes neither clinical indicators of infection, nor indices of the local anatomic alterations of sepsis [16], which are very relevant in IPN patients.

TABLE 5. PRE-OPERATIVE APACHE II SCORE AND MORTALITY OF PATIENTS WITH IPN. COMPARISON OF LITERATURE REPORTS.

Author	No. of Patients	Mean Age (Years)	Mean APACHE II Score of All Patients	Mean APACHE II Score of Non-Survivors	Mortality (%)
Van Goor et al., 1996 (21)	10	51	19	23	30
Doglietto et al., 1994 (20)	42	59	17	22	25
Fugger et al., 1991 (4)	63	N.A.	17	22	32
Larvin et al., 1989 (3)	14	51	16	28	21
Beger et al., 1995 (*)	77	N.A.	12	N.A.	21
Wilson et al., 1990 (22)	38	N.A.	11	14	34
Dominioni et al., 1996	16	54	11	14	19

(*) Reported by B.Rau at the VIIIth Post-graduate Course of Pancreatic Surgery, held in Ulm (Germany), June 12-14, 1995. N.A.: not available.

To assess the severity of the septic state in the present study, we used the sepsis score of Elebute and Stoner [13,16]; the pre-operative mean sepsis score of 16±4 in our patients correlated well with a predicted mortality of approximately 25%, based on previous retrospective studies [16]. The pre-operative sepsis score value of 16±4 in our group, moreover, is identical to that of the IPN patients reported by Larvin et al. [3]; the mortality rates in these two patient series are remarkably similar (19% and 21%, respectively).

The severity of MOF has rarely been taken into consideration, in assessing patients at the beginning of treatment of IPN; different levels of MOF might account for the great differences in death rates reported for the same disease,"infected pancreatitis", by different authors. The mean MOF score of 5±2 in our series is high [14]; this score provides a further quantification of IPN severity, not previously reported in literature on IPN.

According to our sequential surgical technique, peritoneal explorations were carried out every 24-48 hours during the first week of treatment; subsequently, longer intervals were observed (usually 72 hours), based on the individual patient's clinical course. With this surgical strategy, the clinical outcome of patients compared favourably with other literature reports, in terms of both complication rate and survival [3,4,20,22]. The technical complications that we observed (2 pancreatic fistulae, 2 enteric fistulae and 3 severe bleedings) were treated successfully during hospital stay; the limited number of enteric fistulae, as compared to other reports, is probably due to special care in avoiding intestinal damage while debriding adhesions and necrotic tissue.

Mortality in our series of patients with IPN was 19%, ranking among the lowest reported (Table 5). The mean length of hospital stay in our study was 73±33 days, remarkably similar to the 78 days reported by Doglietto et al. with the open abdomen method of treatment [20] and to the 79 days reported by Larvin et al. with the technique of debridement and closed irrigation [3].

The question of the superiority of one over other surgical treatments of IPN remains unsettled, in spite of numerous reports on the subject [9]. The controversy remains mainly because it is very difficult, and perhaps impossible to compare results obtained with different techniques of treatment of IPN. In fact, a clear distinction between the results obtained in patients with IPN, and in pancreatic abscess cases, is not available for most reported series of necrotic pancreatitis treated surgically.

Moreover, it has already been underlined by others [2] that the wide range of IPN survivals achieved by different authors with various approaches, could be due not only to the facilities and surgical skills available in the various centers, but also to important differences in the severity of IPN.

To our knowledge, the presently reported series of 16 IPN cases is the first that stages the severity of IPN in each patient, not only by means of CTCE grading, but also by the sepsis score and the MOF score; hopefully these scores should facilitate comparison between results of different methods of treatment of IPN.

References

1. Widdison AL, Karanjia ND. Pancreatic infection complicating acute pancreatitis. *Br J Surg* 1993; 80: 148-54.

2. D'Egidio A, Schein M. Surgical strategies in the treatment of pancreatic necrosis and infection. *Br J Surg* 1991; 78: 133-7.

3. Larvin M, Chalmers AG, Robinson PJ et al. Debridement and closed cavity irrigation for the treatment of pancreatic necrosis. *Br J Surg* 1989; 76: 465-71.

4. Fugger R, Schulz F, Rogy M et al. Open approach in pancreatic and infected pancreatic necrosis: laparostomies and preplanned revisions. *World J Surg* 1991; 15: 516-21.

5. Kemppainen E, Sainio V, Haapiainen R et al. Early localization of necrosis by contrast-enhanced computed tomography can predict outcome in severe acute pancreatitis. *Br J Surg* 1996; 83: 924-9.

6. Urbach DR, Marshall JC. Pancreatic abscess and infected pancreatic necrosis. *Curr Opinion Surg Infections* 1996; 4: 57-66.

7. Fedorak IJ, KO TC, Djuricin G et al. Secondary pancreatic infections: are they distinct clinical entities? *Surgery* 1992; 112: 824-30.

8. Bradley EL III. Management of infected pancreatic necrosis by open drainage. *Ann Surg* 1987; 206: 542-50.

9. Bradley EL III. A fifteen year experience with open drainage for infected pancreatic necrosis. *Surg Gynecol Obstet* 1993; 177: 215-22.
10. Frey CF, Bradley EL III, Beger HG. Progress in acute pancreatitis. *Surg Gynecol Obstet* 1988; 167: 282-6.
11. Balthazar EJ, Ranson JHC, Naidich DP et al. Acute pancreatitis prognostic value of CT. *Radiology* 1985; 156: 767-72.
12. Ranson JHC, Balthazar E et al. Computed tomography and the prediction of pancreatic abscess in acute pancreatitis. *Ann Surg* 1985; 201: 656-63.
13. Elebute EA, Stoner HB. The grading of sepsis. *Brit J Surg* 1983; 70: 29-31.
14. Goris RJA, Boekhorst TPA, Nuytinck JKS et al. Multiple-organ failure. *Arch Surg* 1985; 120: 1109-15.
15. Knaus WA, Draper EA, Douglas P et al. APACHE II: a severity of disease classification system. *Crit Care Med* 1985; 13: 818-29.
16. Dominioni L, Dionigi R. The grading of sepsis and the assessment of its prognosis in the surgical patient: a review. *Surg Res Comm* 1987; 1: 1-11.
17. Beger HG, Bittner R, Block S et al. Bacterial contamination of pancreatic necrosis. A prospective clinical study. *Gastroenterology* 1986; 91: 433-8.
18. Bittner R, Bloch S, Büchler M et al. Pancreatic abscess and infected pancreatic necrosis. Different local septic complications in acute pancreatitis. *Dig Dis Sci* 1987; 32: 1082-7.
19. Ranson JHC, Rifkind KM, Turner JW. Prognostic signs and non-operative peritoneal lavage in acute pancreatitis. *Surg Gynecol Obstet* 1976; 143: 209-19.
20. Doglietto GB, Gui D, Pacelli F et al. Open vs closed treatment of secondary pancreatic infections. A review of 42 cases. *Arch Surg* 1994; 129: 689-93.
21. Van Goor H, Sluiter WJ, Bleichrodt RP. Early and long term results of necrosectomy and planned reexplorations for infected pancreatic necrosis. *Eur J Surg*, in press.
22. Wilson C, Heath DI and Imrie CW. Prediction of outcome in acute pancreatitis: a comparative study of APACHE II, clinical assessment and multiple factor scoring systems. *Br J Surg* 1990; 77: 1260-4.

CHAPTER 2

CORRELATION BETWEEN PERI-OPERATIVE BLOOD TRANSFUSION AND POST-OPERATIVE INFECTIVE COMPLICATION.

LORENZO DOMINIONI, ANGELO BENEVENTO, GIULIO CARCANO, GIUSEPPE PELONI, FRANCESCA A.ROVERA, and RENZO DIONIGI

Department of Surgery, University of Pavia in Varese, Varese, Italy

Introduction

Nosocomial infections are the most frequent complications observed in surgical patients. In recent years reductions of post-operative infections have been mostly due to a correct use of prophylactic measures such as pre-operative selective bowel decontamination, adequate antibiotic prophylaxis, and better anaesthetic and intensive care management.
Epidemiology of post-operative infection is mainly related to wound infections (1-40% depending on the type of surgical procedure), pulmonary infection (10%) and urinary tract infection (5%).
Blood transfusion carries numerous potential risks concerning the transmission of infective diseases and immunodepression, that can facilitate the occurrence of post-operative sepsis.
The possibility of transmission of bacterial and viral organisms is well documented.
Three mechanisms are involved in blood transfusions associated with infections:
1) Direct transmission of the infection from donor to recipient through blood micro-organisms;
2) Activation of pre-existent or latent recipient infection;
3) Activation of recipient immunitary defence.
Explanation of connections between pre-operative blood transfusion and post-operative septic complication is not well-documented.
The aims of this prospective study, undertaken on 212 patients operated for oesophageal, gastric, pancreatic and colo-rectal cancer, are:
to set up a data bank on surgical infections observed in our Department, in order to register systematically such infectious complications;

E. Zanella (ed.), Advances in Abdominal Surgery, 13–18.

to observe the incidence of post-operative infections related to peri-operative blood transfusion, in patients who underwent surgical resection for cancer.

Patients and methods

In the period from December 1993 to May 1997 we enrolled 2437 patients who underwent surgery in our Department. Among these patients, we selected 267 patients with oesophageal, gastric, pancreatic and colo-rectal cancer, 212 of whom underwent resective surgery for cancer.

In all 212 patients we recorded personal data, anamnestic, and clinical data, number of transfusions, number of wound, pulmonary and urinary tract infections, as well as the presence of abdominal abscess and anastomotic leakage.

Average age was 64.5 years (range 25-91); 59% male and 41% female. Elective surgery was performed in 95.8% of the patients. Twenty-eight patients (13.2%) had oesophageal cancer, 51 (24.1%) gastric cancer; 16 (7.5%) pancreatic cancer and 117 (55.2%) colo-rectal cancer.

The different types of cancer observed had been TNM staged as follows: stage I: 16.3%; stage II: 33.7%; stage III: 34.2%; stage IV: 15.8%.

Altemeier's classification of surgical procedure was: 3 (1.4%) clean ; 91 (42.9%) clean-contaminated; 109 (51.5%) contaminated e 9 (4.2%) heavily contaminated.

Variables recorded for every patient were: haemoglobin and haematocrit values, lymphocyte number, plasma albumin, pre and post-operative stay, and total time of surgery.

Results

Out of 212 patients , 101 (47.6%) developed post-operative infections: (21.7%) wound infections; (10.8%) pulmonary infections; (23.6%) urinary tract infections; (6.1%) intra-abdominal abscess and anastomotic leakage.

Regarding cancer localization, the incidence of post-operative infection was: 62.5% (10 patients) in surgery for pancreatic cancer; 50.4% (59 patients) in surgery for colo-rectal cancer; 41.2% (21 patients) in surgery for gastric cancer and 39.3% (11 patients) in surgery for oesophageal cancer.

Tables 1 and 2 show biochemical data related to the development of surgical infections.

Wound infections were significatively correlated to Altmeier's classification of surgical procedures, post-operative stay and presence of risk factors.

In the group of 212 patients selected, 64 (30.2%) underwent blood transfusion; in this group post-operative infections occured in 60.9% compared to 41.9% of infections which occurred in non-transfused patients. This difference was statistically significative: $p= 0.01$ (Table 3).

Table 1. Association between continous variables and post-operative development of infection.

	Patients who developed infection (Mean+SD)	**Patients who did not develop infection (Mean+SD)**	**p-Value**
Haemoglobin(g/dl)	12,5±1,9	13±2	0,1
Haematocrit (%)	37,1±4,6	37,9±5,3	0,2
Serum albumin (g/dl)	3,6±0,5	3,6±0,5	0,6
Blood lymphocytes level/mm^3	1760±730	1820±800	0,5
Weight loss ≥10%	18 (46,2%)	21 (53,8%)	0,54
Pre-operative hospital stay (gg)	8,6±6,5	9±7,4	0,8
Post-operative hospital stay (gg)	19,3±15,1	15,4±6,4	0,2
Length of operation (min)	226,6±99,3	217,2±86,6	0,8

Table 2. Association between discreet variables and post-operative development of infection

	N° (%) of patients who developed infection	**N° (%) of patients who did not develop infection**	**p-Value**
Site of tumour			
Oesophagus	11/28 (39,3)	17/28 (60,7)	
Stomach	21/51 (41,2)	30/51 (58,8)	0,38
Pancreas	10/16 (62,5)	6/16 (37,5)	
Colon and rectum	59/117 (50,4)	58/117 (49,6)	
Intra-operative contamination			
Clean	3/3 (100)	0/3 (0)	
Clean-contaminated	38/91 (41,8)	53/91 (58,2)	0,2
Contaminated	53/109 (48,6)	56/109 (51,4)	
Dirty	5/9 (55,6)	4/9 (44,4)	
Tumour stage			
I	12/31 (38,7)	19/31 (61,3)	
II	30/64 (46,9)	34/64 (53,1)	0,4
III	30/65 (46,2)	35/65 (53,8)	
IV	18/30 (60)	12/30 (40)	

Table 3. Incidence of post-operative infection in transfused and non-transfused patients

	Patients who received transfusion (n=64)	**Patients who did not receive transfusion (n=148)**	**p-Value**
Post-operative infections	60,9%	41,9%	0,01
Wound infections	29,7%	18,2%	0,06
Respiratory infections	25%	4,7%	0,001
Urinary infections	26,6%	22,3%	0,5
Abscess	15,6%	2%	0,001

Average number of blood units transfused per patient were: 3.2 (range 1- 14). Necessity of blood transfusion was also correlated to cancer staging: 19% of stage I patients received blood transfusion, 26% stage II-III patients, and 35% stage IV patients.

Discussion

In recent years the immunosuppressive effect of blood transfusion has been discussed. This effect is supported when considering the lower degree of allogeni transplant rejection, and a higher frequency of cancer recurrence in patients who underwent blood transfusion.
Opelz and Terasaki demonstrated that blood transfusion before surgery for kidney transplant may prolong graft survival. The direct relationship between the number of blood units transfused and better survival was also documented [5-6].
On the other hand, blood transfusion could delay wound and anastomotic healing by the same mechanism.
In Europe, during the early nineties, 60 to 80% of patients who underwent major surgical procedures received blood transfusions [7]. During the last ten years, several papers concerning the high incidence of post-operative infection related to blood transfusion have been published.
In this study we considered patients who underwent major abdominal surgery for cancer: 47,6% of our patients suffered from at least one post-operative infective complication. We must underline that this was a very select group of patients affected with cancer, that is considered a major risk in the development of post-operative complications. Moreover in these patients endogenous contamination

during surgery was related to the fact that 50% of the surgical procedures were classified as contaminated or highly contaminated.
Blood transfusion was strictly connected with the incidence of post-operative infections in our study (p = 0.01).
Immunological alterations associated with blood transfusion were observed in various clinical situations. Blood transfusions in patients who underwent nephrodyalisis blocked the lymphocytic response towards different mitogenic and antigenic molecules; suppressor lymphocytes were enhanced and an inverted ratio between T-helper and T-suppressor lympohocyte was observed [16,17,18]. Prolonged T-lymphocytic suppression after blood transfusion in patients with chronic inflammatory bowel disease was reported [19]. Lymphocytic response to phitohaemo-agglutinin, concavalin A and such antigen was seen for a period of 4 weeks following blood transfusion in abdominal and thoracic surgery [20,21]. Blood transfusion has been identified as a higher risk factor of complications in emergency surgery for bowel perforation related to abdominal blunt trauma [10].
Immunological alterations following blood transfusion can produce a clinical effect. Usually, a period of post-operative anergy is associated with a higher risk of septic complication.
Blood transfusion may interfere with the immunological response interacting with macrophages and with lymphocytes. These cells play a primary role in wound and anastomotic healing. In an experimental animal model, blood transfusions delay bowel anastomosis healing in the post-operative period, and raise the incidence of peri-anastomotic abscess and generalized peritonytis [22].
In the present study these data are confirmed: we observed a higher number of abdominal, thoracic and cervical abscesses, fistulas, and anastomotic leakage in patients that received blood transfusion (10/64, 15.6%) compared with patients that did not (3/148, 2%) (p = 0.001). Ten out of 13 patients (76,9%) who developed this kind of post-operative complication received blood transfusions.
The incidence of wound infections was not correlated to transfusion, except for those patients who received red blood cells only. It is nowadays confirmed that wound infection is strictly connected with the rate of endogenous contamination, that is, in other words, Altmeier's surgical procedures contamination.
Pulmonary infections are correlated to peri-operative blood transfusion (p=0.001), while urinary tract infections are not, but are mainly due to contamination by bladder catheter.

References

1. Donowitz LG. High risk of Hospital acquired infection in the ICU patient. *Crit Care Med* 1982;10:355.
2. Haley RW. Nationwide nosocomial infection rate. *Am J Epidem* 1985;121:159-67.
3. Chiappa A, Dominioni L, Bianchi M and Dionigi R. Le infezioni nel paziente chirurgico. In: Pagano A, Privitera G: Le Infezioni Ospedaliere. Clinica e Terapia. *Intramed Comunications* 1993;108-23.

4. Studio Nazionale di Prevalenza delle Infezioni Ospedaliere. Boll. Epidemiol. Naz. Ist. Sup. Sanità 1985; N. 6-7.
5. Opelz G, Sengar DPS, Mickey MR, Terasaki P. Effect of blood transfusions on subsequent kidney transplants. *Transplant Proc* 1973; 5: 253.
6. Salvatierra O Jr, Vincenti F, Amend W, Potter D, Iwaki Y, Opelz G, Terasaki P, Duca R, Cochrum K, Hanes , Stoney R, Feduska NJ. Deliberate donor-specific blood transfusions prior to living related renal transplantation. *Ann Surg* 1980;192:543-8.
7. Nystr^m PO, Tadros T, Wobbes T, Waymack JP, Goris RJA, Hau T. Transfusion-induced infection in surgery: a review of incidence, mechanisms, and prevention. *Working Party of the Surgical Infection Society of Europe* 1995;1-26.
8. Agarwal N, Murphy JG, Cayten CG, Stahl WM. Blood transfusion increases the risk of infection after trauma. *Arch Surg* 1993;128:171-7.
9. Dellinger EP, Oreskovich MR, Wertz MJ, Hamasaki V, Lennard ES. Risk of infection following laparotomy for penetrating abdominal injury. *Arch Surg* 1984; 119: 20-7.
10. Nichols RL, Smith JW, Klein DB et al. Risk of infection after penetrating abdominal trauma. *New Engl J Med* 1984;311:1065-70.
11. Spence RK, Carson JA, Poses R et al. Elective surgery without transfusion: influence of preoperative hemoglobin level and blood loss on mortality. *Am J Surg* 1990;159:320-4.
12. Kerman RM, VanBuren CT, Payne W. Influence of blood transfusions on immune responsiveness. *Transplant Proc* 1982;14:335-7.
13. Fischer E, Lenhard V, Seiffert P, Kluge A, Johannsen R. Blood transfusion-induced suppression of cellular immunity in man. *Hum Immunol* 1980;1:187-94.
14. Proud G, Shenton BU, Smith BM. Blood transfusion and renal transplantation. *Br J Surg* 1966;66:678-82.
15. Gascon P, Zoumbos NC, Young NS. Immunologic abnormalities in patients receiving multiple blood transfusions. *Annals of Internal Medicine* 1984;100:173-7.
16. Kaplan J, Sanaik S, Gitlin J, Lusher J. Diminuished helper/suppressor lymphocyte ratios and natural killer activity in recipients of repeated blood transfusion. *Blood* 1984;64:308-10.
17. Luban NLC, Kelleher JKJr, Zaloudek J,Reaman GH. Chronic transfusion alters T lymphocyte subpopulations in children in sickle cell disease (abstract). *Blood* 1983;621:114.
18. Wang W, Herrod H, Presbury G, Wilimag J. Immunologic studies in chronically transfused children (abstract). *Blood* 1983;62:241.
19. Tartter PI, Heimann TH, Aufses AH Jh. Blood transfusion, skin test reactivity, and lymphocytes in inflammatory bowel disease. *Am J Surg* 1986;151:358-61.
20. Dominioni L, Dionigi R, Zonta A, Scarponi A. Lymphocyte blastogenic response following different types of operation for cancer. Abstract pag.136, 14th Congress European Society for Surgical Research, Barcellona, 1979.
21. Roth JA, Golub EA, Grimm BA, Eilber MD, Morton DL. Effects of operation on immune response in cancer patients: sequential evaluation of in vitro lymphocyte function. *Surgery* 1976;79:46-51.
22. Tadros T, Wobbes T, Hendriks TH. Blood transfusion impairs the healing of experimental intestinal anastomoses. *Ann Surg* 1992;215:276-81.

CHAPTER 3

IN VITRO ANTIMICROBIAL ACTIVITIES OF β-LACTAMS, AMINOGLYCOSIDES, QUINOLONES, GLYCOPEPTIDES AND TRIMETHOPRIM-SULFAMETHOXAZOLE AGAINST GRAM-NEGATIVE AND GRAM-POSITIVE BACTERIA ISOLATED FROM PATIENTS WITH INTRA-ABDOMINAL INFECTIONS.

GIOVANNA BRANCA, TERESA SPANU, FIAMMETTA LEONE, PATRIZIA MAZZELLA, GIUSEPPE VELARDI, and GIOVANNI FADDA

Institute of Microbiology, Catholic University of the Sacred Heart, Rome, Italy

Summary

Objective To determine the *in vitro* activity of β-lactams, aminoglycosides, fluoroquinolones, glycopeptides and trimethoprim-sulfamethoxazole against Gram-negative and Gram-positive organisms, isolated from patients with intra-abdominal infections.

Design Observational study from 1994 to 1997

Subjects 730 patients with intra-abdominal infections having undergone surgery.

Setting Surgery wards.

Results Staphylococcus aureus, Pseudomonas aeruginosa, Enterococcus spp, Escherichia coli , Enterobacter spp, Klebsiella pneumoniae and Proteus mirabilis were the most frequently isolated bacteria. Anaerobes were 2.72%. The activities of all drugs were species-dependent. Of Staphylococcus aureus isolates, 48% were meticillin-resistant strains. For enterococci, ampicillin resistance was significantly more prevalent for E. faecium than for E. faecalis. No strains resistant to vancomycin were isolated.

Among Gram-negative rods, β-lactams activity varied considerably. Overall, imipenem, ceftazidime and piperacillin-tazobactam showed the broadest spectrum of activity against all bacteria except *Stenotrophomonas maltophilia* isolates. Ciprofloxacin was active against most Gram negative isolates, but was inactive against most strains of *Acinetobacter* spp *and Enterobacter* spp. *In vitro* both amikacin and gentamycin were active against most species except *Enterobacter* spp; amikacin was in all cases more active than gentamycin. Trimethoprim-sulfamethoxazole was active against most enterobacteriaceae and all *S. maltophilia isolates*, but was inactive against most strains of *P. aeruginosa*

Conclusion In our study many pathogens responsible for intra-abdominal infections were resistant to many antimicrobial agents used for therapy, since no empiric treatment is adequate to deal with all episodes of intra-abdominal infections. These problems underline the need for continued and timely surveillance of resistance among bacteria responsible for intra-abdominal infections, and for developing more reliable criteria for the selection of the most effective therapy for intra-abdominal infections.

Key words: Antimicrobial resistance, intra-abdominal infections.

E. Zanella (ed.), Advances in Abdominal Surgery, 19–29.

Introduction

Infections in intra-abdominal organs are an important cause of illness worldwide [1,2]. The microbial etiology is diverse and influenced by several factors. In addition these infections are often polymicrobial. Treatment of the patient with intra-abdominal infections is based on information about the host, the organism and antimicrobial agent. Changes in antimicrobial susceptibility govern the choice of antimicrobial agents. Therefore, it is of great concern that pathogens responsible for these infections have become increasingly resistant to many antimicrobial agents used for therapy. The incidence of resistant bacteria varies considerably according to the site of infection, patient's age, type of micro-organism, type of hospital and local epidemiological factors.
Our aim was to evaluate the activity of β-lactams, aminoglycosides, fluoroquinolones, glycopeptides and trimethoprim-sulfamethoxazole against organisms isolated in patients with intra-abdominal infections from 1994 to 1997.

Materials and Methods

Organisms
The micro-organisms studied included 1312 bacterial strains isolated from patients with infections, following abdominal surgery at the University Hospital "A.Gemelli" in Rome. Specimens were placed in a suitable anaerobic transport container (Portagerm Bio Merieux) and promptly transported to the microbiological Laboratory. All clinical samples were plated onto sheep blood agar, enriched chocolate agar, Mac Conkey agar for Gram-negative bacteria, sheep blood agar supplemented with colistin and nalidixic acid for Gram-positive cocci, mannitol salt agar for *Staphylococcus* spp., Schaedler blood agar and thioglicollate broth medium for anaerobes. All media were immediately incubated in aerobic and anaerobic atmosphere at 35 °C. Identification was obtained by standard methods [3,4].

Susceptibility tests
The minimum inhibitory concentrations (MICs) of penicillin, ampicillin, amoxicillin-clavulanic acid, cephalotin, cefotetan, ceftazidime, ticarcillin-clavulanic acid, piperacillin, piperacillin-tazobactam, imipenem, amikacin, gentamicin, ciprofloxacin, trimethoprim-sulfamethoxazole, erytromycin, clindamycin, rifampin, vancomycin and teicoplanin were determined by a standardized broth microdilution method. Selection of antimicrobial agents to be tested was dependent on bacterial species. Recommended control strains, and breakpoint for defining susceptibility were used according to the National Committee for Clinical Laboratory Standards [4].

Results and Discussion

The 1312 micro-organisms isolated from patients who underwent abdominal surgery at the University Hospital "A.Gemelli" from 1994 to 1997 are listed in Table 1.

Pseudomonas aeruginosa, *Escherichia coli*, *Klebsiella pneumoniae*, *Proteus mirabilis* , *Enterobacter* spp, were the most frequently isolated Gram-negative bacteria. The most prevalent Gram-positive organism was *Staphylococcus aureus* followed by *Enterococcus* spp, and coagulase negative *Staphylococcus* spp. Another Gram-positive organism was *Streptococccus* spp. Anaerobic bacteria account for 2.72% of all strains.

Results of MIC susceptibility are presented in Table 2. Gram- negative non-fermentative rods are important nosocomial pathogens because of their natural resistance to many antimicrobial agents [5,6,7]. In addition, the emergence of multiple-drug-resistant strains is becoming increasingly apparent. Among the β-lactams studied, imipenem and ceftazidime yieded the highest activity against Gram -negative non-fermentative isolates, followed by piperacillin-tazobactam. In the present study, tazobactam enhanced the activity of piperacillin against *P.aeruginosa* isolates. Aztreonam was reported to be moderately active against *P.aeruginosa* and *Acinetobacter* spp but inactive against other Gram-negative non-fermentative bacteria. Its activity against our Gram-negative non-fermentative bacteria was variable and usually less consistent than the activity of other β-lactams. Amikacin was the most active aminoglycoside against *P.aeruginosa*; most strains of *Acinetobacter* spp were resistant. The fluoroquinolones, primarily ciprofloxacin and ofloxacin, were reported to be active against Gram-negative bacteria. Several authors reported increased resistance rates among *P.aeruginosa* and *A.baumannii*[8]. Among our Gram-negative non-fermentative rods, ciprofloxacin was active against 67% of *P. aeruginosa* isolates, but inactive against *A.baumannii*.

Stenotrophomonas maltophilia exibited the antimicrobial susceptibility patterns typical of this organism, including susceptibilities to quinolones, ticarcillin-clavulanate and trimethoprim-sulfamethoxazole, and a high level of resistance to imipenem. Cefatizidime was active against 50% of *S. maltophilia* isolates.

In recent years, increasing rates of enterobacteriaceae, primarily *Klebsiella pneumoniae* strains, resistant to all cephalosporins except cephamycin, due to "estended spectrum" β-Lactamases (ESBLs), have been reported. In our study 25% of *K.pneumoniae*, 20% *E. coli* and 17% of *P.mirabilis* had "extended spectrum" β-Lactamases (ESBLs). Furthermore, high rates of multiple resistance were shown by *Enterobacter* spp and *Proteus* spp isolates. Therapeutic regimens for patients infected with these multiple-resistant strains have become limited. Carbapenems or fluoroquinolones were a reliable treatment for these infections. In our isolates resistance to both classes occurred (Table 2). More specifically, resistance to imipenem and ciprofloxacin occurs respectively in 5% and 100% of *Enterobacter* spp isolates. Of the 48 *Proteus mirabilis* isolates, 84% were resistant to ciprofloxacin. In addition, 34% of strains showed reduced susceptibility to imipenem (CMI= 8ug/ml).

The emergence of antimicrobial resistance in Gram-positive bacteria has become dramatic. Prior to 1990-1991 there were sporadic cases of methicillin-resistant *S.aureus* (MRSA). The importance of methicillin-resistant *S aureus* as nosocomial pathogen is now well-established. Because MRSA is often resistant to many antibacterial agents, infections due to this organism are difficult to treat. The recent appearance of strains of *S.aureus* with reduced susceptibility to vancomycin (CMI= 8ug/ml) causes serious consequences, since there are limited alternative antimicrobial agents for treating serious MRSA infections [9]. Previous reports documented high MICs of teicoplanin, but not of vancomycin, for *S. aureus* and coagulase negative staphylococci clinical isolates [10-12]. In our study, *S. aureus* is the most frequently isolated organism (Table 2): 48% were MRSA strains exhibiting multiple antimicrobial resistance. No strains with reduced susceptibility to glycopeptides were isolated from patients with intra-abdominal infections during the time of the study.

By 1994 - 1995, resistance rates began to increase in other species, including aminoglicoside sinergy-resistant enterococci and vancomycin-resistant enterococci (VRE). The rapid increase in the incidence of infections with vancomycin-resistant enterococci in Europe and in the United States is cause for great concern [13]. In the present study *Enterococcus* spp accounts for 15% of all organisms. Resistance of *E. faecium* isolates to ampicillin is high (83%). All strains were susceptible to vancomycin.

Our data are consistent with previous reports which showed the extensive resistance of Gram-posistive and Gram-negative organisms to several antibiotics, and stress that the activities of different antimicrobial agents are species-dependent. Therefore no single antimicrobial agent is adequate to deal with all episodes of intra-abdominal infections.

Treatment regimens of these infections are empirically chosen to try to eradicate the most likely etiologic agents, in the hope that the choice can be modified as soon as possible on the basis of culture results and other subsequent information. Recent studies report that survival in patients with intra-abdominal infections is diminished, if initial therapy is inadequate, regardless of the adequacy of subsequent treatment [14].

Appropriate antimicrobial therapy is an essential component of more effective management of intra-abdominal infection. It is critical that steps be taken to provide *in vitro* susceptibility results as soon as possible, and thus limit failure of treatment, by continuing to generate quality susceptibility testing data to guide empiric chemotherapy. Further studies are needed to monitor the spectrum of pathogens responsible for intra-abdominal infections, the evolution or the spread of resistance to major antibiotics, and to develop criteria for the most effective selection of treatment regimens.

Table 1. Gram-negative and Gram-positive bacteria isolated from patients with intra-abdominal infection at University Hospital "A. Gemelli" from 1994 to 1997

Organism	N. (%) isolated
Pseudomonas aeruginosa	225 (17.14)
Stenotrophomonas maltophilia	28 (2.13)
Acinetobacter spp	16 (1.21)
Enterobacter aerogenes	34 (2.59)
Enterobacter cloacae	38 (2.89)
Escherichia coli	143 (10.89)
Klebsiella pneumoniae	55 (4.19)
Morganella morganii	21 (1.60)
Proteus mirabilis	48 (3.65)
Staphylococcus aureus	263 (20.04)
Staphylococcus epidermidis	153 (11.66)
Staphylococcus haemolyticus	35 (2.66)
Enterococcus faecalis	150 (11.43)
Enterococcus faecium	44 (3.35)
Streptococcus agalactiae	5 (0.38)
Streptococcus bovis	6 (0.45)
Streptococcus mitis	9 (0.68)
Streptococcus salivarius	3 (0.22)
Bacteroides thetaiotaomicron	2 (0.15)
Bacteroides distasonis	2 (0.15)
Bacteroides fragilis	24 (1.82)
Bacteroides vulgatus	2 (0.15)
Clostridium perfrigens	4 (0.30)
Clostridium innocuum	2 (0.15)

Table 2. Susceptibilities of Gram-negative and Gram-positive bacteria

Organism	Antimicrobial agent	CMI 90 (μg/ml)	S %	I %	R %
Pseudomonas aeruginosa	Amikacin	≥32	88		12
	Aztreonam	≥32	10		90
	Ceftazidime	≥32	60		40
	Ciprofloxacin	≥4	67		23
	Gentamicin	≥16	70		30
	Imipenem	≥16	65		35
	Piperacillin	≥128	12		88
	Piperacillin - tazobactam	≥128	50		50
	Ticarcillin- clavulanic acid	≥128	36		64
	Trimethoprim-sulfamethoxazole	≥4	15		85
Stenotrophomonas maltophilia	Amikacin	≥32	80		20
	Aztreonam	≥32			100
	Ceftazidime	≥32	50	10	40
	Ciprofloxacin	≥4	80		20
	Gentamicin	8	73		27
	Imipenem	≥16	8		92
	Piperacillin	≥128	15		85
	Piperacillin-tazobactan	16	20		80
	Ticarcillin- clavulanic acid	32	60		40
	Trimethoprim-sulfamethoxazole	2	100		
Acinetobacter spp	Amikacin	≥64	40		60
	Aztreonam	≥32			100
	Ceftazidime	≥32			100
	Ciprofloxacin	≥4			100
	Gentamicin	≥16	20		80
	Imipenem	4	92	3	5

Table 2. continue

	Piperacillin	≥128	50		50
	Piperacillin- tazobactam	≥128	50		50
	Ticarcillin- clavulanic acid	≥128			100
	Trimethoprim-sulfamethoxazole	≥4	6		94
Escherichia coli	Amikacin	≥64	81	3	16
	Amoxicillin-clavulanic acid	≥16	78	4	18
	Ampicillin	≥32	48		52
	Aztreonam	8	100		
	Cefotetan	≤0.5	100		
	Ceftazidime	≥32	80		20
	Cephalothin	≥32	78		18
	Ciprofloxacin	1	88		12
	Gentamicin	≥16	74		26
	Imipenem	4	100		
	Piperacillin-tazobactam	≤2	100		
	Trimethoprim-sulfamethoxazole	≥4	83		17
Enterobacter spp	Amikacin	≥32	80		20
	Amoxicillin-clavulanic acid	≥32			100
	Ampicillin	≥32			100
	Aztreonam	≥32			100
	Cefotetan	≥32			100
	Ceftazidime	≥32			100
	Cephalothin	≥32			100
	Ciprofloxacin	≥4			100
	Gentamicin	4	20		80
	Imipenem	4	95		5
	Piperacillin-tazobactam	≥128		20	80
	Trimethoprim-sulfamethoxazole	2	100		

Table 2. continue

Klebsiella pmeumoniae	Amikacin	8	100		
	Amoxicillin-clavulanic acid	≥32	64		36
	Ampicillin	≥32		72	28
	Aztreonam	8	91		9
	Cefotetan	8	100		
	Ceftazidime	≥32	75		25
	Cephalothin	≥32	50	25	25
	Ciprofloxacin	1	100		
	Gentamicin	4	80		20
	Imipenem	4	100		
	Piperacillin-tazobactam	4	100		
	Trimethoprim-sulfamethoxazole	0.5	100		
Proteus mirabilis	Amikacin	32	88		12
	Amoxicillin-clavulanic acid	≥32	90		10
	Ampicillin	≥32	10		90
	Aztreonam	≥32	83		17
	Cefotetan	0.5	100		
	Ceftazidime	≥32	83		17
	Cephalothin	≥32	40		60
	Ciprofloxacin	≥4	16		84
	Gentamicin	≥16	17		83
	Imipenem	8	66	34	
	Trimethoprim-sulfamethoxazole	2	75		25
Morganella morganii	Amikacin	8	100		
	Amoxicillin- clavulanic acid	≥32			100
	Ampicillin	≥32			100
	Aztreonam	8	100		
	Cefotetan	1	100		

Table 2. continue

	Ceftazidime	$\geq$32	29	71
	Cephalothin	$\geq$32		100
	Ciprofloxacin	1	100	
	Gentamicin	$\geq$16	29	71
	Imipenem	4	100	
	Piperacillin-tazobactam	$\leq$2	100	
	Trimethoprim-sulfamethoxazole	0.5	100	
Enterococcus faecalis	Ampicillin	2	100	
	Penicillin	8	100	
	Teicoplanin	1	100	
	Vancomycin	4	100	
Enterococcus faecium	Ampicillin	16	17	83
	Penicillin	16		100
	Teicoplanin	1	100	
	Vancomycin	1	100	
Staphylococcus aureus	Ciprofloxacin	4	50	50
	Clindamycin	$\geq$4	60	40
	Eritromycin	8	60	40
	Gentamicin	4	58	42
	Ofloxacin	$\geq$8	50	50
	Oxacillin	4	52	48
	Penicillin	>0.25	21	79
	Rifampin	1	50	50
	Teicoplanin	1	100	
	Trimethoprim-sulfamethoxazole	2	94	6
	Vancomycin	1	100	

Table 2. continue

Staphylococcus epidermidis	Ciprofloxacin	4	50	50
	Clindamycin	0.5	75	25
	Eritromycin	4	58	42
	Gentamicin	≥16	38	62
	Ofloxacin	2	50	50
	Oxacillin	4	27	73
	Penicillin	≥0.25	19	81
	Rifampin	1	81	19
	Teicoplanin	4	100	
	Trimethoprim-sulfamethoxazole	4	44	56
	Vancomycin	2	100	
Staphylococcus haemolyticus	Ciprofloxacin	4	20	80
	Clindamycin	4	40	60
	Eritromycin	8	30	70
	Gentamicin	≥16	25	75
	Oxacillin	4	25	75
	Penicillin	0.25	25	75
	Rifampin	1	75	25
	Teicoplanin	8	100	
	Trimethoprim-sulfamethoxazole	4	50	50
	Vancomycin	2	100	

References

1. McClean KL, Sheehan J, Harding GKM. Intraabdominal infection: A Review. *Clin Infec Dis* 1994;19:100-16.
2. Nichols RL, Smith JW. Wound and intraabdominal infections: microbiological considerations and approaches to treatment. *Clin Infect Dis* 1993; 16: (Suppl4) 266-72.
3. Isenberg HD. Clinical microbiology procedures handbook. Washington, DC: American Society for Microbiology, 1992: 1.0.1-2.12.6
4. National Committee for Clinical Laboratory Standards. Performance standards for antimicrobial susceptibility testing. Vol. 14 No. 16. Villanova PA. National Committee for Clinical Laboratory, 1994: M100-S5
5. Fass RJ, Barnishan J, Solomon MC, Ayers LW. In vitro activities of quinolones, B-lactams, tobramycin and trimethoprim-sulfamethoxazole against non-fermentative gram-negative bacilli. *Antimicrob Agents Chemother* 1996; 40: 1412-8
6. Fuchs PC, Barry AL, and Brown SD. Survey of antimicrobial activities of four commonly used third-generation cephalosporins tested against recent bacterial isolates fron ten American medical centers, and assessment of disk diffusion performance. AST Surveillance Group. Diagn Microbiol Infect Dis 1996; 24: 213-9
7. Bergogne-Berenzin E and Towner KJ. Acinetobacter spp. as nosocomial pathogens: microbiological, clinical, and epidemiological features. *Clin Microbiol Rev* 1996; 9: 148-65
8. Acar JF, Goldstein FW. Trends in antibacterial resistance to fluoroquinolones. *Clin Infect Dis* 1997; 24 (Suppl 1) : 67-73
9. Hiramatsu K, Aritaka N., Hanaki H., Kawasaki S, Hosoda Y., Satoshi Y, Yoshinosuke F, Intetsu K. Dissemination in Japanese hospital of strains of Staphylococcus aureus heterogeneosly resistant to vancomycin. *Lancet* 1997; 350: 1670-3
10. Kaatz G, Seo SM, Dorman NJ, Lerner SA. Emergence of teicoplanin resistant during therapy of Staphylococcus aureus endocarditis. *J Infect Dis* 1990; 162: 103-8
11. Mainardi JL, Shlaes DM, Goering RV, Acar JF, Goldstein FW. Decreased teicoplanin susceptibility of methicillin-resistant strains of Staphylococcus aureus. *J Infect Dis* 1995; 171: 1646-50
12. Pagano L, Tacconelli E, Tumbarello M, Laurenti L, Mele L, Spanu T, Cauda R, Fadda G, Leone G. Teicoplanin-resistant coagulase negative staphylococcal bacteraemia in patients with haematological malignancies: a problem of increasing importance. *J Antimicrobial Chemother* 1997, 40: 738-40
13. Murray BE. Editorial response: what can we do about vancomycin resistant enterococci? *Clin Infect Dis* 1995; 20:1134-6.
14. Masdell DM, Morrs DM, Voltura A et al. Antibiotic treatment for surgical peritonitis. *Am Surg* 1991; 214: 543-9

CHAPTER 4

ACUTE ACALCULOUS CHOLECYSTITIS. CLINICAL AND EXPERIMENTAL REMARKS.

FRANCESCO RULLI, *MARIO SIANESI, and EVERARDO ZANELLA

*Department of Surgery, University of Rome "Tor Vergata", Rome, and *Chair of Surgical Pathology, University of Parma, Parma, Italy*

Summary
Acute acalculous cholecystitis is an entity on the increase. The disease causes high rates of morbidity such as those normally observed in critically ill patients. Acute acalculous cholecystitis should be promptly suspected and diagnosed, for timely surgical treatment. This chapter will deal with the experimental and clinical work out that has led to better knowledge of this topic.

Key words: Acute cholecystitis, acute acalculous cholecystitis, multiple organ failure, cholecystectomy.

Introduction

Acute acalculous cholecystitis (AAC) is a rare clinical entity, which has lately increased in frequency [1,2]. Reports of such cases were rare before 1960. The first published case was due to Duncan [3] who in 1811 reported a fatal case of perforated acalculous gallbladder complicating an incarcerated femoral hernia. Few cases were reported in the subsequent century, many of which were caused by congenital anomalies such as kinking or fibrosis of the cystic duct, as well as other less common etiologies such as polyarteritis nodosa or infection [4,5]. More recently, a review of 28621 cholecystectomies performed in Ohio between 1962 and 1966, indicated that 7 percent of all surgically treated cases of acute cholecystitis represented acalculous disease [6]. Thereafter, Glenn and Becker [1] reported that the total number and the percentage of cases of AAC had increased progressively from 1955 untill 1979, reaching 9.5 percent. Furthermore they established a number of predisposing conditions such as trauma, previous surgery, sepsis, parenteral nutrition, and cardiovascular disease.

E. Zanella (ed.), Advances in Abdominal Surgery, 31–38.

Clinical remarks

Reports of AAC complicating surgery, trauma, or burns are now widespread [7], and it can be expected that its incidence will grow as increasingly ill patients are hospitalized, or undergo complex diagnostic or surgical procedures. For example, a striking association of AAC with surgery for ruptured aortic aneurysms, was noted in comparison with elective procedures [8]. AAC after cardiac surgery is uncommon, but certain subgroups of patients may be at particular risk, especially patients undergoing cardiac valve replacement. This observation implicates diminished left ventricular function in the pathogenesis, suggesting that visceral hypoperfusion during and immediately after cardiopulmonary by-pass support, could be of critical importance [7]. The association of ruptured aortic aneurysms with AAC also supports this hypothesis because of the high incidence of shock in these patients. In our published clinical series [9], 2 of the 16 cases described (12%) developed AAC in the clinical context of impairment of the left ventricular function, and one (6%) after having experienced a haemorrhagic shock.

AAC has been observed after trauma and burns [10-12], but its development is not limited to injured or post-operative patients, and may complicate a number of diseases. AAC occurs in patients with diabetes mellitus, congestive heart failure, haemorrhagic shock, prolonged hypotension, and systemic vasculitis [7,9]. It has also been reported in patients with neoplasms, as the result of metastatization of the porta hepatis with cystic duct obstruction; epithelial tumors, including carcinoma of the breast and melanoma, have been reported to produce the clinical setting for AAC [13]. In neoplastic patients with liver metastasis treated with intra-arterial (hepatic artery) chemotherapy, prophylactic cholecystectomy has been recommended in order to prevent AAC [14]. The disease may also complicate diagnostic and therapeutic invasive intervention, such as percutaneous transhepatic decompression of extrahepatic biliary obstruction [15].

Whatever is the primary disease, AAC seems to be a complication in patients with multiple organ dysfunction or failure [16]. In this setting it is conceivable that systemic infections with both bacteria, fungi and sepsis represent the ideal ground for the development of AAC.

Acalculous cholecystitis has occurred in patients with disseminated fungal infections caused by *Candida* species and , as observed by us in one case, in patients with *Salmonella* infections [9,17].

More recently, acute acalculous disease has been reported in patients with the acquired immunodeficiency syndrome (AIDS) and has been associated with *Cytomegalovirus* or *Cryptosporidium* infections [7,18].

Cholecystitis is the most frequent indication for urgent laparotomy in these patients [18], and may represent, as in one case observed by us (unpublished data), a sign of progression of the primary disease. In fact, cholecystectomy has been reported to improve dramatically some patients, but the clinical improvement is transient because the *Cytomegalovirus* or *Cryptosporidium* infections are invariably systemic. There is high post-operative mortality (30-40%), which is similar to the mortality rate for emergency cholecystectomy for AAC in other clinical settings [18].

In the pediatric patient, AAC is the most frequent form of acute biliary disease, not only in older but also in younger children and neonates [19,20]. Even if the pathophysiology of AAC in these little patients has not been completely understood, acute dehydratation from bacterial or viral infections may predispose this lifethreatening complication [20], while in patients without concomitant illness, congenital anomalies of the biliary tract may be responsible for the onset of acalculous cholecystitis.

It has to be underlined that data from literature may differ because of different selection of the patients. Clinical data from intensive care units, surgical departments, and outpatient settings are not comparable. The pathogenesis of AAC is complex and multifactorial, and any case contribution may appear as anecdotal. The following report summarizes data concerning 16 published cases observed by us between 1970 and 1990 [9]. The clinical settings in which we observed the onset of AAC were diabetes (9 cases), chronic obstructive pulmonary dysfunction (5 cases), heart failure (2 cases), multidistrectual atherosclerosis (2 cases), dyslipemia (1 case), haemorrhagic shock from hepatic artery aneurysm rupture (1 case), acute lymphatic leukemia (1 case), thrombocytopenic purpura (1 case), systemic collagenopathy (1 case), and inflammatory bowel disease (1 case). The signs and symptoms did not differ markedly from those normally found when acute cholecystitis is associated with cholelithiasis. Pain and tenderness in the right upper abdominal quadrant, fever, vomiting, and jaundice were common. All patients underwent cholecystectomy. At pathology, nine gallbladder specimens (56%) had focal gangrene, and perforation occurred in 7 instances (44%). Bacteria were cultured from 13 of 16 bile specimens and *E. Coli* was the most common organism (69%). A 31% morbidity and a 25% mortality rate were registered. These data collected in two surgical units clearly show how different the clinical setting can be in which the disease can develop.

Pathogenesis and experimental remarks

The pathogenesis of AAC is complex and not completely understood. Bile stasis, ischemia, and infections have been alleged in order to understand the pathophysiology of AAC. Gastrointestinal hypomotility and functional obstruction (adynamic ileus) do result in biliary stasis as well as post-operative fasting [21,22]; in this context a striking association has been observed between refeeding and onset of post-operative AAC, and it has been postulated that the impact of stone or viscous bile into the cystic duct could represent the primum movens of the disease. Experimentally, studies in cystic duct ligated dogs did not confirm these clinical hypotheses, since the animal model failed to produce cholecystitis, while the introduction of pancreatic juice into the gallbladder produced acute inflammation with or without cystic ligation [23]. On the contrary, Myers et al [24] produced an animal model of acute cholecystitis induced by common bile duct ligation in the rabbit. These authors observed cholecystic histological changes nearly identical to those of acute human cholecystitis. These changes included subserosal oedema, haemorrhage, white cell infiltration, and dilatation of lymphatic. Undoubtedly bile stasis results in alterations of the chemical composition of bile. For example the lysophosphatidylcholine (lysoPC) is a phospholipid which is found in the gallbladder bile of patients with acute cholecystitis. LysoPC is known to produce necrosis of the mucous membrane, edema, and inflammation [25] in the animal model, and Neiderhiser [26] showed that acute cholecystitis, induced in the rabbit gallbladder by perfusion with LysoPC, causes histological changes that are identical to those observed in man, with the exception of extensive haemorrhage and/or gangrene and perforation.

The role of bile stasis in the pathogenesis of AAC has been claimed also in the setting of total parenteral nutrition even if, on the other hand, enteral nutrition of critically ill patients, which preserves a normal gallbladder empyting, does not prevent acute cholecystitis [27].

Recently several authors have postulated a role for gallbladder ischemia in the pathogenesis of this disease. This may be secondary to shock from hypovolemia and/or sepsis. It has to be stressed that total parenteral nutrition is often indicated for hypovolemic and septic patients, thus representing not more than one specific therapeutic support, in patients that anyway are at risk of developing AAC.

Visceral vasoconstriction due to increased sympathetic tone characteristic of the post-operative state, or from administration of inotropic drugs, may further exacerbate this ischemia. The reduction in gallbladder blood flow may render the mucosa more susceptible to the noxious effects of bile, and thereby further predispose the development of cholecystitis. Shaked et al [28] induced acute cholecystitis in dogs by the ligation of the cystic artery. These authors demonstrated that secondary biliary infection is constantly associated in their experimental model of ischemic cholecystitis.

The relationship between bile stasis and ischemia is supported by clinical and also experimental observations: chronic hypotension in critically ill patients may be associated with bile stasis and inspissated bile from prolonged fasting, or by ampullary spasm from analgesics. In this hypothesis bacterial invasion of the ischemic tissue may be the result of bacteriemia or intestinal bacterial translocation.

Gallbladder ischemia may be caused by a number of clinical low-flow states. As reported above, the association of acalculous cholecystitis with ruptured aortic aneurysms and cardio-pulmonary by-pass is highly representative of the possible pathogenesis of AAC. In haemorrhagic as well as in septic shock patients, the vasoconstrictor response mediated by sympathetic efferents may be relevant, since sympathectomy has been shown to play a protective effect in preventing acute

cholecystitis in the dog [29].
The role of localized or systemic infections in the pathophysiology of AAC has been analysed in clinical and experimental studies. Although bacterial invasion of the gallbladder seems to be a secondary phenomenon, the humoral response to Gram-negative bacteriemia may be of some importance in the pathogenesis of AAC. Products from a bacterial wall such as lipopolysaccarides (LPS) induce a marked host response, including the activation of the coagulation cascade. Injection of *E.Coli* endotoxin into dogs and monkeys produces AAC and lung inflammation [30]. Why the gallbladder and lung appear to be target organs for injury consequent to activation of factor XII dependent pathways, is unknown, even if trauma, sepsis, blood transfusion products and cancer, which are common pre-existing factors or conditions in patients with AAC, are all conditions in which activation of factor XII might occur [1]. Kaminski et al [31] showed that the response of cats to bolus LPS administration produces systemic pressure lowering and an "acute response" with pulmonary hypertension, followed by acidosis and circulatory failure; since in the same experimental model LPS induces gallbladder inflammation, this supports the theoretical relationship indicating that sepsis and septic shock could produce AAC.

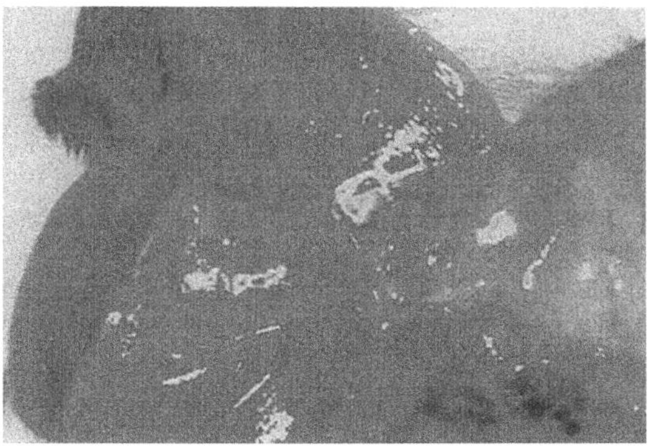

Figure 1. Acute cholecystitis in the Guinea pig. Note the intense redness of the viscus post mortem specimen.
(see Color Plates, p. xvii)

The importance of sepsis in the development of AAC was also confirmed in our experimental studies in the guinea pig [32]. We studied a model of animal AAC induced by intra-abdominal sepsis. The model included ligation and prick of the caecum. Histological studies of the specimen from animal gallbladder revealed various degrees of cholecystitis (Fig.1); bile cultures were positive in only 33% of the gallbladder's bile, and the pathogen cultured were *Streptococcus Faecalis* and *Streptococcus Sp.*. Our study suggested that intra-abdominal sepsis induces AAC, and confirmed the relationship above-mentioned between alithiasic cholecystitis and sepsis. Moreover, our experimental work proved that AAC, in the early stages, is primarily induced by inflammatory processes, while infection of the bile represents a later event [32].
One interesting observation is that the pathological findings in human AAC are similar to those in animal models [1]. There is diffused infiltration of the vascular structures and the gallbladder wall by polymorphonuclear leucocytes. The serosa and the muscularis of the gallbladder are markedly edematous and focally necrotic

(Fig.2). Focal necrosis of the wall of the arteries and veins is also observed, and

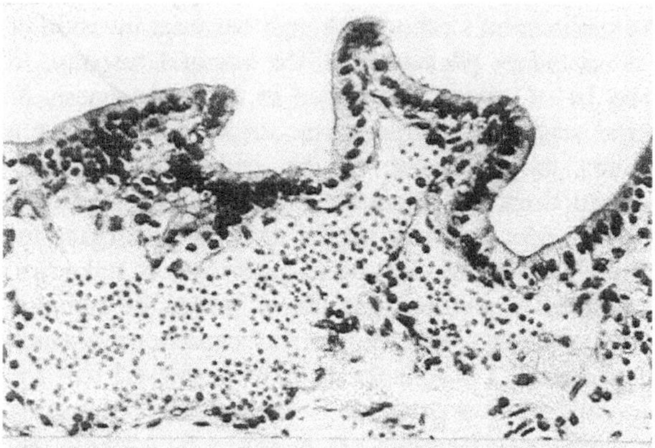

Figure 2. Guinea pig gallbladder with acute cholecystitis.
Note vascular dilatation, edema, and granulocyte infiltrate. Haematoxylin and eosin (x 280).

thrombosis is seen occasionally as well. Furthermore, focal necrosis of gallbladder mucosa or transmural gangrene of the gallbladder may also be observed. AAC is associated with multiple arterial occlusions and minimal to absent venous filling, suggesting that vascular occlusion is central to the pathogenesis of alithiasic cholecystitis.

Conclusions

Several findings reported in the present review are of clinical interest. The well-known association of AAC with multiple clinical conditions might be explained by the multiple etiological factors that could be involved. The fact that AAC might be induced by several factors, in varying degrees of severity, is important in understanding its variable clinical course. In fact, AAC is considered by some authors [33,34] as being a mild disease, while others perceive it as a fulminant one. The importance of determining the probable cause of AAC is mainly for the selection of appropriate treatment. While surgery is the treatment of choice, the controversy is cholecystectomy versus cholecystostomy.

Mortality following cholecystostomy for AAC was found by Howard [33] to be 46 percent, while that of cholecystectomy was 16 percent. In a similar clinical contribution Becker et al [30] found the respective results to be 10 and 4 percent. Although cholecystectomy apparently has a lower mortality rate for AAC than cholecystostomy, it should be remembered that patients selected for cholecystostomy are normally at high operative risk. Recently Yang and Hodgson proposed laparoscopic cholecystostomy for acute cholecystitis, a further step after using laparoscopy for the diagnosis of AAC [35]. In our opinion, the selection of operation for AAC should be influenced by the clinical history and the gross appearance of the gallbladder at ultrasounds, since cholecystostomy is not sufficient for the treatment of acute gangrenous cholecystitis, due to the presence of extensive inflammatory changes and thick viscous bile.

In conclusion, AAC is a clinical entity of variable clinical appearance that might be induced by several factors, including severe infections and shock. Diagnosis, which is not within the scope of the present review, may be difficult, because most patients are critically ill and may be unable to comunicate their symptoms.

References

1. Glenn F, Becker CG. Acute acalculous cholecystitis. An increasing entity. *Ann Surg* 1982; 195:131-6
2. Savoca PE, Longo WE, Zucker KA, McMillen MM, Modlin IM. The increeasing prevalence of acalculous cholecystitis in outpatients. *Ann Surg* 1990;211:433-7
3. Duncan J. Femoral hernia: gangrene of the gallbladder; extravasation of bile; peritonitis; death. *North Med J*; 1811; 2:151
4. Hoerr SO, Hazard JB. Acute cholecystitis without gallbladder stones. *Am J Surg* 1966;11:47-55
5. Shwartz IS, Mendelow H, Winkler I. Polyarteritis nodosa presenting as acute cholecystitis. *Am J Clin Path* 1966;45:468-71
6. Gallbladder Survey Committee. Ohio Chapter, American College of Surgeons. 28,621 cholecystectomies in Ohio. *Am J Surg* 1970; 119:714-7
7. Barie PS, Fischer E. Acute acalculous cholecystitis. *J Am Coll Surg* 1995; 180:232-43
8. Scher KS, Surap D, Jaggers RL. Acute acalculous cholecystitis complicating abdominal aortic aneurysm repair. *Surg Gynecol Obstet* 1986; 168:475-8
9. Sianesi M, Rulli F, Muzi M, Tarasconi P. Aspetti patogenetici della colecistite acuta alitiasica. *Chirurgia* 1993;6:544-7
10. Shields MA. Acute cholecystitis: an important complication of trauma. *J R Coll Surg, Edinb* 1973;18:83-6
11. Flancbaum L, Majerus TC, Cox EF. Acute post-traumatic acalculous cholecystitis. *Am J Surg* 1985; 150: 252-6
12. Alawneh I. Acute non-calculous cholecystitis in burns. *Br J Surg* 1978; 65:243-5
13. Andry G, Turnbull AD, Botet J et al. Cholesonographic charachteristics of cystic duct metastases causing acute acalculous cholecistitis. Case report. *J Surg Oncol* 1986; 31:178-81
14. Lafon PC, Reed K, Rosenthal D. Acute cholecystitis associated with hepatic arterial infusion of floxuridine. *Am J Surg* 1985; 150:687-9
15. Lillemoe KD, Pitt HA, Kaufman SL et al. Acute cholecystitis occurring as a complication of percutaneous transhepatic drainage. *Surg Gynecol Obstet* 1989; 168:348-56
16. Orlando R, Gleason E, Drezner A. Acute acalculous cholecystitis in the critically ill patients. *Am J Surg* 1983; 145:472-6
17. Hughes WT. Systemic candidiasis; a study of 109 fatal cases. *Pediatr Infect Dis J* 1982;1: 11-8
18. LaRaja RD, Rotherberg RE, Odom JW et al. The incidence of intra-abdominal surgery in acquired immunodeficiency syndrome: a statistical review of 904 patients. *Surgery* 1989;105:175-9
19. Dronner AW, Stewart CF. Cholecystitis in children. *Rev Surg* 1964;21:327-34
20. Washburn ME, Barcia P. Uncommon cause of a right upper quadrant abdominal mass in the newborn: acute cholecystitis. *Am J Surg* 1980;140:893-5
21. Sparkmann RD. Abdominal emergencies following unrelated surgical procedures. *Ann Surg* 1952, 135:863-74
22. Glenn F, Wantz GE. Acute cholecystitis following the surgical treatment of unrelated disease. *Surg Gynecol Obstet* 1956;102:145-53
23. Wagner DE, Elliot DW, Endhal CL et al. Specific pancreatic enzymes in the etiology of acute cholecystitis. *Surgery* 1962; 52: 259-65
24. Myers SI, HaleyRussel D, Parks L, Husband K. Common bile duct ligation in rabbit: a new model of acute cholecystitis description of histology and bile analysis. *J Surg Res* 1988; 45:556-64
25. Gottfries A. Lysolecithin: a factor in the pathogenesis of acute cholecystitis. An experimental study on rabbits based on clinical findings in humans. *Acta Chir Scand* 1969;135: 213-7
26. Neiderhiser DH. Acute cholecystitis induced by lysophosphatidylcholine. *AJP* 1986; 124:559-63

27. Merrill RC, Miller-Crotchett P, Lowry P. Gallbladder response to enteral lipids in injured patients. Arch Surg 1989;124: 301-302

28. Shaked G, Ovnat A, Eyal A, Fraser D, Klain J, Peiser J, Charuzi I. Acute acalculous cholecystitis-Experimental and clinical observations. Is J Med Sci 1988;24: 401-404

29. Howard J, Milford MT, DeBakey MF. The significance of the sympathetic nervous system in acute cholecystitis. Surgery 1952; 32:633-644

30. Becker CG, Dubin T, Glenn F. Induction of acute cholecystitis by activation of Factor XII. J Exp Med 1980; 151: 81-90

31. Kaminski DL, Feinstein WK, Deshpande YG. The production of experimental cholecystitis by endotoxin. Prostaglandinis 1994;472:33-239

32. Rulli F, Muzi M, D'Antini P, Melissari M, Sianesi M, Zanella E. Aspetti istopatologici e microbiologici in un modello di colecistite acuta alitiasica: studio sperimentale. Acta Bio-Medica de "L'Ateneo Parmense" 1996;67:61-67

33. Howard RJ. Acute acalculous cholecystitis. Am J Surg 1981;141:194-198

34. Andersson A, Bergdhal L, Boquist L. Acalculous cholecystitis. Am J Surg 1971;122:37

35. Yang HK, Hodgson WJB. Laparoscopic cholecystostomy for acute acalculous cholecystitis. Surg Endosc 1996; 10:673-675

CHAPTER 5

SMALL DIAMETER PORTA-CAVAL SHUNT WITH RINGED PTFE PROSTHESIS FOR THE TREATMENT OF PORTAL HYPERTENSION

FRANCESCO TONELLI, SIMONE PASSINI, and GIACOMO BATIGNANI

Department of Clinical Pathophisiology, Surgical Unit, University of Florence, Florence, Italy

Introduction

Surgery should still play a major role for bleedings due to portal hypertension, even if the majority of patients at first have been treated endoscopically with sclerotherapy or elastic band ligation of the oesophageal varices. Porto-systemic shunts are more effective for the overall therapy of oesophageal varices than other procedures as oesophageal transection, sclerotherapy or elastic band ligation [1-3], even if encephalopathy and hepatic failure often are major drawbacks. Selective shunts were thought to affect liver function less than non-selective shunts [5,11], but they appeared, in the long run, to be as associated as the non-selective ones to a similar incidence of encephalopathy [15]. Recently Sarfeh and co-workers [54,55] pointed out that the use of partial shunts revealed a lower incidence of encephalopathy than the total shunts, because of the preservation of a hepatopethal flow, thus avoiding liver failure [16]
Liver function is an important parameter that can be used to adopt proper treatment in patients with bleeding oesophageal varices, because patients with good liver function showed extremely good results [3,13]. To better understand the relationship between partial shunts and liver functions, we reviewed retrospectively a group of patients who underwent partial shunt operations at different stages of their liver disease.

Patients and methods

During the last 4 years 29 patients with a mean age of 63.5±5.3 years (range 54-75) have undergone "partial" portacaval shunt operation with a ringed

E. Zanella (ed.), Advances in Abdominal Surgery, 39–44.

polytetrafluoroethylene (PTFE) prosthesis 8 or 10 mm in diameter.
All patients were cirrhotics. Six patients were alcoholics (3 of them were also C positive) and 1 had autoimmune cirrhosis. Viral status was B and C positive in 6 patients and C positive in 16.
Three patients (10.3%) had a known pre-operative hepatocellular carcinoma (HCC) that was treated respectively with resection, alcoholization and crioablation. Eleven patients had pre-operative porto-systemic encephalopathy (PSE), classified as light in 8 and moderate in 3 patients. It was due to massive variceal haemorrhage (6 patients), to chronic alcohol abuse (2 patients), and to a careless diet (3 patients).
Twenty-three patients had documented previous variceal haemorrhage and 16 patients had portal hypertensive gastropathy. In 2 patients the indication was refractory ascites.
Nine patients underwent 4.3±2.4 endoscopic sclerotherapies.
All patients received the following pre-operative medications: beta-blockers in 9 patients (31.3%), nitroderived drugs in 6 patients (20.7%) and somatostatin or its analogues in 10 patients (34.9%). In order to obtain an improvement of the haemodynamic state and the haematic crasys we used the following haemoderivates: blood in 3 patients, plasma in 6 patients, platelets in 3 patients and fibrinogen in 1 patient.
Twelve patients were operated as an emergency, and in this situation we used a 10 mm graft in 6 patients and an 8 mm in the others. Indication to surgery were: refractory ascites in 2 patients (16.7%), unsuccessful emergency sclerotherapy in 2 patients (16.7%) and in the others (66.8%) the operation was performed because of an unresponsiveness to drug therapy.
The mean post-operative follow-up was 18.2±4.1 months (range 4-48).
We divided patients using Child's scale in order to obtain their 3-years' survival, evaluated by actuatial curve of Kaplan-Meier.

Results

Using a 23G needle introduced into the portal vein and into the inferior vena cava, after their exposure in the hepatoduodenal ligament, we were able to demonstrate that intra-operative portacaval gradient fell significantly less than 12 mmHg in all patients but one (either using an 8 or a 10 mm prosthesis). When a 10 mm graft was used the decrease in portal pressure was even more evident, but this difference was not evident if it was considered as a portacaval gradient. To accomplish the anastomosis between the PV and the IVC, these vessels were clamped. Then we performed a venotomy and a continuous over-and-over suture

using a 5/0 PTFE on IVC and 6/0 PTFE on PV. I.v. heparin (10.000 IU/24h) was initiated before releasing the two clamps. Heparin was also given after operation.
Post-operative complications were divided into early and late phases. Early complications occurred in 12 patients (41.4%). Seven patients re-bled because of gastric or duodenal ulcers. There were no bleeding episodes from variceal rupture. Other complications were: 1 neuropathy probably related to crioglobulinemia, 2 pleural effusions, 1 bronchopneumonia, 2 acute renal failures and 3 liver failures. On the other hand, late complications were: hepatocellular carcinoma in 7 patients (24.1%), gastro-oesophageal variceal ruptures in 3 patients (10.3%), shunt thrombosis, which happened in 4 patients out of 29 (13.8%) and shunt stenosis which occurred in 2 patients (6.9%).
Gastro-intestinal re-bleeding from varices occurred in 3 patients with shunt thrombosis. One patient was treated with a L-L spleno-renal shunt, 1 patient underwent a distal spleno-renal shunt, and in the last one we utilized an "H" meso-caval shunt with an 8 mm PTFE graft that developed a new thrombosis of the shunt, and for this reason the patient underwent a distal spleno-renal shunt. One patient died in a provincial hospital because of massive gastro-intestinal bleeding. In this patient there was a slight drop in the intra-operative porta-caval pressure gradient, which settled at the post-shunt upper limit (12 mmHg).
Patients with shunt stenosis underwent angiographic shunt dilatation (1 is still alive and free from varices, while the second one died because of progressive hepatocellular dysfunction).
Post-operative EGDS was done, showing the disappearance of gastro-oesophageal varices in all patients. Portal perfusion and shunt patency were demonstrated using a Doppler US and making a cavoportography, which was also used to measure pressures and gradients.
Post-operative evaluation of liver function tests were done to obtain new information about hepatocellular functions and PSE appearance. Fourteen patients were Child A (48.3%), 11 Child B (37.9%) and 4 Child C (13.8%), in comparison with pre-operative hepatocellular functions which were: Child A 41.4%, Child B 37.9% and Child C 20.7%
PSE was observed in 7 patients (24.1%): in 4 patients we used an 8 mm graft and in 3 patients we used a 10 mm prosthesis. Five patients out of 29 (17.2%) had one or more episodes of acute PSE, while chronic encephalopathy was identified in only 2/29 patients (6.9%). These patients were also encephalopathic prior to operation. The incidence of chronic and acute PSE was no different using either a 10 or an 8 mm prosthesis.
Early mortality was 13.9% (4/29). In 2 patients it was due to liver failure, while in the others it was a consequence of multi-organ failure. All these patients were Child C. Three of these patients were operated in an emergency setting.

5 other patients died later from shunting procedure (late mortality 20.7%), because of hepatocellular carcinoma in 2 patients, and progressive liver failure in 3 patients.
One patient died after he received an orthotopic liver transplantation. Eighteen patients are still alive. If we look at the actual survival rate we have obtained the following results: 85.7% of Child A, 65% of Child B and 20% of Child C were alive after 3 years.

Conclusions

The introduction of the portacaval shunt and of the mesocaval shunt with a ringed polytetrafluoroethylene (PTFE) produces a low incidence of encephalopathy, because of the mantenance of hepatopethal flow, with only a partial deviation of portal flow away from the liver [15,17]. An eight or ten millimetres prosthesis has been shown to answer these requirements [14], decreasing the portacaval gradient to the same extent using both a 10 or an 8 mm prosthesis, and reporting a similar incidence of PSE. We have demonstrated a PSE incidence of about 24%, which is like that pointed out in other series [15]. On the other hand, the incidence of the acute form was about 17%, which was well-controlled by using restricted diet, laxatives and antibiotic therapy. Only 7% of the patients showed a chronic form after operation. However these patients had suffered from the acute form prior to operation.
Post-operative complications occurred mainly in patients requiring surgery in an emergency setting (75%).
Early mortality was significantly higher in emergencies, and it also happened exclusively in Child C patients.
Shunt occlusion is the most important late complication. It happened in about 20% of our patients. Partial thrombosis took place in about 7% of patients, and it was treated by angiographic dilatation, while total thrombosis was treated surgically with a peripheric porto-systemic shunt. Our experience shows that shunt thrombosis occured only in patients with good liver function (Child A: 3 patients). These results might suggest that patients with good liver function should be treated with chronic anticoagulant therapy, or perhaps with some form of direct shunt, without the use of prosthesis.
Late mortality was due to liver failure and to the appearance of hepatocellular carcinoma. If we consider total survival our results are similar to those reported by Bismuth et al. [3] and Rypins et al. [13,14], who pointed out a significant difference related to liver function, according to the Child-Pugh classification. These results show that patients with good liver function and variceal bleeding

should not be treated by OLT, because the 5-years' survival in transplanted patients is lower than that of shunted patients.

The problem is different if we consider Child B patients. These patients may be affected more frequently by complications and the expected survival is around 60%. However, organ shortage and restricted criteria for transplantation still represent the main reason for considering shunt surgery for these patients.

It is important to notice that the carrying out of a shunt does not preclude OLT, and on the other hand shunt procedure could be used as "a bridge" to liver transplantation.

On the contrary poor liver function represents a contra-indication to shunt surgery, especially if it is performed in an emergency setting, because of high morbidity and mortality. In these cases TIPS should be used as an elective treatment.

References

1. Adam R, Diamond T, Bismuth H. Partial Porta-caval Shunt: Renaissance of an Old Concept. *Surgery* 1991;111:610-6.
2. Avgerinos A, Armonis A, Manolakopoulos S et al. Endoscopic sclerotherapy (ES) versus endoscopic ligation (EVL) for the prevention of recurrent esophageal variceal haemorrage in cirrhotics. *Gastroenterology* 1994;106:A891.
3. Bismuth H, Adam R, Mathur S, Sherlock D. Options for elective treatment of portal hypertension in cirrhotic patients in the transplantation era. *Am J Surg* 1990;160:105-10.
4. Borgonovo G, Costantini M, Grange D, Vons C, Smadja C, Franco D. Comparison of a modified Sugiura procedure with portal systemic shunt for prevention of recurrent variceal bleeding in cirrhosis. *Surgery* 1996;119:214-20.
5. Capussotti L, Vergara V, Polastri R, Marucci MM, Bouzari H, Fava C. A critical appraisal of the small-diameter porta-caval H-graft. *Am J Surg* 1995;170:10-4.
6. Capussotti L, Vergara V, Polastri R, et al. L'anastomosi porto-cava parziale: indicazioni e risultati a breve e lungo termine. *Chirurgia* 1993;8:27-32.
7. Collins JC, Conroy RM, Sarfeh IJ. Collateral Ablation Improves Portal Perfusion After Partial Porta-caval Shunt. *Am Surg* 1995;10:868-73.
8. Gimson AES, Ramage JK, Panoz MZ et al. Hemodynamic events in a prospective randomized trial of propranolol versus placebo in the prevention of first variceal hemorrage. *Gastroenterology* 1990;99:1401-7.
9. Orloff MJ, Orloff MS, Orloff SL, Rombotti M, Grard B. Three decades of experience with emergency portacaval shunt for acutely bleeding esophageal varices in 400 unselected patients with cirrhosis of liver. *J Am Coll Surg* 1995;180:257-72.
10. Rikkers LF, Burnett DA, Valentine GD, Buchi KN, Cormier RA. Shunt surgery versus endoscopic sclerotherapy for long term treatment of variceal bleeding. *Ann Surg* 1987;207:430-6.
11. Rosemurgy AS, McAllister EW, Kearney RF. Prospective study of a prosthetic H-graft porta-caval shunt. *Am J Surg* 1991;161:159-64.
12. Rosemurgy AS, Normann JG, Goode SE. Does the direction of portal blood flow determine outcome with small-diameter prosthetic H-graft porta-caval shunt? *Surgery* 1997;121:95-101.
13. Rypins EB, Sarfeh IJ. Influence of portal hemodynamics on long-term survival of alcoholic cirrhotic patients after small-diameter prosthetic H-graft. *Am J Surg* 1988;155:152-6.
14. Rypins EB, Mason RG, Conroy RM, Sarfeh IJ. Predictability and maintenance of portal flow patterns after small-diameter H-graft in man. *Ann Surg* 1984; 200:706-10.

15. Sarfeh IJ, Rypins EB, Conroy RM, Mason JR. Porta-caval H-graft: relationship of shunt diameter, portal flow patterns and encephalopathy. *Ann Surg* 1982; 197:422-6.
16. Sarfeh IJ, Rypins EB, Mason GR, et al. A systemic appraisal of portacaval H-graft diameters. Clinical and hemodynamic prospective. *Ann Surg* 1986;204:356-62.
17. Sarfeh IJ, Rypins EB, Fardi M, Conroy RM, Mason GR et al. Clinical implications of portal hemodynamics after small-diameter portacaval H-graft. *Surgery* 1984; 96:223-9.

CHAPTER 6

RENAL FAILURE COMPLICATING OBSTRUCTIVE JAUNDICE. AN UPDATING.

ATTILIO M. FARINON, FRANCESCO RULLI, and EVERARDO ZANELLA

Department of Surgery, University of Rome "Tor Vergata", Rome, Italy

Summary

The association between renal failure and obstructive jaundice is a well-known clinical setting. Despite numerous clinical and experimental contributions on this topic we are still far from defining the etiology and pathogenesis of renal failure complicating obstructive jaundice. The aim of this chapter is to assess the current extent of the problem, with a close analysis of pathophysiological data concerning the "hepato-renal syndrome".

Introduction

Impairment of renal function is a known consequence of total obstruction to the outflow of bile. Although the pathogenesis of renal failure in jaundiced patients is not completely understood, several factors are considered as predisposing to this life-threatening complication.

Jaundiced patients undergoing invasive diagnostic and surgical procedures are at increased risk of subsequent morbidity and mortality compared with non-jaundiced cases [1]. Among recognized complications associated with obstructive jaundice (sepsis, gastro-intestinal bleeding, impaired wound healing), renal failure is responsible for the most significant rates of morbidity and mortality [2,3].

Knowledge of the association between obstructive jaundice and renal failure is long-standing. In 1911, Clairmont and von Haberer [4] reported the occurrence of renal failure developing after surgery for obstructive jaundice in five patients, all of whom died from acute renal failure. Later, Helwig and Schutz [5] in 1930, and Heyd [6] in 1931 introduced the term "hepato-renal syndrome" in order to better describe the possible relationship between liver disfunction and renal failure. This term is now reserved for patients with liver disease who develop renal disfunction in the absence of other causes of renal disease [3].

This chapter deals with the incidence and extent of the problem, and investigates some

E. Zanella (ed.), Advances in Abdominal Surgery, 45–54.

pathogenetic and diagnostic aspects, assessed on the basis of experimental and clinical data.

Epidemiology

Renal impairment is extremely common in the presence of obstructive jaundice, and up to 75% of patients show a decrease in post-operative glomerular filtration rate [7]. The incidence of acute renal failure in different series of patients is as high as 18% but, overall, the mean incidence is approximately 8% [3]. In a series of elderly patients we registered an incidence of 34% [8]. Patient populations are not similar in age, risk, and selection, and the overall post-operative mortality rate for jaundiced patients ranges from 0 to 27%, with renal failure as a major contributing cause in 30-40% of cases. When the mortality rate for jaundiced patients with acute renal failure is examined, the mean rate is 68% with some series reporting a rate of 100% [8,9,10,11,12]. In our series mortality from renal failure was 12.5% with an overall mortality of 18.7%. It is thus apparent that the development of post-operative renal failure is common, and is associated with an unacceptably high mortality rate.

Pathogenetic factors

Many factors are claimed to be of pathogenetic importance: a direct effect of bile acids and bilirubin on the kidney, endotoxins, disseminated intra-vascular coagulation, and impaired haemodynamics. Concerning bile acids, Aoyagi and Lowenstein [13] found that a reversible form of acute renal failure can be induced in rats by infusion of bile acids, combined with a 30 min. renal ischemia. Furthermore, they outlined that kidney insufficiency did not develop by employing unassociated ischemia or bile acids infusion. High doses of bile acids infused in the rat induce neuromuscolar hyperexcitability and myocardial toxicity resulting in hypotension and arrhythmia [14]. In vitro bile acids cause inhibition of the adenosinotriphosphatase activity, oxigen intake and protein synthesis in the rat jejunum [15], disruption of lysosomes [13,16], production of haemolysis [17], and increase in the permeability of the aortic endothelium of rabbits to Evans blue [18].
The real influence of increased serum bilirubin and bile acids levels on renal ischemia has never been demonstrated, even if our clinical and experimental findings led us to suspect that the duration of jaundice plays a role in the onset of renal failure. In our clinical series [8], a close correlation was seen between duration of jaundice and very low urinary sodium levels, showing predictability of the possible development of renal

failure. Experimentally, we observed reduced sodium excretion and urine osmolality in jaundiced rats, with a significant decrease 5 to 30 days after bile duct ligation [19].
The role of endotoxins from intestinal Gram- bacteria in the genesis of renal failure appears also questionable. Endotoxins in the portal bloodstream have been considered as vasoconstrictors, although experimental data have failed to confirm their role in the development of renal failure [20,21]. A prostaglandins deficiency was also indicated, but even their administration does not improve the course of renal insufficiency [22,23,24,25].
Although renal impairment seems to be associated with major post-operative complications, such as intra-abdominal and respiratory infections [26,27,28], it is not always present, as confirmed by our own experience [8]. Nevertheless, endotoxins may activate platelets, leucocytes, and complement, thus promoting intra-vascular coagulation [29,30]. Endotoxins may, therefore, be responsible for renovascular fibrin deposition [31,32] and that has been confirmed in a number of animal studies. Sagar and Shields [33] found that fibrinogen deposition was confined to the kidney, following common bile duct ligation in rats, and this was also the case after injection of endotoxins [34]. It has been suggested that obstructive jaundice leads to impaired clearance of endotoxins, which in turn causes a low-grade disseminated intra-vascular coagulation, and so contributes to renal insufficiency [35,36]. Intra-vascular coagulation is a dynamic process, whereby procoagulant activity is countered by fibrinolysis, and this may be impaired in obstructive jaundice [18]. The attenuated fibrinolytic response may be secondary to the endotoxin itself, or to the action of endotoxins on the release of other mediators, such as cytokines and prostaglandins [34]. Increased serum concentration of bile salts produces endothelial damage, possibly reducing their fibrinolytic capacity, and hence promoting intra-vascular coagulation [18].
Haemodynamic and body fluid disturbances may be responsible for the onset of renal failure as observed in cirrhotic decompensated patients. Severe hepatic insufficiency is responsible for changes in the aminoacidemic pattern, with alterations of the normal aromatic and branched-chain aminoacid ratio [37]. The encephalopathy due to false neurotransmitters has been related to these biochemical changes, and particularly to increased aromatic aminoacidemic levels. The presence of high levels of false neurotransmitters could be responsible for the decreased cortical renal flow [8,38]. The combination of severity of hepatic impairment and cerebral neurotransmission, damaged by aminoacidemic pattern alterations, seems to explain cerebral and peripheral vascular disorders in cirrhotic patients [37,38].
Williams et al. [9] showed experimentally that jaundiced dogs suffered from hypovolemic shock much more than non-jaundiced animals. Thus pre-operative fluid depletion in jaundiced patients may represent a *primum movens* in the pathogenesis of

renal failure. On the contrary, Cattell and Birnsting [39] did not find volume depletion in jaundiced patients nor in experimentally jaundiced animals. Bomzon et al. demonstrated [40] in jaundiced baboons, animals phylogenetically close to humans, a decrease in total peripheral resistances in the presence of a slight and non-statistically significant hypotension. In jaundiced dogs, Finberg et al. [41] observed a sharp reduction in the pressor response to angiotensin II; they suggested that the overall cardiovascular effects of obstructive jaundice may be due to decreased peripheral resistance associated to slight hypotension in non depleted subjects.

Attempts at prevention and early diagnosis

Even if the association of renal disfunction and obstructive jaundice is a well-established issue, the underlying pathophysiological mechanisms are still not understood. From a practical point of view, the aim of the surgeon is to prevent renal impairment. Since elevated bilirubin levels seem to correlate with morbidity and mortality, it has been postulated that a lowering of bilirubin levels prior to operation might be beneficial. Nakayama [42] demonstrated a decrease in post-operative morbidity and mortality after percutaneous drainage; however, this study incorporated historical controls, and has been subjected to criticism. Prospective randomised studies on this topic failed to confirm benefit from pre-operative biliary drainage [43,44]. More recently, biliary endoscopic stenting showed the prevention of complications associated with percutaneous insertion, and Speer et al. [45] demonstrated a lower mortality rate after endoscopic decompression of the biliary tract, as compared with the percutaneous technique.

Although some studies have revealed fewer post-operative complications in patients submitted to pre-operative internal drainage [46,47], namely reduced incidence of sepsis and gastro-intestinal bleeding, there is a lack of data regarding renal insufficiency. A definitive answer on the utility of biliary drainage in preventing renal failure has not yet been given.

Considering that no single or specific treatment for jaundiced patients at risk of developing renal failure has been generally accepted [3,28], only the improvement of the clinical course in severely compromised patients remains as a reliable prognostic sign [48]. In fact, blood volume expansion resulted ineffective in decreasing mortality in these patients, even if pre-operative assessment and balance of fluid and electrolyte disturbances may be of some help [3].

The need for careful differentiation of renal function impairment derives from these considerations, thus distinguishing organic (i.e. acute tubular necrosis) from functional failure in order to plan adequately treatment for the kidney in the former case, and for the liver in the latter. To solve this problem, pre- and post-operative monitoring of patients is undoubtedly fundamental, in leading to early recognition of the disorder. The need for early detection of functional failure should be moreover underlined, considering that its natural evolution is towards acute renal failure [48]. In this respect, a method was tested by us in a clinical series, based on the correlation between urinary sodium levels and jaundice duration [8]. We observed that patients at risk of developing renal failure were those with long-standing jaundice, and low urinary sodium levels. In fact, we registered four deaths among patients with jaundice lasting more than 25 days and urinary sodium levels lower than 21 mEq/l. These data were clearly defined by the mathematical transformation of the obtained data into a logarithmic scale, providing a linear correlation between urinary sodium levels and jaundice duration. The regression curve obtained (Fig. 1) shows the location of patients along it, and two different portions, characterized respectively by positive

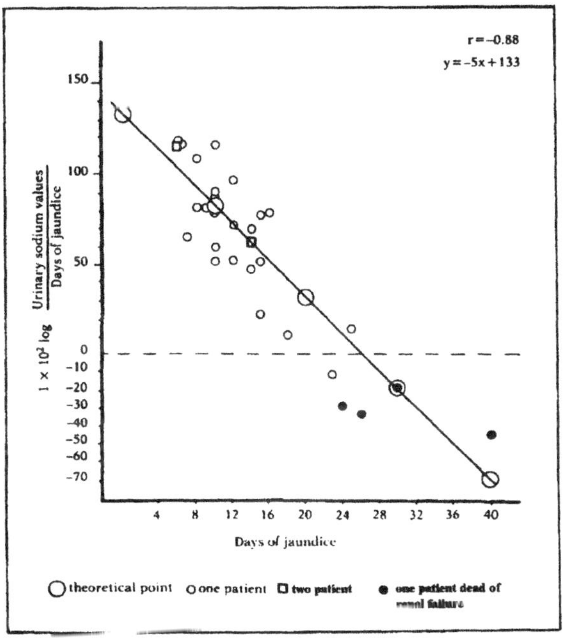

Figure 1. Regression curve deriving from the correlation between 1 x 10^2 log of urinary sodium values/days of jaundice, and jaundice duration. The four patients who died of HRS were included in the section characterized by negative values; one patient was located in a theoretical point. *After Furlnon et al.* [8].

or negative logarithmic values. Five patients were located in the negative portion, with 4 deaths from renal failure. The statistical analysis shows a significant correlation ($r = -0.88$), confirming a clear relationship between long-standing jaundice and urinary sodium levels. This method not only allowed early diagnosis of renal impairment, but also demonstrated high accuracy in predicting the outcome in jaundiced patients who underwent surgical treatment for biliary obstruction.

Our clinical data were confirmed in animal experiments [19]; in bile duct ligated rats we observed a reduced sodium excretion, with a significant decrease from the 5th to the 30th day after the bile duct ligation, with a minimum peak of 0.20 ± 0.1 mEq/24h. This low renal sodium excretion may be due to progressive proximal tubular damage [49] or, as we believe, to an early impaired tubular function with unaltered reabsorptive capacity. In subsequent experimental studies from our group (unpublished data) we evaluated the role of enzymuria in the early detection of renal impairment. The increased excretion of these enzymes is related to their leak from the damaged tubular cells, and it accounts for the presence of an anatomic lesion [50,51]. Among these enzymes, a-glucosidase (AGL), a lysosomal enzyme of tubular cells [52], and alanine-amino-peptidase (AAP), a protease widely represented in the brush border of the renal tubular cells [53], may be considered as highly specific indicators of proximal tubular damage.

These studies were undertaken to evaluate the reliability of urinary enzymes assay in jaundiced rats, and to assess its relationship with biochemical data of renal function and pathological findings of kidney damage.

Diuresis showed a marked rise in the jaundiced animals; this was statistically significant ($p < 0.01$) when compared with the urine volume of sham-operated and non-operated rats. Although no change in blood urea nitrogen and plasma creatinine was observed in the experimental animals, a significant variation of creatinine clearance was recorded. As previously observed clinically and experimentally, a progressive decrease in sodium and potassium urinary excretion was noted from the 5th to 30th post-operative day. Light microscopic examination of kidney specimens mainly revealed tubular cell degeneration, as well as the presence of biliary thrombi and bile deposits in cells. Concerning sham-operated animals, kidney histology showed minimal vacuolar lesions of tubular cells. Significant correlations were obtained by comparing laboratory parameters connected to kidney damage score [49] (urinary osmolality vs score: $r=0.59$, $p<0.05$; urinary sodium vs score: $r=0.53$, $p<0.05$; urinary potassium vs score: $r=0.62$, $p<0.05$).

In bile duct ligated rats a significant correlation was also found between the severity of tubular lesions and the fractional excretion of urinary enzymes (Ufr AGL/24h: $r = 0.77$, $p<0.001$; Ufr AAP/24h: $r = 0.69$, $p<0.01$). These experimental observations were confirmed in our clinical experience, in which we failed to find a clear relationship between high levels of bilirubin, duration of jaundice, BUN, and creatinine levels. In other terms, normal parameters of renal function are never predictive of renal failure in jaundiced patients. The differential diagnosis of renal failure in its early stage may be difficult, but it is of paramount importance to identify the "prerenal" forms, which may be associated with acute hypotension, hypovolaemia and infection, and followed by acute tubular necrosis. Moreover, even if the so-called "hepato-renal syndrome" has been associated with advanced cirrhosis, the term was originally introduced to outline renal disfunction, developing after surgery for mechanical biliary obstruction in patients with severe hepatic insufficiency [53,54]. This syndrome, that is to be considered a perfect clinical model of multiple organ failure, should be clinically suspected in a patient with liver disease, in the absence of laboratory or other known cause of renal failure [55]. It is to be stressed that patients with hepato-renal syndrome are often in the terminal stages of liver failure and the mortality rate is extremely high, although spontaneous recovery has been reported.

The differential diagnosis among "prerenal", "renal" or acute tubular necrosis, and "hepato-renal syndrome" being mandatory, on the basis of our clinical and experimental experiences, we consider urinary sodium levels and enzymuria as two important parameters for an early diagnosis of renal failure in jaundiced patients. In fact, the increased excretion of urinary enzymes (parenchymatous enzymuria) is related to their leak from the damaged tubular cells [50,51] and it accounts for the presence of anatomic lesions that we confirmed in our experimental work. On the other hand, low levels of urinary sodium, associated with "functional" rather than "organic" renal failure, may be useful in the assessment of volume depletion, as well as in the recognition of "hepato-renal syndrome".

Anyway, our experience led us to assume that a "pure" form (functional or organic) of renal failure complicating obstructive jaundice represents a rare occurrence. Even in the experimental animal it is difficult to delineate a sharp differentiation between functional and organic forms on the basis of biochemical and pathological data (unpublished data).

Conclusions

In this review we have examined some of the important issues of renal impairment and failure in obstructive-jaundice patients. Despite a significant amount of clinical and experimental research, no single pathophysiological mechanism or sequence has been identified. Since the failure to identify any specific pathophysiological mechanism is evident, it is also obvious that no single therapeutic agent or strategy has been identified. It is then logical to suggest greater attention regarding pre-operative assessment and management of fluid balance. Early detection of renal impairment seemed in our experience to be an important instrument in the need to differentiate among the different forms of renal failure, with the aim of early treatment, when possible.

References

1. Pain JA, Cahill GJ, Bailey ME. Perioperative complications in obstructive jaundice: therapeutic considerations. *Br J Surg* 1985; 72:942-59.
2. Wait RB, Kahng KU. Renal failure complicating obstructive jaundice. *Am J Surg* 1989; 157:256-63.
3. Fogarty BJ, Parks RW, Rowlands BJ, Diamond T. Renal dysfunction in obstructive jaundice. *Br J Surg* 1995;82:877-84.
4. Clairmont P, von Haberer H. Ueber anurie nach gallensteinoperationen. *Grenzgeb Med Chir* 1911; 159-72.
5. Helwig FC, Schutz CB. A liver kidney syndrome. Clinical pathological and experimental studies. *Surg Gynecol Obstet* 1930;55:570-80.
6. Heyd CG "Liver deaths" in surgery of the gallbladder. *JAMA* 1931; 97: 1847-8.
7. Cahill CJ. Prevention of postoperative renal failure in patients with obstructive jaundice – the role of bile acids. *Br J Surg* 1983; 70:590-5
8. Farinon AM, Rulli F, Percudani M, Muzi M, Baratta V. Urinary sodium levels related to jaundice duration in the assessment of postoperative risk of hepato-renal syndrome in eldely patients undergoing surgery for biliary obstruction. *It J Surg Sci* 1989;19:11-7.
9. Willimas RD, Elliot DW, Zollinger RM. The effect of hypotension in obstructive jaundice. *Arch Surg* 1960; 81:334-40.
10. Dawson JL. The incidence of postoperative renal failure in obstructive jaundice. *Br J Surg* 1965;52:663-5.
11. Wittenstein BH, Giacchino JL, Pickleman JR et al. Obstructive jaundice: the necessity for improved management. *Am Surg* 1981; 47:116-20.
12. Armstrong CP, Dixon JM, Taylor TV, Davies GC. Surgical experience of deeply jaundiced patients with bile duct obstruction. *Br J Surg* 1984; 71:234-8.
13. Aoyagi P, Lowenstein N. The effects of bile acids and renal ichemia on renal function. *J Lab Clin Med* 1968; 71:686-92.
14. Emerson WC. The toxic constituents of bile. *J Lab Clin Med* 1929; 14: 635-41.
15. Parkinson TM, Olson JA. Inhibitory effects of bile acids on adenosin triphophatase oxigen consumption and the transport and diffusion of water-soluble substances in the small intestine of the rat. *Life Sci* 1964;3:107-19.
16. Weissman G. Studies of lysosomes. The effects of neutral steroids and bile acids on lysosomes in vitro. *Biochem Farmacol* 1965; 14:525-36.
17. Weissman G, Kaiser H. Hemolysis and augmentation of hemolysis by neutral steroids and bile acids. *Biochem Farmacol* 1965;14:537-46.
18. Wardle EN. Renal failure in obstructive jaundice. Pathogenetic factors. *Postgrad Med J* 1975;51:512-4.
19. Farinon AM, Rulli F, Muzi M, Torquati A, Villani A, Bosco M, Bonomo V, De Sole P, Antenucci M. Effects of common bile duct ligation on the renal function in rats. *Progress Report* 1991; 3:45-55.
20. O' Connor M. Mechanical biliary obstruction. A review of the multisystemic consequence of obstructive jaundice and their impact on perioperative morbidity and mortality. *Am Surg* 1985; 51: 245-51.
21. Wilkinson SP, Moodie H, Stamatakid JD. Endotoxinemia and renal failure in cirrhosis and obstructive jaundice. *Br Med J* 1976;2:1415-8.

22. Arieff AL, Chidsey CA. Renal function in cirrhosis and the effects of prostaglandine A. *Am J Med* 1974;56: 695-703.

23. Fichman MP, Littenburg G, Horton R. Effect of prostaglandin A on renal and adrenal function in man. *Circ Res* 1972; 30:19-35.

24. Staudacher V, Nespoli A, Chiara O, Bigatello L, Loda M, Di Pace C. Ipertensione portale: cenni di terapia ragionata. *Federazione Medica* 1982; 9:939-52.

25. Zusman RM, Axelrod L, Tolkoff-Rubin N. The treatment of the hepato-renal syndrome with intra-renal administration of prostaglandins. *Prostaglandins* 1977;13:819-30.

26. Kennedy AC, Burton JA, Luke RG, Bridges JD, Lindsay RM, Ellison MEM, Edwards N, Dargie HS. Factors affecting the prognosis in acute renal failure: a survey of 251 cases. *Quart J Med* 1973; 42:73-86.

27. Koppel MH, Coburn JV, Matlock M, Mims MM, Goldstein H, Boyle J, Rubini ME. Transplantation of cadaveric kidneys from patients with hepato-renal syndrome. Evidence for the functional nature of renal failure in advanced liver diseases. *N Engl J Med* 1969;280:1367-70.

28. Marshall VC. Acute renal failure in surgical patients. *Br J Surg* 1971;58:17-21.

29. Morrison DC, Ulevic TCHJ. The effect of bacterial endotoxins on host mediation system. A review. *Am J Pathol* 1978;93:527-617.

30. Muller-Berghaus G. The role of platelets, leucocytes and complement in the activation of intravascular coagulation by endotoxin. In: de Gaetano G, Garattini S, eds. Platelets: a multidisciplinary approach. New York:Raven Press, 1978: 303-20.

31. Wardle EN, Wright NA. Endotoxin and renal failure associated with obstructive jaundice. *Br Med J* 1970;4:472-4.

32 Wardle EN. Endotoxaemia and the pathogenesis of acute renal failure. *Quart J Med* 1975;44:389-98.

33. Sagar S, Shields R. Fibrinogen in the hepato-renal syndrome: an experimental study. *Br J Surg* 1980;67:562-4.

34. Fletcher MS, Westwick J, Kakkar VV. Endotoxins, prostaglandins and renal fibrin deposition in obstructive jaundice. *Br J Surg* 1982;69:625-9.

35. Wardle EN. Fibrinogen disease. *Arch Surg* 1974;109:741-6.

36. Wilkinson SP, Arroyo V, Gazard BG, Moodie H, Williams R. Relation of renal impairment and haemorragic diathesis to endotoxaemia on fulminant hepatic failure. *Lancet* 1974; i:521-4.

37. Fisher JE, Baldessarini RJ. False neurotransmitters and hepatic failure. *Lancet* 1971; ii:74-79.

38. Nespoli A, Bevilacqua G, Staudacher G, Rossi N, Salerno F, Castelli MR. The role of false neurotransmitters in the pathogenesis of hepatorenal encephlopathy and hyperdinamic syndrome in cirrhosis. *Arch Surg* 1981; 116:1129-38.

39. Cattell WR, Birnsting MA. Blood-volume and hypotension in obstructive jaundice. *Br J Surg* 1967; 54:272-8.

40. Bomzon L, Wilten PB, McCalden TA. Impaired skeletal muscle vasomotor response to infused noradrenaline in baboons with obstructive jaundice. *Clin Sci* 1978; 55:109-12.

41. Finberg JPM, Syrop HA, Better OS. Blunted pressor response to angiotensin and sympathomimetic amines in bile duct ligated dogs. *Clin Sci* 1981;61:535-9.

42. Nakayama T, Ikeda A, Okuda K. Percutaneous transhepatic drainage of the biliary tract technique and results in 104 cases. *Gastroenterology* 1978;74:554-9.

43. Hatfield ARW, Terblanche J, Fataar S. Preoperative external biliary drainage in obsructive jaundice. *Lancet* 1982; ii:896-9.

44. Pitt HA, Gomes AS, Lois JT, et al. Does preoperative percutaneous biliary drainage reduce operative risk or increase hospital cost? *Ann Surg* 1985;201:545-53.

45. Speer AG, Russell RCG, Hatfield ARW et al. Randomised trial of endoscopic versus percutaneous stent insertion in malignant obstructive jaundice. *Lancet* 1987;ii:57-62.

46. Lygidakis NJ, van der Heyde MN, Lubbers MJ. Evaluation of preoperative biliary drainage in the surgical management of pancreatic head carcinoma. *Acta Chirurgica Scandinavica* 1987;153:665-8.

47. Trede M, Schwall G. The complications of pancreatectomy. *Ann Surg* 1988; 207:39-47.
48. Better OS, Chaimovitz C. The hepato-renal syndrome. In: disease of the kidney. Edited by R.W. Scrier, CW, Gohschalk. Boston-Toronto, Little Brown, 1988, 1489-500.
49. Amodio P, Rigotti P, Bazzerla G, et al: Are urinary enzymes useful markers of kidney damage in obstructive jaundice? *Nephron* 1985; 39: 377-81.
50. Burchard U, Haschen RJ, Krosch H: Clinical usefulness of enzyme determinations in urine; in Dubach, Schidt (ed): Diagnostic significance of enzyme and proteins in urine. Bern, Huber, 1979, pp 106.
51. Bonini PA, Guarnieri GF, De Nadai-Frank A, et al: Significato fisiopatologico e applicazioni cliniche degli enzimi urinari. *Quad Sclavo Diagn* 1973; 9:419-41.
52. Ceriotti G, Bonini PA: Specificita dell'alfa-glucosidasi urinaria nelle lesioni citolitiche del tubulo renale. *Minerva Nefrol* 1971; 18:126.
53. Peters J.E., Mampel E, Schneider SI. Alaninaminopepptidase (L-Alanyl-Peptidhydrolase) im Urin bei Nierenrkrankungen. *Clin chim Acta* 1972; 37:213.
54. Mirouze D, Michel H. Le syndrome hépatorénal. *Presse Med* 1983;12:36-40.
55. Papper S. Hepatorenal syndrome. *Contrib Nephrol* 1980; 23: 55-74.

CHAPTER 7

HEPATOLITHIASIS, CYSTIC DILATATION OF BILE DUCTS AND THE VARIABLE RISK OF CHOLANGIOCARCINOMA. RE-EVALUATION OF AN OLD PROBLEM.

FRANCESCO CETTA, GIULIA MONTALTO, CLAUDIO BALDI, MICHELE ZUCKERMANN, and *GENNARO NUZZO.

*Institute of Surgical Clinics, University of Siena, Siena, and *Institute of Surgical Pathology, Catholic University of the Sacred Heart, Rome, Italy*

Summary

Patients and methods A review of the most recent findings concerning hepatolithiasis, cystic bile duct dilatation and the variable risk of cholangiocarcinoma is reported. In particular, data are reported concerning an Italian series of 107 out of 6745 consecutive patients with bile tract surgery, who had gallstones (GS) within the intrahepatic ducts. Fifteen of them had cystic dilatation of bile ducts (CBDD). All these patients had systematic bile culture and stone analysis by IR spectroscopy. The 107 patients underwent a follow-up period ranging between 1 and 20 years.

Results Intrahepatic GS were: concomitant with GS in the common duct and/or in the gallbladder, in the absence of evident CBDD, in 57 patients; cranially to a post-surgical stricture in 35. One of them had cholangiocarcinoma (CLC) associated with CBDD either in the presence or absence of previous bile tract surgery. Two of these patients had cholangiocarcinoma. Finally, 8 patients had Caroli's disease (i.e. CBDD restricted to the intrahepatic duct) which was bilateral in 1 case, involving the left lobe in 6, and the right in 1 case, respectively. None had CLC. In particular GS associated with "pure" Caroli's disease were cholesterol in 5 cases, and mixed pigment in 3.

Conclusions Most patients with intrahepatic gallstones in Western countries have secondary hepatolithiasis (HL), i.e. associated with gallbladder and/or common duct stones or with a post-surgical stricture. True "primary" HL, usually associated with cystic dilatation of the bile ducts, in the present series accounted for only 13,9% of cases. In particular, patients with "pure" Caroli's disease, having cystic dilatation restricted to intrahepatic ducts, more frequently had cholesterol stones (5 of 8) and more rarely positive bile culture (25%) ($p < 0.01$) than patients with extrahepatic cystic bile duct dilatation. These patients also seem to have a lower incidence of cholangiocarcinoma (0 out of 8) than those with CBDD affecting extrahepatic ducts, or both intra- and extrahepatic ducts.

Introduction

Hepatolithiasis (HL) means the presence of gallstones within the intrahepatic ducts, above the main biliary confluence between the right and left ducts. HL is currently considered as a peculiar entity, that is typical of the East, and is

E. Zanella (ed.), Advances in Abdominal Surgery, 55–67.

characterized by the constant presence of infection related to brown pigment stones [1-5]. However, the presence of cholesterol gallstones within the intrahepatic ducts has been reported with increasing frequency both in Eastern and Western countries [1-2, 6-12].

At the moment, there are some doubts as to whether cholesterol stones found within the intrahepatic ducts have actually formed primarily above the main biliary confluence or are, on the contrary, secondary intrahepatic stones, i.e. they originally formed within the gallbladder (where other similar gallstones still persist) and subsequently migrated through the cystic duct, into the common duct and then into the intrahepatic ducts, cranially to the main biliary confluence.

Our original studies have recently documented that bile duct stricture precedes, not follows the occurrence of gallstones within the intrahepatic ducts [11]. This means that gallstones can initially form in the liver, only if there is an antecedent bile duct stricture, which determines local bile stasis, i.e. an impairment to the free flow of bile.

Intrahepatic gallstones both for pathogenetic and classificative purposes can be subdivided into 3 groups:

1) Gallstones, mainly cholesterol or mixed, but also pigment stones, which are found in concomitance with stones of similar aspect and structure in the common duct and/or in the gallbladder. These stones must be considered as "secondary" hepatolithiasis, since they are likely to have initially formed within the gallbladder.

2) Gallstones of various types, but frequently brown pigment, i.e. "infectious" stones [3-5], which are found cranially to a post-surgical stricture, i.e. in patients with previous operations on the bile tract and/or biliary-enteric anastomoses. In this case, stones have initially formed within the intrahepatic ducts, but as a consequence of a biliary stasis (and/or biliary infection), determined by iatrogenic factors [3-5].

3) "True" primary hepatolithiasis, due to local bile stasis, usually associated with dilatation of the intrahepatic bile ducts. In this case there are 3 different possibilities: a) HL associated with cystic bile duct dilatation, either of extrahepatic ducts or of both intra- and extrahepatic ducts; b) recurrent HL in patients with cystic duct dilatation and still dilated ducts, after partial or incomplete removal, usually including only the extrahepatic ducts. This finding is usually associated with a "relative" post-operative stricture at the site of the previous biliary-enteric anastomosis; c) HL associated with congenital bile duct dilatation restricted to the intrahepatic ducts (Caroli's disease), either diffuse or sectorial [6-8].

The aim of the present study has been to analyze the data from 107 consecutive patients with "intrahepatic" gallstones, that have been observed in 2 different Institutions: the Institute of Surgical Clinics of Siena and the Institute of Surgical Pathology of Rome, Catholic University of the Sacred Heart, since 1979 and 1976, respectively. In particular, the following aspects have been investigated: (i) prevalence of the various groups of HL; (ii) prevalence of the various morphological and structural types of gallstones (cholesterol, mixed, pigment) [9] within each group; (iii) prevalence of associated bile infection; (iv) incidence of associated cholangiocarcinoma, either already present at the time of the first operation, or subsequently detected during the follow-up period.

Material and methods

Six thousand – seven hundred – ninety five consecutive patients, who underwent surgery for bile tract diseases, were analyzed.
Patients belonged to 2 different Institutions: 2050 patients to the Institute of Surgical Clinics of Siena and 4745 patients to the Institute of Surgical Pathology and then Geriatric Surgery of the Catholic University of the Sacred Heart of Rome.
All of the patients belonging to the Siena series had systematic bile and stone analysis.
Among patients belonging to the Rome group, only those presenting hepatolithiasis had bile culture and stone analysis, wich was performed in the Siena laboratory.
In all of the patients, clinical, radiological, and laboratory data were recorded. Histological examination of the gallbladder was always performed. In some patients with biliary tract and liver surgery, bile duct and liver specimens were also examined. In addition to routine histological examination, scanning electron microscopy (ISI SX-25 SEM Pabish, Milan, Italy) at 7 KV and transmission electron microscopy (Zeiss EM 109 TEM, Karl Zeiss, Oberkochen, FRG) at 80 KV, of gallbladder, common duct and liver specimens, were also performed in selected cases. Bile samples were always obtained at operation and, in patients with T tubes or percutaneous transhepatic biliary drainage (PTBD), every 2 days in the post-operative period. Bile specimens were obtained at operation both from the gallbladder (except in patients with previous cholecystectomy) and from the common duct. Gallbladder specimens were taken by direct puncture before cholecystectomy. Common duct specimens were obtained using Caroli's cannula inserted into the common duct through the cystic duct, before routine intra-operative cholangiography, or by direct puncture of the common duct in patients with previous cholecystectomy. Avoiding contamination, part of the bile was placed in sterile tubes to perform bile culture according to standard methods, and part was used to determine bile pH and bile composition. Bile pH was always measured within 1 hour after operation, using microelectrodes at constant temperature by a pH M61 pHmeter (Radiometer, Copenhagen, Denmark). Bile lipid analysis was performed according to previously published methods [3-5]. Stones obtained at operation were washed, dried, and photographed. After cross-section, they were classified according to previously reported morphological and structural criteria [9]. If all stones from the same patient appeared similar, only one was analyzed. If different types of stones were present in the same patient, one

specimen from each subgroup of stones was analyzed. In particular, in stones with a central nucleus, that was different from the periphery at visual inspection, specimens from both sites were taken and examined separately. The analysis of stone composition was performed by X-ray diffractometry, using a Siemens D 500 diffractometer (Siemens, Milan, Italy), and infrared spectroscopy, using a Perkin-Elmer 1600 FTIR, (Perkin-Elmer, spectrophotometer Norwolk CT, USA). Identification of the various compounds was made by comparing the observed spectra and diffraction angles with those reported in the literature [3-5]. In a subset of patients, stone culture, stereomicroscopy, and scanning electron microscopy of stones (ISI SX-25 SEM Pabisch, Milan, Italy) were also performed. In order to evaluate the role of pancreato-biliary reflux in patients with cystic bile duct dilatation, in some patients bile phospholipase activity (according to Goswami and Frey) and bile trypsin content, by radioimmunoassay (test kit from CEA Sorin Saluggia, Vercelli, Italy) were also determined.

The follow-up interval ranged between 1 and 20 years; 92% of patients had at least one control after 6 months; 53% of patients were followed-up for an interval greater than 3 years. 61% of subjects had at least one contrastographic examination (IV cholangiography, ERCP, CT, MR cholangiography) after operation.

Statistical analysis: data were expressed as mean $\pm$ SD. Groups of data were analyzed for statistical significance using either students' test unpaired data, or one-way analysis or variance (ANOVA) followed by the Newman-keuls procedure. A p value of < 0.05 was considered statistically significant. The distribution of discrete variables in different groups was compared, using X^2 analysis including Yates correction, or Fisher's exact test when appropriate. The data were analyzed using the program "Primer of Biostatics" (version 3.0) (Mc Graw-Hill Inc., New York).

Results

One hundred and seven patients had gallstones within the intrahepatic ducts (1,57%). There were 65 females and 42 males. The mean age was 61 years (range 18-85). Data concerning types of associated gallstones, bile culture and associated cholangiocarcinoma, according to the various groups of intrahepatic gallstones are shown in Table 1.

Fifty-seven patients (51,4%) had intrahepatic stones concomitant with similar common duct and/or gallbladder stones. Gallstones were cholesterol in 21 cases, mixed in 34 and brown pigment in only 2 patients. Bile culture was positive in 19 of these patients (33%). There was no patient with associated cholangiocarcinoma either already present at operation or occurring subsequently during the follow-up period.Thirty-five patients (32,7%) had intrahepatic stones cranially to a post-surgical stricture.

Table 1. Types of gallstones, bile culture and associated carcinoma in patients with intrahepatic gallstones

INTRAHEPATIC GALLSTONES	N°	BROWN GS	MIXED GS	CH GS	POSITIVE BILE CULTURE N°	%	CHOLANGIO CARCINOMA N°	%
CONCOMITANT GALLBLADDER + COMMON DUCT	57	2	34	21	19	33	--	--
POST-SURGICAL STRICTURE	35	19	11(+1)	5	33	94✧	1	3*
CBDD	4	2	1	1	3	75	1	25*
CBDD + POST-SURGICAL STRICTURE	3	2	1	--	3	100✧	1	33*
CAROLI'S DISEASE	8	--	3	5	2	25✧	--	--
TOTAL	107							

GS = gallstones; CH = cholesterol; CBDD = congenital bile duct dilatation

* $p < 0.001$ ✧ $p < 0.001$

Gallstones were brown in 19 cases, mixed in 11 and cholesterol in 5 patients. The last patient had a black intrahepatic common duct stone containing suture material, cranially to a stricture at the confluence between cystic duct and common duct after cholecystectomy for black gallstones. Bile culture was positive in 33 cases (94%). There was only one patient, a 61-year-old female, who had associated cholangiocarcinoma (3%).

The third group of patients, who had intrahepatic gallstones associated with congenital cystic bile duct dilatation (n = 15, 13,5%), was subdivided into 3 subgroups, according to the previously reported criteria. Patients with congenital dilatation of the extrahepatic bile ducts (n= 4) had brown stones in 2 cases, mixed in 1 and cholesterol in the last case. Bile culture was positive in 3 patients (75%). One of these patients, a 61-year-old woman with Todani type IV cystic dilatation, had cystic cholangiocarcinoma in the left duct detected at operation. Three patients with previous surgery for cystic bile duct dilatation had, in one case a cysto-jejunostomy performed elsewhere 9 years before, with recurrent stones, but not cholangiocarcinoma, whereas the 2 remaining patients had a previous hepatico-jejunostomy after complete removal of the choledochal cyst. Two of these patients had brown stones, the third-one had mixed stones, also associated with brown mud. All 3 patients had positive bile culture (100%). One of the 2 patients with complete removal of the common duct, a 55-year-old man, with Todani type IV cystic

dilatation had cholangiocarcinoma, 11 years after operation.
Eight patients (6 F, 2 M) had "pure" Caroli's disease, i.e. with cystic dilatation restricted to the intrahepatic ducts, in the absence of common duct dilatation or concomitant common duct stones. Caroli's disease was diffuse in 1 case, restricted to the right lobe in one, and to the left lobe in 6 cases. Five patients had typical cholesterol stones, with radiate structure on cross section . All of them had negative bile culture.Three patients had mixed cholesterol stones, which in two cases were also associated with mixed brown stones in the same patient. Two of the 3 had positive bile culture. Therefore, only 25% of patients with Caroli's disease and hepatolithiasis had positive bile culture versus 94% and 100% of those with cystic dilatation also involving the extrahepatic ducts ($P < 0.01$) (Table 1). None of the patients with Caroli's disease had brown stones as unique stones. None had associated cholangiocarcinoma. In particular, 6 patients had neither gallbladder, or common duct stones, one had previous cholecystectomy and the latter had a "porcelain gallbladder". Interestingly, the 2 patients with brown microconcrements associated with cholesterol stones both had positive biliary culture. Both had suffered from repeat episodes of cholangitis, complicated in one case by septic shock, after performing ERCP. None of the 3 patients with Caroli's disease who had ERCP showed an abnormal pancreato-biliary junction. Two of these patients also had values of biliary trypsin within the normal range, 10 excluding evident pancreato-biliary reflux.

Discussion

In a consecutive series of surgical patients with HL, occurrring in a Western country such as Italy, the relative prevalence of the 3 types of intrahepatic lithiasis was the following: 51.4% had HL associated with concomitant gallbladder or common duct stones; 32.7% had HL, which had formed cranially to a bile duct stricture in patients with previous operations on the bile tract; 13.9% had HL associated with various types of congenital cystic dilatation of the bile ducts.
Present data show that HL cannot any longer be considered synonimous with brown pigment gallstones, which are typically related to bile infection, mainly by Escherichia Coli [3-7]. In fact, even excluding the 57 patients of the first group, showing gallstones, which probably had initially formed within the gallbladder, in patients belonging to group 2 and 3 (i.e. those with gallstones primarily formed within the intrahepatic ducts) stones resulted brown pigment in 19 cases, and cholesterol or mixed in 16 patients in group 2 (i.e. the group with gallstones formed above a post-surgical bile duct stricture). On the contrary, stones were brown pigment in only 4 cases, in comparison with 11 cases with cholesterol or mixed stones, in the last group with congenital bile duct dilatation. In particular, in patients with Caroli's disease, which was sectorial in 7 cases and diffuse in 1 patient, "pure" cholesterol stones were found in 5 cases and mixed stones were

found in 3 cases. In 2 of the 3 cases, mixed stones were also associated with some brown stones, i.e. there was a double stone population. It must be outlined that in 6 of these patients the gallbladder was acalculous, whereas the remaining 2 patients had previous cholecystectomy in one case and "porcelain gallbladder" in the last case. It is also noteworthy that the 2 patients with bile infection associated with a double stone population, including some "earthy" brown stones, had repeat episodes of cholangitis, after ERCP. On the basis of these findings, we suggest not to perform ERCP in patients with "pure" Caroli's disease, i.e. with cystic dilatation restricted to the intrahepatic ducts, because of the risk of severe septic complications, in subjects with previously "sterile" bile ducts.

This high prevalence of primary cholesterol stones in patients with "pure" Caroli's disease is new, and is neither in agreement with common belief, nor with most opinions currently reported in literature. However, it is only apparently difficult to explain. In fact, in the 5 patients with cholesterol stones and in 1 of the 3 with mixed stones (the one not associated with concomitant brown stones), bile culture resulted negative. Therefore, the basic requirement for brown pigment stone formation, i.e bile infection, was lacking [6]. In all patients with Caroli's disease a stricture of at least a small portion of the intrahepatic bile ducts was always evident. This stricture in most cases was located at the main bile duct confluence, in the left hepatic duct, or in the more cranial ducts. This finding gives further evidence to the view that [10-11] gallstones do not form primarily within the intrahepatic ducts in the absence of bile stasis, that is usually but not always also associated with an evident bile duct stricture. In addition, the cumulative data obtained in patients with Caroli's disease also confirm that brown stones usually form, mostly in old patients, if bile stasis is also associated with bile infection, namely by Escherichia Coli [4]. On the contrary, if only sectorial bile stasis is present, without infection, and in particular if the normal function of the sphincter of Oddi is preserved (as usually occurs in patients with bile duct dilatation restricted to the intrahepatic ducts, in the absence of common duct dilatation and/or common duct or gallbladder stones) then mixed cholesterol or also "pure" cholesterol stones can form primarily within the intrahepatic ducts [4-5].

We have recently documented in the course of a prospective study that stricture of intrahepatic bile ducts precedes, not follows, the occurrence of intrahepatic stones, and is the main factor responsible for their formation [11]. However, it must be stressed that: bile duct stricture, in particular in patients with previous biliary-enteric anastomosis, can be a "relative" stricture, i.e. the anastomosis can be sufficiently wide to permit the passage of balloons, probes and other surgical instruments of large diameter [4]. There is, however, a marked dilatation of bile ducts above the anastomosis, clearly suggesting bile stasis. In addition, this stricture is not always detectable by common diagnostic procedures, because it can be borderline, even if it actually determines a marked impairment to the free flow of bile in the affected liver segments [4-5].

Therefore, the type of gallstone (in terms of both outer aspect and structure) [9] which is going to occur above the intrahepatic stricture will be determined more by the presence or absence of local infection (i.e. in that segment or micro-environment) than by metabolic factors, such as bile supersaturation with cholesterol or other bile constituents [12-13]. In fact, if metabolic disorder were mainly responsible for intrahepatic lithiasis, gallstones would form everywhere within the intrahepatic ducts, and not only in the district located cranially to a bile duct stricture [10-11]. The suggested pathophysiological mechanism for the occurrence of all types of hepatolithiasis is the following: if patients are old, and bile infection is present and relevant, brown stones usually occur; on the contrary, if infection is absent or not relevant at the time of gallstone formation, mixed or cholesterol stones can frequently occur [12-15].

Both hepatolithiasis and congenital cystic bile duct dilatation (either with or without concomitant gallstones) can be associated with cholangiocarcinoma [17-26]. Recent studies, in particular from Eastern countries, have shown that most patients with cystic bile duct dilatation are usually associated with having an abnormally long common channel outside the control of the sphincter of Oddi [18-19], and that in these patients there is an increased risk of both cholangiocarcinoma in the dilated bile ducts [19], and/or of gallbladder carcinoma (mostly of the papillary histotype, usually in the absence of gallbladder stones) [27-29]. Several cases of patients with congenital cystic bile duct dilatation undergoing cancerous changes have been reported, after the first description of cholangiocarcinoma associated with a choledocal cyst in 1944 [20]. Kasai et al. were the first to report the increased incidence of carcinoma arising in choledocal cysts, and advocated primary cyst excision [21]. It must be noted that hepatobiliary malignancy in patients with congenital bile duct dilatation, is neither always intracystic nor prevented completely by cyst excision [22]. However, it should be pointed out that the majority of cases reported have involved dilated intrahepatic ducts and not those of normal size.

Present data show that hepatolithiasis and cystic bile duct dilatation are distinct entities in terms of subsequent occurrence of cholangiocarcinoma. Unfortunately, despite the apparently large number of consecutive patients in the present series, numbers are too small, in particular when stratified for subgroups, to draw definitive conclusions. However, at least for the largest subgroups, data seem to be evident enough. The simple presence of stones within the intrahepatic ducts, in particular when they are cholesterol, or are associated with similar stones within the gallbladder and/or the common duct, doesn't seem to be a main risk factor for subsequent development of cholangiocarcinoma.

In fact, no patient with cholangiocarcinoma was observed among the 57 patients belonging to group 1. Whether this could be due to the fact that in these patients intrahepatic lithiasis was just an episodic condition of short duration, and not a chronic disease, is speculative. Only one of the 35 patients with HL associated with post-surgical stricture developed cholangiocarcinoma (3%). On the contrary, cholangiocarcinoma was more frequently associated with HL, when intrahepatic stones were formed as a complication of cystic duct dilatation of bile ducts (25%). However, caution must be suggested in the interpretation of this finding concerning this subgroup, since numbers are too small. However, present data together with cumulative observations reported in literature, suggest that the risk of malignant change could be even greater after incomplete surgical treatment, i.e. in patients with both extra- and intrahepatic dilatation, in whom only a portion of dilated ducts is removed (usually the extrahepatic ducts). Preliminary observations suggest that surgery could be an adequate procedure if all the strictures have been removed. On the contrary, if some strictured segments still persist within the intrahepatic ducts, this will lead to recurrent intrahepatic cholelithiasis [14-15]. In most of these patients with biliary enteric anastomosis, bile infection and brown stones almost invariably occur. On the contrary, at least in the present series, in patients with "pure" Caroli's disease, i.e. with bile duct dilatation restricted to intrahepatic ducts (with a "normal" common duct and a well functioning sphincter of Oddi) [5], cholesterol stones were found in about two/thirds of cases (5 out of 8), mixed stones were found in the 3 remaining patients (associated with brown stones in 2 cases) and bile infection was found in only 25% of cases.

The incidence of cholangiocarcinoma in the 8 patients with Caroli's disease of the average present series (length of the follow-up in this subgroup was 2 to 17 years, average 9 years) was null. This finding is apparently in contrast with data from previous series in the literature reporting a risk of cholangiocarcinoma in patients with Caroli's disease, usually variable between 11 and 20%, and even higher, whereas it could be in agreement with the 7% risk reported in the Longmire series in 1983 [24]. It must be outlined, however, that: most of the cases reported in the literature are single cases, and in literature reviews concerning Caroli's disease patients, showing both intra- and extrahepatic cystic bile duct dilatation, or developing cholangiocarcinoma after previous "incomplete" surgical removal, are often included [25-26]. Present data, even if numbers are still small, suggest a distinction between the 2 entities, both in terms of associated HL and incidence of cholangiocarcinoma. A possible pathophysiological explanation is the following: in patients with both intra- and extrahepatic cystic dilatation, that is usually associated with a "long common channel", or other abnormalities of the lower portion of the common duct, there is usually pancreatobiliary reflux, and often bile infection associated with brown stones, likely to determine an increased risk of malignant transformation [30-45]. It has been hypothesized that the reflux of the pancreatic juice into the bile tract, leading to constant inflammation, and epithelial denudation of the bile duct wall, could cause cyst formation and, subsequently, cancerous changes. On the contrary, in "pure" Caroli's disease, the sphincter of Oddi is functioning normally, there is no bile infection and associated gallstones are frequently cholesterol, as present findings clearly show. Therefore, the risk of cholangiocarcinoma, even if present, doesn't seem to be as high as in the Todani I and IV types of cystic bile duct dilatation [19-20].

What's the clinical message emerging from the analysis of the present series? In

Western countries,the great majority of gallstones that are found within intrahepatic bile ducts are of gallbladder origin. Therefore, for therapeutic purposes, the complete removal of all gallstones, in particular if they are cholesterol, mixed or even black pigment stones, should prevent recurrence, because the gallbladder, i.e. the site of their original formation, is always removed during the same operation, and there are no residual factors facilitating stone reformation. This statement is valid only from a theoretical point of view. In fact, in clinical practice, in particular in patients with complete repletion of the common duct and intrahepatic ducts with gallstones, there is a high risk of missing some residual stones in the smallest ducts, or of reformation of true "recurrent" stones (i.e. of the brown subtype [4-5]) because of strictures determined by concomitant cholangitis. Therefore, in most of these patients it will be safer to anastomose a Roux-en-Y loop to the abdominal wall after performing hepaticojejunostomy, in order to facilitate repeated endoscopic procedures, to remove residual stones and/or drain residual areas of focal cholangitis. This treatment is the only possible treatment, excluding liver transplantation, in patients with diffuse hepatolithiasis cranially located to a post-surgical stricture, or complicating congenital cystic dilatation involving both liver lobes.

It must be stressed once again that there is no chance of radical treatment or persistent cure of hepatolithiasis occurring cranially to an intrahepatic stricture, if the stricture itself is not removed. In fact, despite initial positive results obtained by dissolution, lithotripsy or even endoscopic and/or surgical removal of gallstones, stones formed cranially to a stricture, particularly brown stones, are going invariably to recur, if the stricture persists [6]. Therefore, in these cases, therapeutic success often means "best palliative" .

On the contrary, in patients with sectorial Caroli's disease, i.e. restricted to one liver lobe or even to a liver sector (usually including II and III, or II, III and IV segments), it is possible to obtain definitive treatment of HL by liver resection, that must include all "strictured" ducts. This strictured tract is sometimes more downstream than was initially estimated on the basis of pre-operative "imaging procedures", and often requires an extension of the initially planned resection (i.e. inclusion of the IV segment, in addition to the removal of segments II and III). Liver resection, if performed in Institutions where operative mortality for benign diseases is close to null, is advisable in all patients with sectorial Caroli's disease, even if the risk of cholangiocarcinoma in these particular cases is not as high as previously estimated. Surgical treatment is even more indicated in patients with cystic bile duct dilatation involving both intra- and extrahepatic bile ducts, because in these cases, in addition to symptoms and complications related to associated gallstones and relapsing cholangitis, there is also an increased risk of cholangiocarcinoma. In these patients, the amount of specimen removal, without leaving any residual diseased tract, is still a matter for discussion. Open questions concern both caudal and cranial extension of the resection. Concerning the caudal limit of the resection, the complete removal of the abnormal common channel at the lower portion of the common duct has been advised. However, an increased risk of major complications, including post-operative hemorrhage, acute pancreatitis, and abdominal abscesses, has recently beeen reported in adults, while trying to remove the intrapancreatic portion of the bile tract. Therefore, because this lower portion is functionally excluded from the passage of the bile flow, many Authors now suggest stopping common duct resection close to, but outside the pancreatic tissue, in the lower margin which is not involved in malignant changes. Concerning the cranial limit of the resection, the specimen should include not only the entire extrahepatic bile tract, but also the liver segments involved in dilatation, with complete removal of all strictures, when the disease also involves the intrahepatic ducts. Complete removal of all intrahepatic strictures, either congenital [15] or secondary, is mandatory. In fact, if residual strictures persist, intrahepatic stones are going to reform, and the patients remain at risk of developing cholangiocarcinoma

References

1. Kim M-H, Sekeijima J, Lee SP. Primary intraheaptic stones. *Am J Gastroenterol* 1995; 90: 540-8.
2. Nakayama F, Soloway RD, Nakama T, Miyazaki K, Ichimiya H, Sheen PC, Ker CG. Hepatolithiasis in East Asia: retrospective study. *Dig Dis Sci* 1986; 31: 21-6.
3. Cetta F. Bile infection documented as initial event in the pathogenesis of brown pigment biliary stones. *Hepatology* 1986; 6: 482-9.
4. Cetta F. The role of bacteria in pigment gallstone disease. *Ann Surg* 1991; 213: 315-26.
5. Cetta F. Do surgical and endoscopic sphincterotomy prevent or facilitate recurrent common duct stone formation? *Arch Surg* 1993; 128: 329-36.
6. Cetta F, Lombardo F, Cariati A. The role of the content (decreased level of apolipoprotein A1) and the container (bile duct stricture, sectorial dilatation of the ducts determining bile stasis) in the pathogenesis of hepatolithiasis, either pigment or cholesterol. *Hepatology* 1994; 19: 1539-41.
7. Cetta F, Lombardo F, Giubbolini M, Malet P. Hepatolithiasis: i) frequency, stone type and composition in a consecutive series of 1350 surgical patients. *Gastroenterology* 1993; 104: A 355.
8. Cetta F, Lombardo F, Baldi C, Cappelli A. Hepatolithiasis: a Western experience. Suggestion for pathogenesis. In Bresadola F Ed. "Proceedings 18° Cong. SIRC" *New Magazine Publ* 1994; 239-46.
9. Cetta F, Lombardo F, Giubbolini M, Baldi C, Cariati A. Classification of gallstones and epidemiologic studies. *Dig Dis Sci* 1995; 40:2189-91.
10. Matsumoto Y, Fujii H, Yoshioka M, Sekikawa T, Wada T, Yamamoto M, Eguchi H, Sugahara K. Biliary strictures as a cause of primary intrahepatic bile duct stones. *World J Surg* 1986; 10: 867-75.
11. Cetta F. Bile stasis due to bile duct stricture precedes, not follows, the formation of primary intrahepatic stones and plays a basic role in their pathogenesis. *Am J Gastroenterol* 1996; 91:2451 2.
12. Shoda J, He B, Tanaka N, Matsuzaki Y, Yamamori S, Osuga T. Primary dual defect of cholesterol and bile acid metabolism in liver of patients with intrahepatic calculi. *Gastroenterology* 1995; 108: 1534-46.
13. Cetta F, Lombardo F, Giubbolini M, Baldi C, Cariati A, Malet P. Hepatolithiasis and cholesterol and bile acid metabolism. *Gastroenterology* 1996; 110: 963-70.
14. Uno K, Tsuchida Y, Kawarasaki H, Ohniya H, Honna T. Development of intrahepatic cholelithiasis long after primary excision of choledochal cysts. *J Am Coll Surg* 1996, 183:583-8.
15. Ando H, Ito T, Kaneko K, Seo T. Congenital stenosis of the intrahepatic bile duct associated with choledochal cysts. *J Am Coll Surg* 1995; 181:426-30.
16. Cetta F, Montalto G, Nuzzo G. Recurrent hepatolithiasis after primary excision of choledochal cysts. *J Am Coll Surg* 1997; 185:197-201.

17. Cetta F, Montalto G, Zuckermann M, Cetta D. Hemobilia, infection, bile stasis and intrahepatic stones in liver transplant recipients. *Surgery* 1998; 123:115-7.
18. Todani T, Watanabe Y, Narusue M, Tabuchi K, Okajima K. Congenital bile duct cysts: classification, operative procedures, and review of thirty-seven cases including cancer arising from choledochal cyst. *Am J Surg* 1997; 134:263-9.
19. Todani T, Tabuchi K, Watanabe Y, Kobayashi T. Carcinoma arising in the wall of congenital bile duct cysts. *Cancer* 1979; 44:1134-41.
20. Irwin ST, Morison JE. Congenital cyst of the common bile duct containing stones and undergoing cancerous change. *Br J Surg* 1944; 32:319-21.
21. Kasai M, Asakura Y, Taira Y. Surgical treatment of choledochal cyst. *Ann Surg* 1970; 172:844-51.
22. Nagorney DM, McIlrath DC, Adson MA. Choledochal cysts in adults. Clinical management. *Surgery* 1984; 96:656-63.
23. Rossi RL, Silverman ML, Braasch JW, Munson JL, Remine SG. Carcinomas arising in cystic conditions of the bile ducts. A clinical and pathologic study. *Ann Surg* 1987; 205:377-84.
24. Dayton MT, Longmire WP, Tompkins RK. Caroli's disease: A premalignat condition? *Am J Surg* 1983; 145:41-8.
25. Barros JL, Polo JR, Sanabia J, Garcia-Sabrido JL, Gomez-Lorenzo FJ. Congenital cystic dilatation of the intrahepatic bile ducts (Caroli's disease): report of a case and review of the literature. *Surgery* 1979; 85:589-92.
26. Ribeiro A, Reddy RK, Bernstein D, Jeffers L, Schiff ER. Caroli's syndrome in twin sisters. *Am J Gastroenterol* 1996; 91:1024-6.
27. Kimura K, Ohto M, Saisho H, Unozawa T, Tsuciya Y, Morita M, Ebara M, Matsutani S, Okuda K. Association of gallbladder carcinoma and anamalous pancreaticobiliary ductal union. *Gastroenterology* 1985; 89:1258-65.
28. Kinoshita H, Nagata E, Hirohashi K, Sakai K, Kobaiashi Y. Carcinoma of the gallbladder with an anomalous connection between the choledochus and the pancreatic duct. *Cancer* 1984; 54:762-9.
29. Tomono H, Nimura Y, Aono K, Nakashima I, Iwamoto T, Nakashima N. Point mutation of the c-Ki-ras gene in carcinoma and atypical epithelium associated with congenital biliary dilatation. *Am J Gastroenterol* 1996; 91:1211-4.
30. Komi N, Tamura T, Miyoshi Y, Kunitomo K, Udaka H, Takehara H. Nationwide surgery of cases of choledochal cysts: analysis of coexistent anomalies, complications, and surgical treatment in 645 cases. *Surg Gastroenterol* 1984; 3:69-73.
31. Baumann R, Wittersheim C, Dron K. Dilatations kystiques congénitales du cholèdoque. Anomalie de la jonction bilio-pancréatique. *Hépato-Gastro* 1997; 4: 281-6.
32. Lipsett P, Pitt HA, Colombani PM, Biotnott JK, Cameron JL. Choledochal cyst disease. A changing pattern of presentation. *Ann Surg* 1994; 220: 644-52.
33. Chijiiwa K, Koga A. Surgical management and long-term follow-up of patients with choledochal cysts. *Am J Surg* 1993; 165:238-42.
34. Schudamore CH, Hemming AW, Teare JP, Fache JS, Erb SR, Watkinson AF. Surgical management of choledochal cysts. *Am J Surg* 1994; 167:497-500.
35. Hewitt PM, Kridge JEJ, Bormann PC, Terblanche J. Choledochal cysts in adults. *Br J Surg* 1995; 82:382-5.
36. Chaudhary A, Dhar P, Sachdev A, Kumar N, Vij JC, Sarin SK, Broor SL, Sharma SS. Choledochal cysts - difference in children and adults. *Br J Surg* 1996; 83:186-8.
37. Lopez RR, Pinson WM, Campbell JR, Harrison M, Katon RM. Variation in management based on type of choledochal cyst. *Am J Surg* 1991; 161:612-5.
38. Nagorney DM, McIlrath DC, Adson MA. Choledochal cysts in adults: clinical management. *Ann Surg* 1994; 94:656-63.
39. Stain SC, Guthrie CR, Yellin AE, Donovan AJ. Choledochal cyst in the adult. *Ann Surg* 1983; 52:2086-8.
40. Todani T, Watanabe Y, Toki A, Urushihara N. Carcinoma related to choledochal cysts with internal drainage operations. *Surg Gynecol Obstet* 1987; 164:61-4.

41. Benhidjeb T., Munster B., Ridwelski K., Rudolph B., Mau H., Lippert H.: Cystic dilatation of the common bile duct: surgical treatment and long-term results. Br. J. Surg. 1994; 81:433-436.
42. Takiff H., Stone M., Fonkalsrud E.W.: Choledochal cysts: results of primary surgery and need for reoperation in young patients. Am. J. Surg. 1985; 150:141-145.
43. Yamaguchi M.: Congenital choledochal cysts. Analysis of 1.433 patients in the Japanese literature. Am. J. Surg. 1980; 140:653-657.
44. Ando H., Ito T., Kaneko K., Seo T., Ito F.: Intrahepatic bile duct stenosis causing intrahepatic calculi formation following excision of a choledochal cyst. J. Am. Coll. Surg. 1996; 183:56-60.
45. Ando H., Kaneko K., Ito T., Watanabe Y., Seo T., Harada T., Ito F., Nagaya M., Sugito T.: Complete excision of the intrapancreatic portion of choledochal cysts. J. Am. Coll. Surg. 1996; 183:317-321.

CHAPTER 8

BILIARY STENT OCCLUSION : A MICROBIOLOGICAL AND SCANNING ELECTRON MICROSCOPY (SEM) INVESTIGATION.

ANTONIO BASOLI, FAUSTO FIOCCA, * ROBERTA DI ROSA, * * LUCILLA BALDASSARRI, and * * GIANFRANCO DONELLI

*2nd Department of Surgery, and * Department of Clinical Medicine, University of Rome "La Sapienza", and * * Laboratory of Ultrastructure, ISS, Rome, Italy*

Summary

In obstructive jaundice the decompression of occluded common bile duct with transhepatic or perduodenoscopic positioning of a biliary stent, represents a valid alternative to surgery because of a lower incidence of morbility and mortality, a shorter mean hospital stay and the rapid regression of jaundice and itching. The main limitation of this procedure is the late occlusion of the stents which requires their removal, with an increased risk for the patient and an additional health care cost.

The aim of this study was to investigate factors involved in plastic biliary stent blockage : the stent, the bile and the micro-organisms.

Immediately after their removal, 5 mm of biliary and duodenal ends of the stents were cut under sterile conditions and then bisected. The 4 samples were soaked in PBS and glutaraldehyde. PBS samples were sonicated for quantitative microbiological analysis. Glutaraldehyde samples were examined by scanning electron microscopy (SEM).

We analyzed the organic material deposited on 30 biliary stents, extracted from 26 patients (mean implantation time,106 days, range 2-380). A quantitative microbiological analysis was performed and a mixed flora obtained from 21 stents. Among the 26 patients, 20 underwent broad-spectrum antibiotic therapy. Several species were identified: 10 Gram positive, 6 Gram negative, 1 anaerobe, 1 mycete. SEM analysis detected the presence of abundant amorphous material and coccoid or bacillary forms on the surface of stents.

Our results are in agreement with those of the literature, and seem to indicate that contamination is the major factor in the pathogenesis of stent occlusion. We also observed that among isolated bacteria, enterococci were predominant, even if an analysis of a higher number of cases is required to better identify micro-organisms most frequently found in the material occluding the stents. To hinder or at least reduce stent blockage additional studies of biomaterials will be fundamental, especially on the interaction between the electrical charges of the stent surface and those of the bacterial membrane.

Introduction

In obstructive jaundice, decompression of occluded common bile duct with the transhepatic positioning or during ERCP of a biliary stent [2,6,7,8] represents a

E. Zanella (ed.), Advances in Abdominal Surgery, 69–80.

valid alternative to surgery in inoperable tumors, as well as in benign stricture of elderly patients and/or in case of high surgical risk.

Stent insertion presents a lower incidence of morbidity and mortality and mean hospital stay after treatment is markedly shorter than after surgery. The rapid regression of jaundice and itching, with consequent marked improvement in the quality of life, is achieved in over 90% of patients [6,8].

Even if in approximately 5% of cases early complications such as bleeding, pancreatitis, stent migration may be present [8], major limitations are late occlusions.

Numerous studies have shown that occlusion is caused by the deposition on the stent surface of amorphous material composed of bacteria, proteins, bilirubinate crystals, calcium palmitate [8,10]. Biliary stent occlusion causes bile flow reduction with consequent acute cholangitis, varying from 4 to 36% in the different series [9,10].

Data of the incidence of stent occlusion is very heterogeneous: while in retrospective studies there was 10-30% incidence of occlusion, higher percentages (21%-54%) have been reported in prospective randomized trials [8] (Table 1).

Table 1. Incidence of stent occlusion in prospective randomized trials

Trials	Year	N	Stent Diameter (French Gauge)	Occlusions N	Occlusions %	Mean Patency (months)
Shepherd	1988	23	10	10	43	N.A.
Davis	1992	56	10	30	54	4.2
Knyrim	1993	28	11.5	12	43	6.0
Sung	1994	67	10	35	52	1.8
Smith	1994	95	10	36	38	4.54.5
Barrioz	1994	10	10-12	7	70	1.4
Ghosh	1994	70	10-12	15	21	9.2
Total		349		145	42	4.9

Once the stent is occluded, it must necessarily be removed and replaced by a new one, and the patient must be hospitalized again. This limits the patient's functional indipendence and quality of life, with higher, hardly sustainable health care costs. Moreover, the positioning of a new stent requires a new endoscopic or percutaneous treatment, and involves various problems such as bile duct traumas, acute cholangitis [10] and a shorter occlusion time as compared with that of the first insertion [7].

While the precise dynamics of occlusion have not been clarified as yet, the most commonly accepted pathogenetic hypothesis is bacterial colonization and subsequent adhesion to the stent with the deposition of a biofilm, which allows tighter bacterial adhesion and protects microorganisms against both the host defenses and antibiotic therapy. Bacterial enzymes apparently act on bile constituents, followed by their precipitation and sludge formation [7,8,10,11].

However, the process is not altogether clear; first, the interaction between the bacteria and the biomaterial of the stent is not exactly known; second, it has not been completely ruled out as yet whether bile pigments may deposit on the stent surface and directly interact with it, and whether bacterial adhesion to the wall is secondary [8,10].

In tackling the problems of biliary stent occlusion, and thus of its prevention, the 3 major factors involved in this process should be considered:

1 The biliary stent; 2. The bile; 3. The micro-organisms.

In recent years, numerous studies have been conducted to design an "ideal" stent which could prevent occlusion [8], the stent characteristics include its diameter, shape, surface and materials. As for materials, possible interactions between the stent and the bile constituents, should be considered.

A. *Diameter.* The most common system for preventing occlusion is the use of a large diameter stent. While a large stent does not inhibit bacterial adhesion or biofilm deposition,it allows more space to sludge; consequently, a longer time is required for stent occlusion. A number of authors have shown a clear advantage, in terms of longer duration of patency and fewer episodes of cholangitis, of stents 10 Fr in diameter, as compared with those of a lower diameter [8,12].

B. *Shape*. It is another factor which conditions sludge formation. The flow of the bile through a straight stent is significantly higher than through a curved or pigtail stent, or with side holes at the level of anchoring edges. These are preferential sites for sludge formation, probably due to the creation of turbulent bile flows that favor clogging [13]. Recently, a pilot study conducted on a new biliary stent without side holes, the tannenbaum stent, has shown very encouraging results; it allows effective bile duct decompression and patency for a longer period as compared to conventional plastic stents [14].

C. *Surface.* Polymers commonly used for biliary stents seem to have a smooth surface; however, by scanning electron microscopy (SEM) it was shown that there are surface irregularities which might facilitate bacterial or biofilm adhesion or both. A new polymer, vivathane, for ultrasmooth-walled stents has been tested in vitro. The achieved results are very encouraging with a marked reduction in bacterial adhesion and stent occlusion; however in vivo results are still lacking [15].

In the past, to reduce bacterial adhesion by acting on the stent inner surface, a hydrophilic polymer coated polyurethane stent (Hydromer) [16] was tested. This was based on the observation that since a hydrophobic environment was previously shown to favour bacterial adhesion, it was thought that a hydrophilic environment could prevent it. The experiment did show a reduction in bacterial adhesion; however this stent was not used in clinical practice due to the excessive mechanical weakness of the hydrophilic polymer [16].

D. *Materials.* As for the interactions between the stent and the bile constituents, there are:

Electrostatic interactions: the translation motion at the two-phase interface (polymer-bile) determines a potential difference which may be responsible for charged solute (lipids, glycolipids, proteins) absorption.

Hydrophobic interactions: they favour aggregation per se.

Chemisorption: most likely, the materials used for stents are not completely inert, and some polymers can be endowed with a certain reactivity which may favour the precipitation of some bile constituents [8].

Bile

The main constituents of the bile involved in the formation of occluding material are bile pigments, bile acids, cholesterol, phospholipids and proteins [11]. Recently, attention has been focused ,in particular, on the latter. It has been shown that the material adhering to the stent plastic surface contains two protein bands, 13kD and 16kD, whose origin is still unknown. These proteins are not commonly present in human bile, and thus it has been hypothesized that they represent either the reflux of pancreatic protein precipitates, or that they are produced by bacterial degradation of some host proteins (as IgA). Although protein adhesion to the stent surface may play a role in the initial sludge formation, its precise role is still unknown [10]. Jung et al. have published the results of an in vitro study where they observed that there are some proteins, fibronectin and vitronectin in particular, adherent to the stent surface. These proteins seem to be able to enhance bacterial adhesion to the stent surface; it was also observed that there was a clear correlation between the quantity of absorbed fibronectin and the amount of adherent bacteria. This was explained by the hypothesis that in vivo some bile proteins might be absorbed on the stent inner surface, while some might be used by bacteria as receptors, thus starting the process of bacterial adhesion to the stent surface [10].

As for the other bile constituents, the importance of bile salts is to be stressed. Some substances such as ursodeoxycholic acid, have a choleretic effect; namely they prevent bile stagnation in biliary stents. Some authors have tested the use of ursodeoxycholic acid to prevent biliary stent occlusion, but results were controversial. A clinical trial conducted by Ghost and Palmer in 1994 did not show any benefit in long-term treatment with ursodeoxycholic acid combined with various classes of antibiotics. In contrast, Barriotz and Ingrand obtained a significantly prolonged stent patency using ursodeoxycholic acid combined with norfloxacin [18].

Micro-organisms

The role played by bacteria seems determininant in sludge formation. Micro-organisms reach the bile ducts through the portal vein, the hepatic artery, and lymphatic vessels, or by ascending route from the duodenum through the papilla of Vater. The latter is favoured by papillotomy, or the presence of a transpapillary stent [19]. In vitro studies have evidenced that stents perfused with sterile bile did not show a significant sludge deposition. When bacteria were introduced into the system, sludge deposition was rapid and resulted in occlusion. Dowidar and Speer have hypothesized that micro-organisms adhere to the stent surface using the pili, or through the production of a mucopolysaccharide membrane acting as "cement". Bacteria grow within the glycocalyx matrix and form a sessile colony and then a biofilm. This structure might enable bacteria to firmly adhere to the surface in spite of the presence of bile flow. The biofilm matrix might supply the bacteria with a physical barrier against the host defenses (leukocytes and IgA) and prevent antibiotic penetration [20].

Bacteria implanted in the bile ducts might be able to synthesize several enzymes, among which a B-glycuronidase, produced mainly by Enterobacter, active in the bile. This enzyme splits glycuronidated bilirubin releasing glycuronic acid, used by bacteria as a source of energy as well as raw material for the formation of glycocalyx where insoluble calcium bilirubinate crystals precipitate. Bacterial phospholipase splits lipids and lecithins and also causes calcium salt and fatty acid deposition. These crystals combine with the already present bacterial mass to form the sludge.

Materials and Methods

Stents

Plastic (polyethylene, polyurethane and teflon) stents were analyzed. They were inserted by endoscopy or transhepatic route and removed from bile ducts of patients with obstructive jaundice, for occlusion or when repositioning of new stents was required. This allowed the study of stents in different phases of the occlusion process. Immediately after removal, 5 mm of the biliary and duodenal ends of the stent were cut under sterile conditions and then bisected. The 4 samples were soaked in PBS (2 ml, pH7.4) and glutaraldehyde,to prevent drying. 2.5% cacodylate-buffered glutaraldehyde was prepared before use. PBS samples were sonicated on ice for 10 min at 20 Mhz to separate bacteria present on the surface or in the biofilm. The obtained suspension was diluted and plated on nonselective media (blood agar plates) for quantitative microbiology. Plates were incubated at different oxygen tensions (aerobes, microaerophils, anaerobes) for at least one week. Isolated strains of anaerobes and aerobes were typed, tested for antibiotic sensitivity and frozen for subsequent in vitro studies.

Samples fixed in 2.5% cacodylate-buffered glutaraldehyde were processed with the standard procedure for SEM by dehydration in increasing ethanol solutions and critical point drying (CPD). To evaluate the effect of exposure to organic solvents on clogging, some samples were dehydrated by drying at 40°C for 2 hours. After gold sputter-coating, samples were examined by SEM. New stents of different materials were also prepared and tested, one of which (Hydroflex) was coated with a hydrophilic layer. This stent was previously soaked for 1 min in sterile water for the hydration of coating material.

Because of the presence of hydrated material, glutaraldehyde and ruthenium red fixation was performed. SEM analysis was aimed at the evaluation of the amount, morphology and specific composition of organic materials. The state of stent preservation was compared to that of new stents of the same type.

Personal series

Thirty 10 Fr stents of different chemical composition (polyethylene, polyurethane and teflon) explanted from 26 patients (14 men, 12 women) ranging in age from 46 to 89 years (mean age: 66.7) were examined. All patients were treated for obstructive jaundice; in 13 it was malignant (5 pancreatic carcinomas, 5 CBD carcinomas, 2 gallbladder carcinomas, and 1 case of metastases of the hepatic portal). 9 patients on stent explantation showed jaundice and fever while the remaining 4 were symptoms-free. 13 patients had a benign form (7 cases of iatrogenic stricture, 3 cases of cholelithiasis, 2 cases of chronic pancreatitis, 1 case of sclerosing cholangitis). Seven patients on stent explantation showed jaundice and fever while 6 were symptom-free. Among the 13 patients with malignant disease, 10 underwent broad-spectrum antibiotic therapy (1 pt for 2 days, 3 pts for 5 days, 1 pt for 6 days, 1 pt for 7 days, 1 pt for 8 days, 1 pt for 10 days, 1 pt for 26 days, 1 pt for 30 days; average 10.4 days), while the remaining 3 patients did not receive any antibiotic therapy.

As for the 13 patients with benign disease, 10 underwent broad-spectrum antibiotic therapy (2 pts for 3 days, 2 pts for 4 days, 2 ptas for 5 days, 1 pt for 6 days, 1 pt for 13 days, 1 pt for 14 days, 1 pt for 19 days: average 7.6 days) while the remaining 3 patients did not receive any antibiotic therapy.

In 3 of the 13 patients with benign disease, the stents were repeatedly removed and examined (twice in 1 pt, once in 2).

Indwelling stents were maintained for from 2 to 380 days (average 106 days). In santibiotic-treated patients, stents were maintanined for a mean of 101.2 days in cases of malignant disease, 91.5 days in those with benign disease. In untreated patients, stents were maintained for 70.6 days on an average in case of malignant disease, and 75 days in case of benign disease. 12 stents were removed without occlusion (average 31.7 days) while 18 stents were replaced for occlusion (average 179.5 days); of these, 3 were from the group of untreated patatients (16.6%) and 15 from that of treated patients (83.4%). All removed stents were examined for quantitative microbiology and SEM.

Results

Bacteriology of removed stents showed that of the 18 stents replaced for occlusion, 13 had a bacterial growth in both ends or in one, while 3 were sterile. 11 were from patients with malignant disease and 7 from those with benign disease.
Of the 12 stents without occlusion on explantation, 6 were contaminated and 6 were sterile. In this group, 4 stents were from patients with malignant disease, 8 from those with benign disease (Table 2).

Table 2. Removed stents and their characteristics

	Stents No.	Contaminated	Sterile	Malignant Stricture	Benign Stricture
Occluded	18	15	3	11	7
Non occluded	12	6	6	4	8
Total	30	21	9	15	15

The bacterial flora presents in the 12 contaminated stents was typed based on morphology, staining culture and biochemistry. Results of isolated strains divided into occluded and non occluded stents on removal, are reported in Table 2. Of the 18 occluded stents, overall, 41 strains were isolated with an average of 2.27 strains/stent. Of the 12 non occluded stents, 9 strains were isolated with an average of 0.75 strains/stent. Among isolated micro-organisms, Gram positives were predominant. Isolation of Enterococci was relevant (predominantly E. faecalis); there were 17 strains out of 41 in the group of occluded stents and 6 out of 9 in the group of non-occluded stents. Strains of Staphylococci were less numerous and present only in occluded stents; coagulase-negative staphylococci were most common. Enterobacteria were also relevant in occluded stents (9 strains). Only one anaerobe, Veillonella parvula, was isolated. Candida species was present in a small number (5) of samples (Table 3).

Table 3. Isolated microorganisms

Aerobic cocci Gram (+)	Occuled Stent	Patent Stent	Total
Enterococcus faecalis	10	4	14
Enterococcus faecium	5	1	6
Enterococcus (others)	2	1	3
Streptococcus bovis	1	0	1

Continue

Table 3.Continue

Staphilococcus aureus	1	0	1
Staphilococcus epidermitis	4	0	4
Staphilococcus capitis	1	0	1
Pediococcus	1	0	1
Bacilli Gram (+)			
Corinebacterium Spp.	1	0	1
Bacillus Spp.	0	1	1
Bacilli Gram (-)			
Escherichia coli	4	0	4
Klebsiella oxytoca	2	0	2
Klebsiella pneumonia	1	0	1
Enterobacter freundi	1	0	1
Enterobacter cloacae	1	1	2
Pseudomonas Spp.	1	0	1
Anaerobies	1	0	1
Veillonella parvula	1	0	1
Mycetes			
Candida Spp.	4	1	5
Total	41	9	50

As for the bacterial counts, altogether they were over 10,000 CFU/ml in 7 out of 18 occluded stents and in only 1 of the 12 non-occluded stents. Counts between 1000 to 10,000 CFU/ml were present in 5 stents of group 1 and in 4 of group 2. Counts of less than 1000 CFU/ml were present in 3 occluded stents and in a single non occluded stent (Table 4).

Table 4. Count of isolated bacterial strains

Counts	Occluded stents	Non occluded stents
> 10000	7	1
1000 – 10000	5	4
< 1000	3	1
Sterile	3	6

The surface characteristics of unused stents were first detected by SEM. Surfaces were essentially smooth (Fig 1a), with a more marked uneveness on the outer side.

Some imperfections might be due to the preparation for SEM. In the case of Hydroflex, coated with a hydrophilic polymeric layer, because of the presence of highly hydrated material, glutaraldehyde or ruthenium red fixation was performed: however this did not seem to improve the preservation of coating which condensed a series of aggregates.
Samples from explanted stents underwent CPD and air-drying In the first case (Fig.1b,Fig.1c), the presence of abundant amorphous material and coccoid or bacillary forms (Fig.1d) was detected. Air-drying, which prevented exposure to chemical solvents, allowed the observation of crystals of various morphology, embedded in the organic matrix (Fig.1e).

Figure 1a

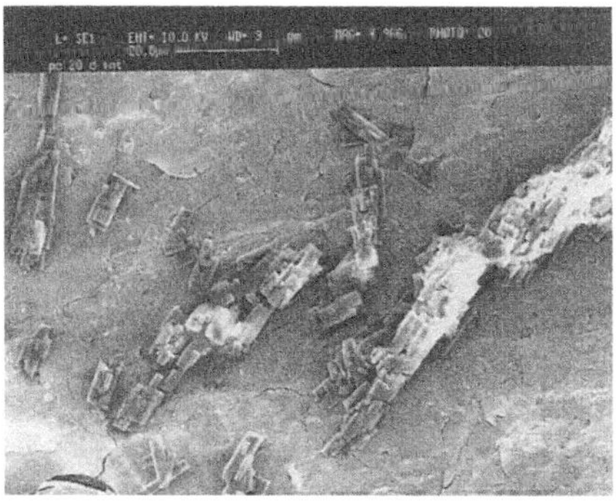

Figure 1b

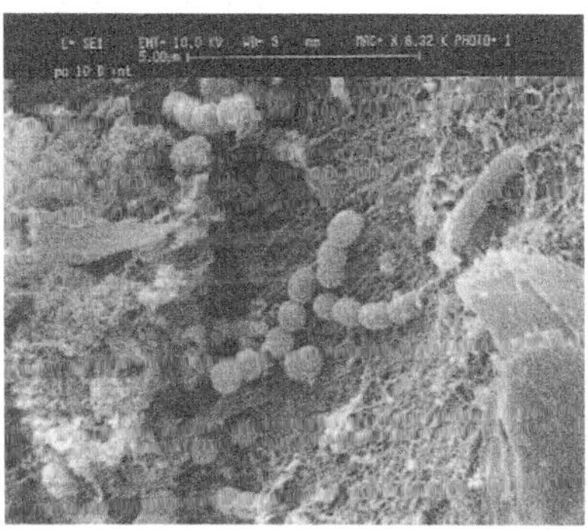

Figure 1c

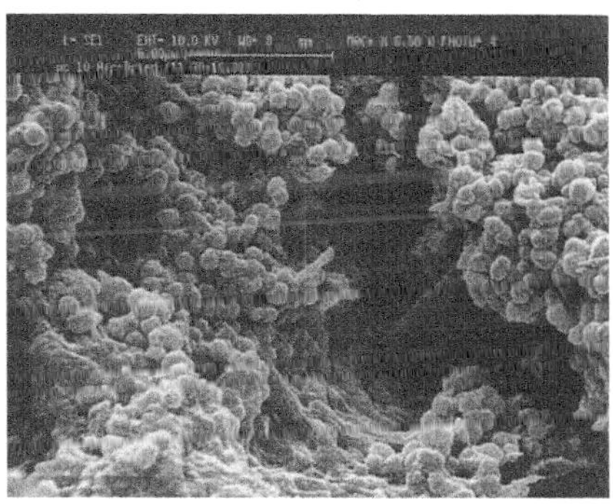

Figure 1d

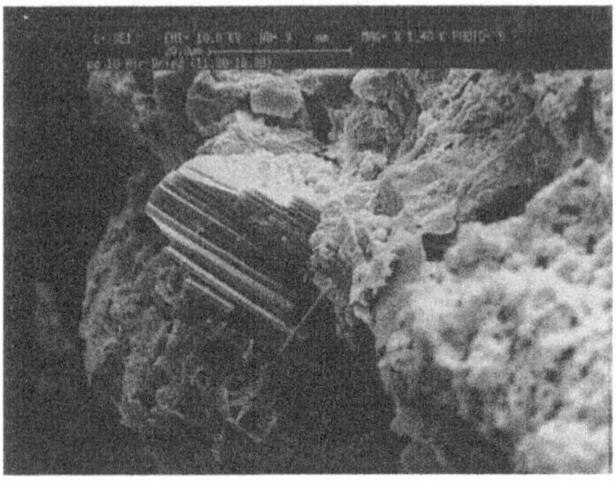

Figure 1e

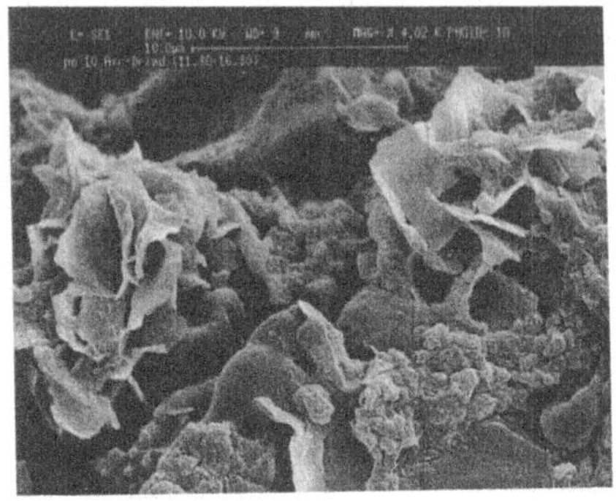

Discussion

Stents are certainly useful in the treatment of obstructive jaundice, the malignant form in particular [8].

Unfortunately, the benefit of indwelling stents is limited by the occlusion, which requires their removal, with an increased risk for the patient and a non negligible additional health care cost [7,8].

Our results are in agreement with those of the literature [8,10,11] and seem to indicate microbial contamination as the major factor in the pathogenesis of occlusion. In fact, microbiology and SEM showed the presence of bacteria with bile precipitates in the occluding material.

Several clinical trials with various antibiotics, isolated or in combination, have been carried out to prevent stent occlusion. Antibiotics were administered to patients or used for stent cleansing; however, no particular benefits were gained [8]. In this respect, Molinari suggested that a suitable therapy should be tailored to the single case, after the isolation of causative agents removed from stents or found in the endoscopically collected bile [21].

In our experience, broad-spectrum antibiotic therapy did not seem to be particularly effective, keeping in mind that among the 18 stents explanted because of occlusion, the majority (83.4%) were from patients treated with antibiotics, and only a minority (16.6%) were from patients who did not receive antibiotic therapy. The indiscriminate use of antibiotics may be hazarduous when it results in the selection of a resistant microbial flora. In our series, there were 5 cases of Candida contamination.

We have also observed that among isolated bacteria, enterococci were predominant; they are often resistant to cephalosporins, quinolones, aminoglycosides, commonly used in biliary infections. Undoubtedly, the analysis of a higher number of cases is required to better identify micro-organisms most frequently found in the material occluding the stents.

To prevent occlusion, additional studies on biomaterials will be fundamental. Donelli and coworkers observed that, after contact with polylysine (a poly-amino acid able to induce a change in the cell membrane conductivity and permeability), experimental K562 cells from leukemia do not grow in suspension as, occurs experimentally, but grow more slowly and adherent to each other. These observations seem to indicate that , as well as the type, amount and distribution of cell membrane components such as lipids, proteins and polysaccharides, membrane active ion transport might be altered. Although the precise mechanism of these changes in K562 cells is unknown, they might cause the change in the growth-pattern of these cells [22].

It is possible to hypothesize that a study on the interaction between the electrical charges of the stent surface and those of the bacterial membrane may lead to the experimentation of new materials able to hinder, or at least reduce, bacterial adhesion to the stent surface.

References

1. Millis JM et al. Management of bile duct strictures. An envolving strategy. *Arch Surg* 1992 ; 127 :1077-84
2. Lillemoe KD, Pitt HA. Surgical palliation and otherwise. *Cancer* 1996 ; 78 :605-14
3. Lee SP, Sekijima J. Gallstones in Yamada. Textbook of gastroenterology. J.B.Lipponcott Company Philadelphia 1991, pp 1975.
4. Cakmakci M, Timaksis B et al. Effects of obstructive jaundice and external biliary diversion on bacterial traslocation in rats. *Eur J Surg* 1996 ; 162 :567-71.
5. Speer AG, Cotton PB. Randomized trial of endoscopic versus percutaneous stent insertion in malignant obstructive jaundice. *Lancet* 1987 :57-62.
6. Smith AC, Dowsett JF et al. Randomized trial of endoscopic stenting versus surgical bypass in malignant low bileduct obstruction. *Lancet* 1994; 344 :1655-60.
7. Sung JJY, Chung SCS et al. Endoscopic stenting for pallation of malignant biliary obstruction. A review of progress in the last 15 years. *Dig Dis Sci* 1995 ;40 : 1167-73.
8. Libby ED, Leung JW. Prevention of Biliary Stent Clogging: A clinical Review. *Am J Gastroent* 1996;91:1302-8.
9. Dowidar N, Moesgaard F, et al. Clogging and other complications of endoscopic biliary endoprostheses. *Scand J Gastr* 1991 ; 26 : 1132-6.
10. Groen AK et al. Characterization of the content of occluded biliary endoprostheses. *Endoscopy* 1987 ; 19 : 57-9.
11. Yu JLF, Andersson R. Protein adsorption and bacterial adhesion to bilary stent materials. *J Surg Res* 1996,62.69-73.
12. Kadakia SS, Starnes E. Comparison of 10 French gauge stent with 11.5 French gauge stent in patients with biliary tract diseases. *Gastrointest Endosc* 1994;38:454-9.
13. Seitz U, Vadeyar H. Prolonged patency with a new design teflon biliary prosthesis. *Endoscopy* 1994 ; 26 : 478-82.
14. Binmoeller KF, Seitz U. The Tannenbaum stent : a new plastic biliary stent without side holes. *Am J Gastroent* 1995 ; 90 :1764-8.
15. McAllister EW, Carey LC. The role of polymeric surface smoothness of biliary stents in bacterial adherence, biofilm deposition, and stent occlusion. *Gastrointest Endosc* 1993;39:422-5.
16. Jansen B, Goodman L P. Bacterial adherence to hydrophilic polymer-coated polyurethane stents. *Gastrointest Endosc* 1993;39:670-3.

17. Davis PH, Groen AK. Randomized trial of self-expanding metal stents versus polyetylene stents for distal malignant biliary obstruction. *Lancet* 1992 ; 340 :1488-92.
18. Barrioz C, Ingrand P. Randomized trial of prevention of biliary stent occlusion by ursodeoxycholic acid plus norfloxacin. *Lancet* 1994;344: 581-2.
19. Gallone L. Patologia del fegato e della vie biliari. In: Patologia Chirurgica. Casa Editrice Ambrosiana, Milano 1986, pp 1651.
20. Speer AG, Cotton PB. Biliary stent blockage with bacterial biofilm. An electron microscopy study. *Ann Int Med* 1988;108:546-53.
21. Molinari G, Pugliese V. Bacteria Involved in the Blockage of Biliary Stents and their Susceptibility to antibacterial agents. *Eur J Clin Microbiol Infect Dis* 1996;15:88-92.
22. Santini M T, Cametti C, Indovina PL, Morelli G, Donelli G. Polylysine induces changes in membrane electrical properties of K562 cells. *J Biomed Mater Res* 1997 ; 35 :165-74.

CHAPTER 9

CYSTIC TUMORS OF THE PANCREAS : SEROUS CYSTADENOMA AND MUCINOUS CYSTIC NEOPLASM.

ATTILIO M. FARINON, MARIO SIANESI *, FRANCESCO RULLI, and EVERARDO ZANELLA

*Department of Surgery of the University of Rome "Tor Vergata",Rome ,and *Chair of Surgical Pathology, University of Parme ,Parme,Italy*

Summary

Serous cystadenoma and mucinous cystic neoplasm are acquired neoplastic cysts, which together account for approximately 10-15% of all pancreatic cysts. When a cystic lesion is encountered, the first priority is to determine whether it is an inflammatory or neoplastic cyst. Failure to recognize the true nature of a neoplastic cyst will lead to an incorrect treatment strategy. Despite progress made in diagnostic techniques, the pre-operative differentiation between benign and malignant cystic neoplasms of the pancreas remains problematic. This chapter aims at an attempt to analyze and discuss these problems.

Introduction

Cystic neoplasms of the pancreas represent a pathologically heterogeneous group of tumors, including serous cystadenoma, mucinous cystadenoma and cystadenocarcinoma, as well as mucinous ductal ectasia, papillary cystic tumor, cystic islet-cell tumor, acinar cystadenocarcinoma, and other neoplastic lesions, that undergo necrosis and cystic degeneration (i.e. ductal adenocarcinoma, sarcoma, and lymphoma) [1]. Anyhow, as outlined by Rosai [2] , secondary cystic changes present in most exocrine or endocrine pancreatic neoplasms, are to be distinguished from tumors characterized by a cystic configuration as part of their definition (i.e. cystadenoma and cystadenocarcinoma).

Cystic tumors account for 10-15% of all pancreatic cystic lesions, and cystadenocarcinoma accounts for about 1% of all pancreatic carcinomas [3]. Nevertheless, this frequently quoted ratio may not be correct today, particularly concerning neoplastic versus inflammatory cystic lesions, these being more frequently detected, albeit asymptomatic, by ultrasonography and computed tomography [1]. Cystadenoma and cystadenocarcinoma of the pancreas are

E. Zanella (ed.), Advances in Abdominal Surgery, 81–93.

relatively frequent in women between the ages of 50 and 60, which is younger than for pancreatic carcinoma [4].

In their landmark reports [5,6] Compagno and Oertel, first classified cystic tumors of the pancreas, from the pathological point of view, into microcystic adenomas (serous glycogen-rich cystadenoma) and macrocystic mucinous neoplasms. The former are to be considered as benign lesions, while the latter are potentially malignant, as is supported by the observation that normal epithelium and abnormal epithelium (or clearly malignant areas) can co-exist within the same lesion.

However, pancreatic cystic lesions represent a diagnostic challenge for the clinician and pathologist, since differentiation between cystic neoplasms and inflammatory pseudocysts or other cystic lesions, or between benign and malignant cystic tumors, is often impossible, if based solely on biopsy or imaging techniques alone. In the report from Warshaw et al [7], 40% of the patients referred to the Massachusetts General Hospital for mucinous tumors had been misdiagnosed as having pseudocysts, and were then inappropriately treated. As Lumsden and Bradley emphasized in their publication [8], although the distinction between a pseudocyst and cystic neoplasm is perhaps the most critical, distinguishing between various types of cystic neoplasms is also subject to error.

Serous cystadenoma

Serous cystadenoma, also known as microcystic or glycogen-rich adenoma, has the gross appearance of a large multiloculated mass, characterized by the presence of numerous and usually tiny cystic cavities filled with a clear serous fluid, ranging in size from less than 1.0 mm to about 2.0 cm. These give to the cut surface of the adenoma, the "spongy" appearance typical of infantile polycystic kidneys [2]. Less frequently, serous cystadenoma shows as a uni- or oligolocular macrocystic lesion [2,9,10]. Lewandrowski et al [9], suggested that cysts larger than 2.0 cm in diameter should be considered macrocysts, and proposed macrocystic serous adenoma as a morphological variant differing from microcystic adenoma. A central stellate scar, occasionally calcified, with radiating fibrous septae may often be observed. About half of cystadenomas are located in the head of the pancreas, and only a few encompass the entire gland [5].

Microscopic appearances are based on the presence of multiple small cysts lined by cuboidal or flat epithelial cells, containing an abundance of glycogen but only a small amount of mucin, hence the name "glycogen-rich cystadenomas" which is also used for these lesions (Fig. 1). A layer of myoepithelial cells is observable beneath the epithelium [11]. The CEA and CA19-9 levels in the cystic lumen are usually low, as compared with mucinous neoplasms [12].

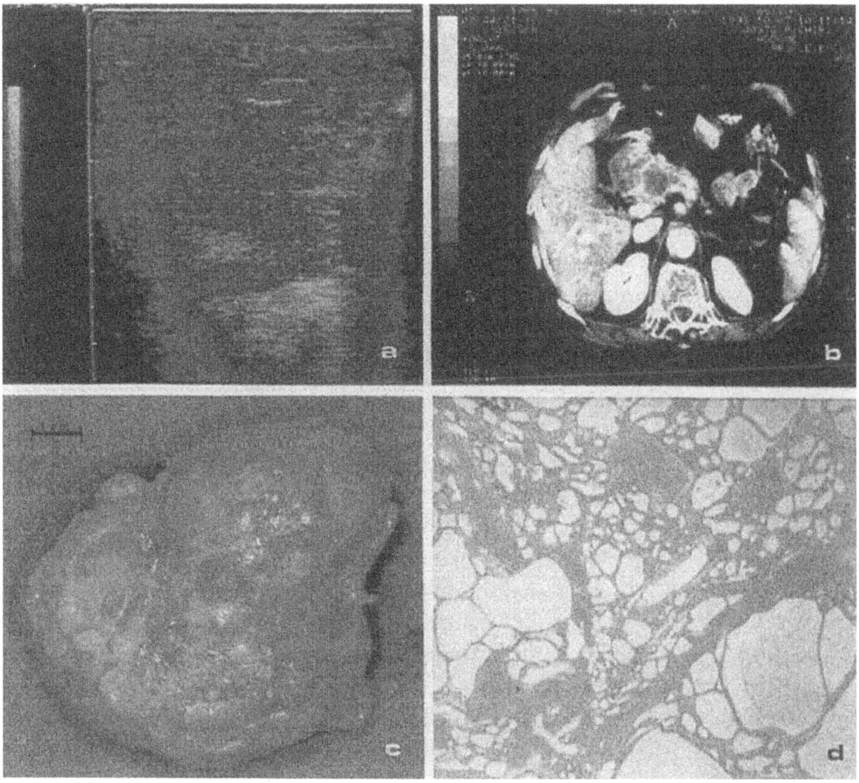

Figure 1. Case n.8 : M.I. , 65 year old female. Ultrasound (a) and C.T. scan (b) show a serous cystadenoma located in the neck and body of the pancreas; the gross appearance of the surgical specimen (c), obtained by middle pancreatic resection, is characterized by numerous small cysts; histological features (d) display cysts containing flocculent material. (see Color Plates, p. xvii)

Malignant transformation of serous cystadenoma should be regarded as an exceedingly unusual event, these neoplasms being virtually always benign. Whenever it occurs, serous cystadenocarcinoma may be similar in appearance to that of microcystic adenoma, in spite of the presence of metastases. Nuclear atypia and aneuploid DNA patterns may be present, albeit aneuploidy may also be found in several microcystic adenomas [13] .

The association of serous cystadenoma of the pancreas with other disorders has been described. Soloway [14] and Pyke et al [15] reported the coexistence of multinodular goiter and a papillary carcinoma of the thyroid. Montag et al [16] and Del Castillo et al [17] observed association with a ductal adenocarcinoma of the pancreas, and Pyke et al [15] with a synchronous ampullary carcinoma. However, a true association probably does exist with von Hippel-Lindau syndrome, an autosomally dominant, inherited, cancer-prone disorder, including retinal angiomatosis, haemangioblastoma of the central nervous system, renal cysts, renal cancer, pheocromocytoma, and epididimal cystadenoma [18,19]. In a recent review [19], pancreatic cystic lesions were demonstrated in 15% (10/55) of patients with the syndrome, and the only resected case presented a serous cystadenoma. Del Castillo et al [17] treated a woman with von Hippel-Lindau syndrome, displaying four confirmed serous cystadenomas of the pancreas.

Mucinous cystic neoplasm

"Mucinous cystic neoplasm with overt or latent malignancy" is the term proposed by Compagno and Oertel [6], in order to distinguish mucinous from serous cystic lesions. The term "cystadenoma" should be reserved for the latter lesion, uniformly benign, glycogen rich and mucine negative. Mucinous cystic tumors are mostly observed at a younger (4th and 5th decades) age, and predominantly in women. Macrocystic neoplasms are larger than serous cystadenomas, and are characterized by large multilocular or, infrequently, unilocular cysts lined by tall columnar cells, rich in mucin but lacking glycogen, and often forming papillae [6]. The underlying stroma may be very cellular, and its appearance closely resembles that of ovarian stroma [2] (Fig.2). Most mucinous cystic tumors are located in the body or tail of the pancreas, rather than in the head (Table 1).
These tumors have been classified as benign (mucinous cystadenoma) and malignant (mucinous cystadenocarcinoma), but the natural evolution of benign lesions towards malignancy is generally admitted [4]. For this reason, it seems more appropriate to consider all these tumors as mucinous cystic neoplasms, recognizing that the majority will present an aggressive behaviour if left untreated, and that within cystadenocarcinomas a great degree of heterogeneity is to be expected in the natural course of the disease [1,6]. Malignant transformation of mucinous cystadenomas has been reported even several years after incomplete excision, or internal drainage performed under the false presumption of pseudocysts [4,6,8,20,21]. The diagnosis of malignancy is essentially based on the presence of invasion of the wall by neoplastic glands, or frank anaplasia of the superficial component [2]. Extensive sampling of the specimen is required, and the absence of epithelial lining in a limited biopsy specimen does not rule out the diagnosis of a cystic tumor. Moreover, the presence of an inner epithelium within the cyst wall is variable: Warshaw et al.[7] found it discontinuous and patchy in 40% of serous cystadenomas, and 72% of mucinous neoplasms, with a denuded area encompassing up to 98% of the cyst wall surface (average involvement of 40%). Sometimes, the outer layer of hyalinized connective tissue may be absent, and the middle zone of densely cellular primitive mesenchymal stroma,

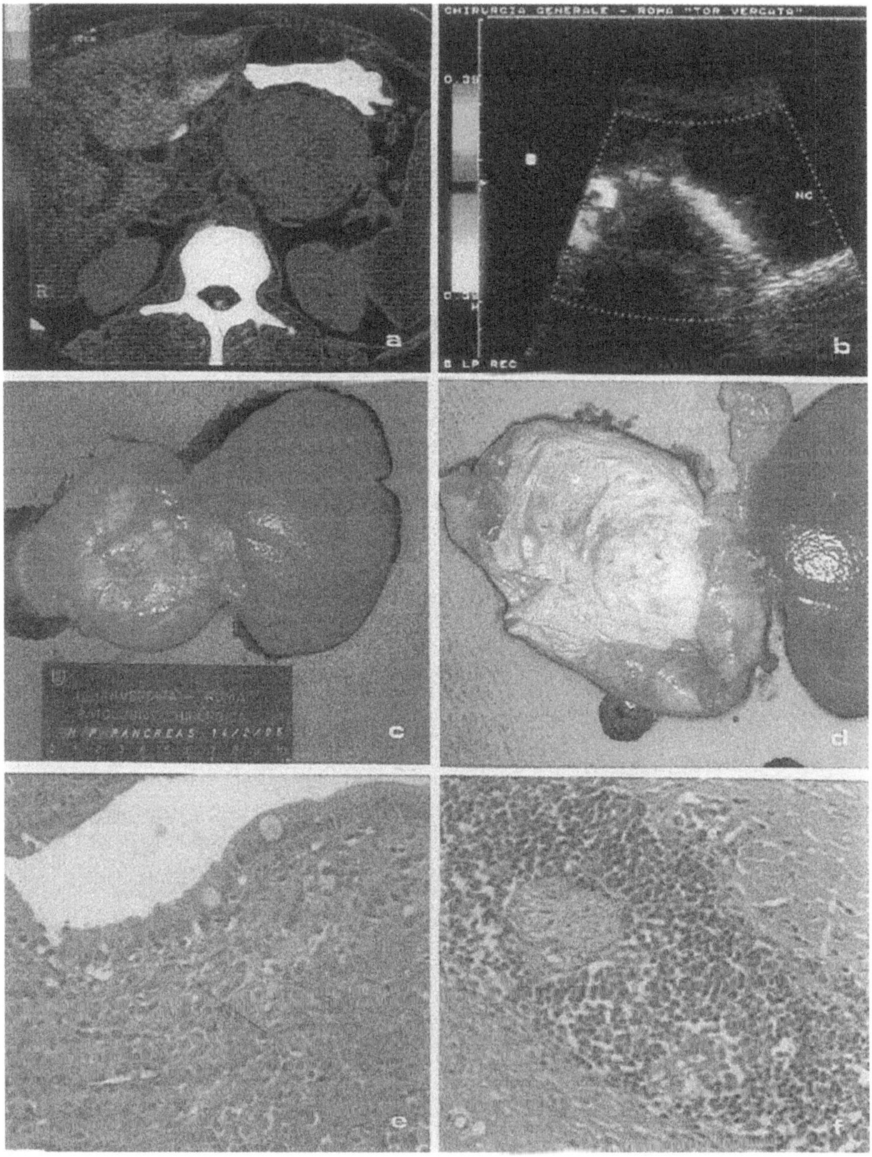

Figure 2. Case n.7 :P.N. 32 year-old female C.T.scan (a) and echo-color-doppler (b) show a cystic biloculated mass of the pancreatic tail; grown features of the outer (c) and cut (d) surface of the surgical specimen are detailed, as well as histological appearances demonstrating a mucinous cystic neoplasm of the pancreas with ovarian-like stroma (e) and with adjacent fibrotic tissue exhibiting focal perineural pseudoinvasion (f)

(see Color Plates, p. xviii)

Table 1. Cystic neoplasms of the pancreas: personal series

Case	Patient		Cystic neoplasm		
n.	Name	Year/sex	Site	Type	Surgical treatment
1	RI	67/F	Head	MCAD	DP
2	MC	72/F	Tail	MCADK	(unresectable because of local extension)
3	FL	58/M	Tail	MCAD	LPS
4	MR	76/M	Tail	MCADK*	(unresectable because of local extension and distant metastases)
5	BP	57/F	Tail	MCADK	(unresectable because of local extension and distant metastases)
6	GG	65/F	Tail	MCADK	LPS
7	PN	32/F	Tail	MCAD	LPS
8	MI	65/F	Body	SCAD	MP
9	AT	73/F	Head	SCAD	(left untreated)
10	GG	63/M	Head	MCADK	DP
11	SG	53/M	Head	MCADK	(unresectable because of local extension and distant metastases)
12	DF	40/F	Tail	SCAD	LPS
13	BL	82/F	Head & Body	MCADK	(unresectable because of local extension and distant metastases)

MCAD = mucinous cystadenoma; MCADK = mucinous cystadenocarcinoma;
SCAD = serous cystadenoma
DP = duodenopancreatectomy; LPS = left pancreatectomy with splenectomy; MP = middle pancreatectomy
*cystojejunostomy twelve years before

resembling ovarian stroma, may appear hypocellular or atrophic. Tumor markers such as CEA and CA 19-9 have been demonstrated immuno-histochemically, in mucinous cystic neoplasms, and their expression seems to be more relevant in malignant lesions [21,22].

Differentiation of pancreatic cystic lesions

In adults cystic lesions of the pancreas are pseudocysts in 80-90% of cases, the remaining cystic lesions being true cysts with epithelial lining. Many of these are neoplastic, including serous cystadenoma, mucinous cystadenoma, and mucinous cystadenocarcinoma.

Pre-operative differentiation between inflammatory and neoplastic cystic lesions of the pancreas, often represents a diagnostic challenge; moreover, considering that management strategy is strictly dependent on the type of cystic lesion.

However, most pseudocysts are characterized by a typical clinical presentation and imaging appearance, that do not pose a diagnostic dilemma. They are unilocular, moderately thin-walled cystic lesions, that follow an episode of acute pancreatitis or trauma (frequently undergoing spontaneous regression), or occur in the setting of chronic pancreatitis. On computed tomography and ultrasonography, solid components, septae, and loculations which are commonly present in cystic tumors, are not to be found in pseudocysts. Calcifications may be present in one third of cystic neoplasms, and are common in chronic pancreatitis, but may never be found in the pseudocyst wall [1]. Likewise, a significant number of cystic tumors show typical aspects that permit a confident diagnosis. The finding of a sharply - marginated, cystic pancreatic mass containing numerous tiny (<2 cm in diameter) well-defined cystic cavities, is consistent with the diagnosis of serous cystadenoma, even more so in the presence of a central scar, sometimes containing calcification. Similarly, most mucinous cystic neoplasms (cystadenomas and cystadenocarcinomas) show a typical appearance, usually based on the presence of a large multilocular cyst (less than six loculations exceeding 2 cm in diameter), with intracystic mural nodules or extracystic solid components, and occasionally peripheral calcification [23].

In spite of this statement, diagnostic errors with pancreatic cystic lesions certainly occur: clinical and radiological criteria do not result as being uniformly reliable, and intra-operative biopsy is to be considered unreliable, as it fails in correctly classifying pancreatic cysts in over 20% of cases [12].

Therefore, cyst fluid-analysis (amylase and lipase content, relative viscosity, tumor markers) and cytological findings have been suggested as being promising and helpful in differentiating pseudocysts from neoplastic cysts, and even in distinguishing potentially malignant mucinous cystadenomas from benign serous

Table 2. Serum and cystic fluid tumor markers measurement

	CEA		CA 19-9		CA 15-3		CA 50		TPA	
	S	C	S	C	S	C	S	C	S	C
7. P.N., 32 y, female MCAD Tail of the pancreas	1.3	>70	6.7	>240	16.5	26.2	14.2	>300	17.3	>2.000
10.G.G., 63 y, male MCADK Head of the pancreas	5.2	49.000	58	229			>300	>300	47	>2.000
11.S.G., 53 y, male MCADK Head of the pancreas	2.7	30.750	>240	>240	17.1	29	>300	>300	52	11.692
12.D.F., 40 y, female SCAD Tail of the pancreas	0.7	1.8	10.5	>240	14.2	27	5.2		43	>2.000
13.B.L., 82 y, female MCADK Head and body of the pancreas	4.1	10.820	98	>240			>300	>300	37	>2.000

MCADK = mucinous cystadenocarcinoma; SCAD = serous cystadenoma; MCAD = mucinous cystadenoma
S = serum; C = cyst; n.v.: CEA < 10 ng/ml; CA 19-9 <37 U/ml; CA 15-3 < 24 U/l; CA 50 < 14 U/ml; TPA <70 UI

cystadenomas [12,24,25,26]. Pancreatic cyst-fluid can be obtained before operation by ultrasound or computed tomography-guided percutaneous needle aspiration, or during operation. Enzyme analysis, relative viscosity, and cytology represent the tests performable on samples collected during operation, because of rapid performance, and being immediately available. Measurement of tumor markers' expression is only practical as a pre-operative procedure on percutaneous needle aspirates.

Concerning enzyme analysis, the amylase and lipase content of pseudocysts is almost always high, whereas the level in neoplastic cysts, is commonly low, although cystic tumors of all types may exhibit high fluid enzymatic content.

Measurement of cyst-fluid relative viscosity may be of significant benefit in differentiating mucinous neoplasms from non-mucinous cysts both prior to operation and during operation. This is supported by results obtained with magnetic resonance techniques, which offer the ability to characterize biological fluids by using magnetic relaxation times, in distinguishing malignant from benign mucinous cystic tumors. The viscosity of cystic fluid showed wide variations, with higher signal intensity on T1-weighted images in cystic neoplasms containing gelatinous mucin, which proved to be histologically malignant in the experience reported by Nishihara et al [27] .

Cytological analysis of aspirated cystic fluid is only helpful if positive, and caution is advised in interpretation to avoid misclassification of the cystic lesions [12]. Although the epithelial cells may appear benign, especially in tumors where the malignant component is focal, a definitive diagnosis is possible in a significative percentage of malignant tumors.

Evaluation of tumor markers' expression in cyst-fluid (as opposed to serum) is based on the observation that marker specificity appears markedly enhanced, when the sample is obtained directly from the tumor secretions [25]. Measurement of carcinoembrionic antigen (CEA) levels seems to allow reliable discrimination between benign lesions (psudocysts and serous cystadenomas) and mucinous and malignant tumors (mucinous cystic neoplasms, mucinous cystadenocarcinomas, and cystic ductal adenocarcinomas) [24,26,27]. As outlined by Lewandrowski et al [12], high cyst-fluid CEA levels do not predict malignancy, but rather indicate that the cyst is either malignant or of the mucinous type. Carbohydrate antigen CA 19-9 levels within the cyst-fluid appeared to be highly variable and non-discriminatory [13] , as we too observed in 5 out of 13 cystic neoplasms of the pancreas (Table 2). A moderately increased concentration of the antigen has been noted in benign pancreatic disease (pseudocyst, pancreatitis) [28], especially in pancreatitis where CA 19 9 levels are correlated with alkaline phosphatase levels [29]. However, determination of CA19-9 serum levels may prove to be a valuable marker in the detection of recurrence, even in a case of local recurrence, after resection of mucinous cystadenoma judged histologically as benign [30].

High CA 125 cyst-fluid levels seem to be predictive of malignancy and low values of a benign lesion, including mucinous cystic neoplasm. Serous cystadenoma showed variable values overlapping with those of malignant and benign cysts, but further experience is required to assess the usefulness of this marker [12,31].
Levels of tumor-associate glycoprotein 72 (TAG-72) in the cyst contents were markedly elevated in mucinous cystadenocarcinomas, as compared with that in pseudocysts and serous cystadenomas, while intermediate values were recorded in benign mucinous cystic neoplasms [25]. It has been hypothized that expression of CA 72-4 occurs at some point during the transformation of a benign into malignant mucinous tumor, and that expression of this antigen, like CA 15.3 [32], may be a marker for the genetic events leading to carcinogenesis in this tumor.
In addition to previously reported cyst-fluid markers, measurement of proliferative antigen TPA (tissue polypeptide antigen) may be considered an aid, in pre-operative differential diagnosis [26]. Markedly elevated or very low values seem to indicate a malignant or benign cystic lesion, respectively.

Surgical considerations

The historical development of the surgical management of cystic neoplasms of the pancreas, including cyst puncture, marsupialization, and internal drainage, has now reached the generally accepted use of resection and total excision, for pancreatic cystic neoplasms [33].
Internal drainage of cystic neoplasms of the pancreas should be discouraged, since symptomatic improvement is rare, and continued tumor enlargement is the rule [34], moreover, considering that drainage procedure withholds the possibility of definitive cure and long-term survival by complete surgical resection [35]. If a cystic neoplasm has been unwittingly drained into an adjacent segment of intestine, under the false presumption of pseudocyst, subsequent clinical behaviour may offer a clue that this has occurred [8]. However, curative resection may not be feasible years after internal drainage of a pancreatic cystic neoplasm, and such delay may be responsible for the development of interval metastases whenever a malignant cyst is present [34]. In our series, that was the case of a patient who previously underwent twelve years' surgical drainage of a cystic neoplasm mistaken for pancreatic pseudocyst, that then proved to be unresectable, because of local extension and distant metastases (Case n. 4). These observations emphasize the necessity for prompt and accurate diagnosis at the initial presentation, and for the avoidance of non-operative drainage of pancreatic pseudocyst, in order to prevent the inappropriate treatment of cystic neoplasms.
In view of current low-operative mortality, and of the difficulty of differentiating prior to operation between serous or mucinous tumors and between benign or

malignant forms of mucinous neoplasms, it is generally advocated that patients who present a lesion consistent with a cystic neoplasm on imaging techniques, should be explored, and the lesion resected. Exceptions could be made in selected patients, who are high surgical risks, such as those few patients with typical radiological findings of a serous microcystic tumor located in the head of the pancreas [3]. That was the case of an elderly woman who presented a mass in the head of the pancreas, incidentally found during celiotomy for gallbladder and common bile duct lithiasis. During the operation the mass, showing ultrasonographic and histopathological appearances (Fig. 3) consistent with a serous cystic neoplasm, was left untreated, and monitored periodically by imaging studies (Case n. 9).

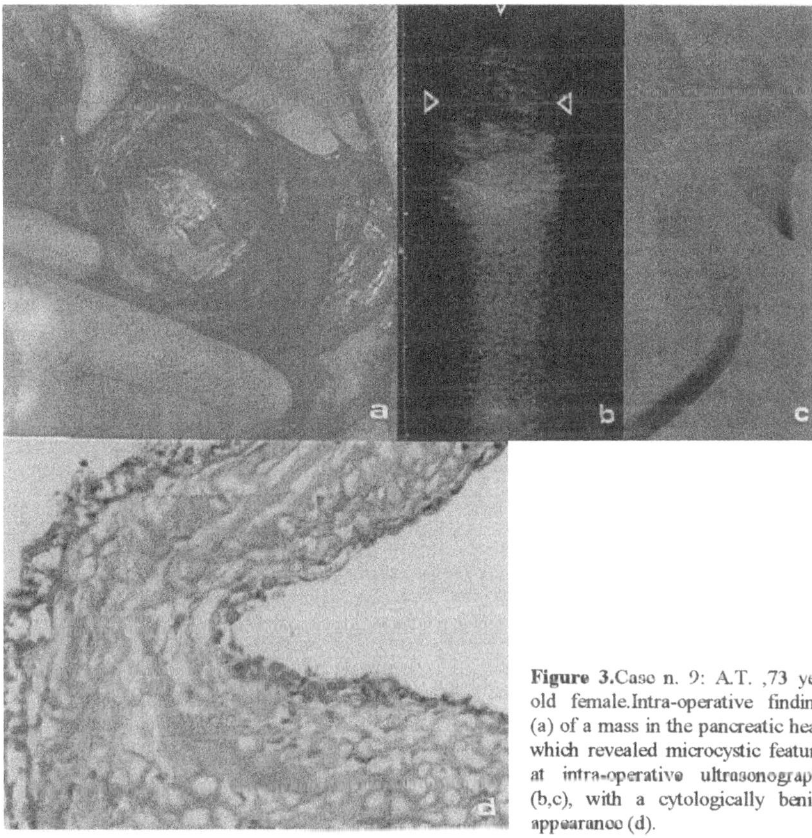

Figure 3. Case n. 9: A.T. ,73 year old female. Intra-operative findings (a) of a mass in the pancreatic head, which revealed microcystic features at intra-operative ultrasonography (b,c), with a cytologically benign appearance (d).
(see Color Plates, p. xix)

However, systematic resection of mucinous tumors appears mandatory, in view of their potential for malignancy. Depending on the location of the tumor, a duodenopancreatectomy, or a left pancreatectomy with splenectomy, should be

carried out, whereas in the treatment of a few cases located in the neck or body of the pancreas, a middle pancreatectomy with drainage of the remaining distal pancreas into a Roux-en-Y jejunal loop, should be advocated [17]. In our experience, only one patient was treated with this technique (Case n. 8).
Although the number of asymptomatic patients diagnosed incidentally by imaging techniques has increased, the results of resection of cystadenocarcinoma are frequently unsatisfactory, because of the advanced stage of the tumor. The prognosis after resection of cystadenocarcinomas is far better than for ductal carcinomas, and 5-year survivals range from 50% to 76% [7,36,37], compared with 5-year survivals higher than 95%, expected for those lesions considered benign or borderline [1]. Actually, no data are available on the results of chemotherapy and radiation therapy following resective treatment, and few reports may be found on the resectability obtained, in unresectable cystadenocarcinoma after neoadjuvant therapy [38,39].

References

1. Fernandez-del Castillo C, Warshaw L. Cystic tumors of the pancreas. *Surg Clin N Amer* 1995;75:1001-16.
2. Rosai J. Ackerman's surgical pathology. Eight edition. St Louis: Mosby,1996:982-9.
3. Katoh H, Rossi RL, Braasch JW, Munson JL, Shimozawa E, Tanabe T. Cystadenoma and cystadenocarcinoma of the pancreas. *Hepato-Gastroenterol* 1989; 36:424-30.
4. Sastre B, Carabalona B, Sahel J, Agostini S, Michotey G. Mucinous cystadenoma and cystadenocarcinoma of the pancreas: possibility for late recurrence and malignant transformation. *Dig Surg* 1991;8: 239-43.
5. Compagno J, Oertel JE. Microcystic adenoma of the pancreas (glycogen-rich cystadenomas): a clinicopathologic study of 34 cases. *Am J Clin Pathol* 1978;69:289-98.
6. Compagno J, Oertel JE. Mucinous cystic neoplasm of the pancreas with overt and latent malignancy (cystadenocarcinoma and cystadenoma). A clinicopathologic study of 41 cases. *Am J Clin Pathol* 1978;69:573-80.
7. Warshaw AL, Compton CC, Lewandroski KB, Cardenosa G, Mueller PR. Cystic tumors of the pancreas: new clinical, radiologic, and pathologic observations in 67 patients. *Ann Surg* 1990;212:432-45.
8. Lumsden A, Bradley III EL. Pseudocyst or cystic neoplasm ? : differential diagnosis and initial management of cystic pancreatic lesions. *Hepato-Gatroenterol* 1989;36:462-6.
9. Lewandrowski KB, Warshaw AL, Compton CC. Macrocystic serous cystadenoma of the pancreas: a morphologic variant differing from microcystic adenoma. *Hum Pathol* 1992;23:871-5.
10. Mori k, Takeyama S, Hirosawa H, Watanabe T, Taniya T, Arakawa H, et al. A case of macrocystic serous cystadenoma of the pancreas. *Int J Pancreatol* 1995;17:91-3.
11. Nyongo A, Huntrakoon M. Microcystic adenoma of the pancreas with myoepithelial cells. *Am J Clin Pathol* 1985;84:114-20.
12. Lewandrowski KB, Southern JF, Pins MR, ComptonCC, Warshaw AL. Cyst fluid analysis in the differential diagnosis of pancreatic cysts. A comparison of pseudocysts, serous cystadenomas, mucinous cystic neoplasms, and mucinous cystadenocarcinoma. *Ann Surg* 1993;217:41-7.
13. Unger PD, Danque PO, Fuchs A, Kaneko M. DNA flow cytometric evaluation of serous and mucinous cystic neoplasm of the pancreas. *Arch Pathol Lab Med* 1991;115:563-5.
14. Soloway HB. Constitutional abnormalities associated with pancreatic cystadenomas. *Cancer* 1965;18:1297-300.
15. Pyke CM, Van Heerden JA, Colby TV, Sarr MG, Weaver AL. The spectrum of serous cystadenoma of the pancreas. *Ann Surg* 1992;215:132-9.

16. Montag AG, Fossati N, Michelassi F. Pancreatic microcystic adenoma coexistent with pancreatic ductal carcinoma: a report of two cases. *Amer J Surg Pathol* 1990;14:352-5.
17. Fernandez-del Castillo C, Rivera JA, Warshaw AL. Cystic tumors. In: Trede M, Carter DC. Surgery of the pancreas. New York: Churchill Livingstone,1997:415-23.
18. Horton WA, Wong V, Elbridge R. Von Hippel-Lindau disease: clinical pathological manifestations in nine families with 50 affected members. *Arch Intern Med* 1976;136:769-77.
19. Neumann HPH, Dinkel E, Brambs H, Wimmer B, Friedburg H, Volk B, et al. Pancreatic lesions in the von Hippel-Lindau syndrome. *Gastroenterology* 1991;101:465-71.
20. Itai Y, Moos AA, Ohtomo K. Computed tomography of cystadenoma and cystadenocarcinoma of the pancreas. *Radiology* 1982;145:419-25.
21. Yamaguchi K, Enjoji M. Cystic neoplasms of the pancreas. *Gastroenterology* 1987;92:1934-43.
22. Motojima K, Tomioka T, Tsunoda T, Kanamatsu T. Immunohistochemical study of pancreatic cystadenocarcinoma. *Am J Gastroenterol* 1992;87:43-7.
23. Mac Carty RL. Cyst fluid analysis and imaging of pancreatic cystic lesions. *AJR* 1995;16:820-1.
24. Lewandrowski K, Lee J, Southern J, Centeno B, Warshaw A. Cyst fluid analysis in the differential diagnosis of pancreatic cysts: a new approach to the preoperative assessment of pancreatic cystic lesions. *AJR* 1995;164:815-9.
25. Alles AJ, Warshaw AL, Southern JF, Compton CC, Lewandrowski KB. Expression of CA 72-4 (TAG-72) in the fluid contents of pancreatic cysts. *Ann Surg* 1994;219:131-4.
26. Tatsuta M, Iishi H, Ichiii M et al. Values of carcinoembryonic antigen, elastase 1, and carbohydrate antigen determinant in aspirated pancreatic cystic fluid in the diagnosis of cysts of the pancreas. *Cancer* 1986;57:1836-9.
27. Pinto M, Meriano F. Diagnosis of cystic pancreatic lesions by cytologic examination and carcinoembryonic antigen and amylase levels of cyst contents. *Acta Cytol* 1991;35:456-63.
28. Sand JA, Hyoty MK, Mattila J, Dagorn JC, Nordback IH. Clinical assessment compared with cyst fluid analysis in the differential diagnosis of cystic lesions in the pancreas. *Surgery* 1996;119:275-80.
29. Nishida K, Shiga K, Kato K et al. Two cases of pancreatic cystadenocarcinoma with elevated CA 19.9 levels in the cystic fluid in comparison with two cases of pancreatic cystadenoma. *Hepato-Gastroenterol* 1989;36:442-5.
30. Paris F, Kerschen A, Jaeck D. Antigen CA19-9 and mucinous cystadenoma of the pancreas. *Brit J Surg* 1990;77:1250-1.
31. Levy M, Hammel P, Zins M, Vilgrain V, Amouyal G, Amouyal P, et al. Diagnostic des cystadénomes et cystadénocarcinomes du pancreas. *Gastroenterol Clin Biol* 1995;19:189-96.
32. Rubin D, Warshaw AL, Southern JF, Pins M, Compton CC, Lewandroski KB. Expression of CA 15.3 protein in the cyst contents distinguishes benign from malignant pancreatic mucinous cystic neoplasm. *Surgery* 1994;115:52-5.
33. Zamora J L. Cystic neoplasms of the pancreas: evolution of a concept. *Am J Surg* 1985;149:819-23.
34. Warshaw A L, Rutledge P L. Cystic tumors mistaken for pancreatic pseudocysts. *Ann Surg* 1987;205:393-8.
35. Andersson R, Ihse I. Cystadenoma and cystadenocarcinomas, serous adenomas. In: Howard J, Idezuki Y, Ihse I, Prinz R. Surgical disease of the pancreas. Baltimore: Williams & Wilkins, 1998:675-9
36. Talamini M A, Pitt H A, Hruban R H, Boitnott J K, Coleman J A, Cameron JL. Spectrum of cystic tumors of the pancreas. *Am J Surg* 1992;163:117-23.
37. Yamaguchi K, Hirakata R, Kitamura K. Mucinous cystic neoplasms of the pancreas: estimation of grade of malignancy with imaging techniques and its surgical implications. *Acta Chir Scand* 1990;156:553-64.
38. Wood D, Silberman AW, Heifetz L, Memsic L, Shabot MM. Cystadenocarcinoma of the pancreas: neoadjuvant therapy and CEA monitoring. *J Surg Oncol* 1990;43:56-60.
39. Doberstein C, Kirchner R, Gordon L. Cystic neoplasm of the pancreas. *Mount Sinai J Med* 1990;57:102-5.

CHAPTER 10

A CRITICAL REVIEW OF CLASSIFICATION SYSTEMS FOR COLORECTAL CANCER.

ANACLETO PERACCHIA, LEOPOLDO SARLI, NICOLA PIETRA, and SARA GOBBI

Institute of Surgical Clinics, University of Parma, Parma ,Italy

Summary

After a chronological overview of the various staging systems for colorectal cancer, presented in an effort to demonstrate the reasons for the current state of confusion, four different systems (Dukes, Astler and Coller, ACPS, TNM) were compared in 791 patients treated at some stage of their disease at Parma University's Institute of Surgery. Life survival table analysis was used to examine survival according to each staging system. From the analysis of the staging systems commonly utilised, Dukes'system modified by Astler and Coller, emerges as the best reference model now available. The system can be fine-tuned to a certain extent, in order to improve its predictive value, by taking into account the number of lymph nodes affected by the tumour; further improvement is also foreseeable, above all by the use of genetic variables. However, no classification system can be correct, if it is not accompanied by an accurate pre-operative diagnosis and a thorough post-operative histological study.

A rational strategy to improve the prognosis of colorectal cancer would be, in addition to earlier detection, a more aggressive treatment of high risk patients. This would require a reliable method of classification into high- and low-risk patients for recurrent disease. In recent years, many attempts have been made to improve the prediction of final outcome. However, although the first attempt at stratification into distinct groups, in terms of extension of the disease and of probability of survival, go back to 1926 [1], the gold standard for staging systems has yet to be identified. One reason for this difficulty is that, side by side with the necessity to adopt a high number of variables in order to improve predictive capacity, there is the need for a classification system which would be easy to understand, to remember and to apply, and which could be reproduced by all researchers.

Pathological classifications

One of the great advantages of the staging system proposed by *Dukes* in 1932 [2] (Table 1) is its easy use, which does not affect its predictive efficacy; thus Duke's staging is still today one of the most important clinicopathological variables of prognostic value [3-5].

Dukes based this system on his conviction that the most important prognostic indicators are the extension of the tumour into the bowel wall and the presence of lymph node metastasis, and that the lymph nodes cannot be affected until the

E. Zanella (ed.), Advances in Abdominal Surgery, 95–106.

Table 1. Anatomopathological classification of colorectal cancer according to *Dukes.*

stage A	*tumour confined within the intestinal wall,*
stage B	*extension of the tumour, by direct continuity,to the perirectal tissues, without metastasis ,*
stage C	*all cases with lymph node involvement.*

neoplasia has reached the serosa of the colon or the perirectal tissues. An important modification to Dukes' system (Table 2) was proposed by *Astler* and *Coller* in 1954 (6), and takes into account the possibility of lymph node metastases, also in the absence of complete parietal penetration of the tumour.

Table 2. Anatomopathological classification of colorectal cancer according to *Astler and Coller.*

A. lesion limited to the mucosa
B1.lesion infiltrating the muscularis
B2.lesion extending beyond the muscularis
C1.lesion not completely penetrating the intestinal wall with lymph node metastasis
C2.lesion completely penetrating the intestinal wall with lymph node metastasis

Clinicopathological classifications

The classical Dukes' and Astler and Coller's staging systems are based on the pathological report, which is a static description of the extent of spread within the surgical specimen. The clinician, however, needs to know how far the tumour has spread. For the radio-therapist the report on rectal cancer must include a detailed account of anatomic location and spread, including its position relative to the peritoneum and the extent of mesorectal involvement [7]. Potentially valuable clinical variables, sometimes associated with better or worse outcome despite the pathological stage of the disease, could improve accuracy of prediction [8-9]. For this reason the need arose for clinicopathological classifications, the first attempt at which was by *Turnbull,* who, in 1967, while conserving Dukes' classical A-B-C subdivisions, added another stage, D, to identify both those tumours with distant metastases, and those not radically resectable on account of their infiltration of adjacent organs or tissues [10,11].
The most well-known and widespread clinicopathological classification is the *TNM system* proposed by the International Union against Cancer in 1978 [12] and subsequently modified by the "*Task Force on the Colon and Rectum of the American Joint Committee on Cancer Staging and End-Results Reporting*" [13] (Table 3). The TNM system is recommended at this time, since it is the most completely descriptive of appropriate prognostic factors [14] and allows for the conversion of other staging systems into a common format [15,16]. Even this

Table 3. Postsurgical TNM system of anatomoclinical classification of colorectal cancer.

0.	*carcinoma in situ*	**Tis N0 M0**
IA.	*neoplasia invading the submucosa*	**T1 N0 M0**
IB.	*neoplasia invading the muscularis itself*	**T2 N0 M0**
IIA.	*neoplasia with invasion, through the muscularis, into the subserosa or into the pericolic or perirectal tissues not covered with peritoneum*	**T3 N0 M0**
IIB.	*neoplasia perforating the visceral peritoneum, or directly invading other organs or structures*	**T4 N0 M0**
IIIA.	*each degree of parietal invasion with metastasis in 1-3 pericolic or perirectal lymph nodes*	**each T N1 M0**
IIIB.	*each degree of parietal invasion with metastasis in 4 or more pericolic or perirectal lymph nodes or in any lymph node along the course of the vascular stems*	**each T N2,3 M0**
IV.	*distant metastasis*	**each T each N M1**

system, however, provokes criticism, linked above all to the complexity of its application, which is accentuated by the constant revisions to which it is subjected [17].

The clinicopathological staging system which has been in use at the Concord Hospital in Australia since 1971 [18,19], known as the *Australian Clinicopathological Staging System (ACPS)*, contains similar prerogatives to the TNM, with the advantage of a simpler applicability. It derives from Dukes' system modified by the addition of clinical and/or pathological information relating to the persistence of tumour foci after surgical intervention (Table 4).

Table 4: Australian Clinico-Pathological Staging System (ACPS) for the classification of colorectal

0.	*neoplasia infiltrating the intramucosa*
A.	*neoplasia infiltrating the submucosa*
A2.	*neoplasia infiltrating the muscularis*
B1.	*neoplasia not infiltrating beyond the serosa and, by the rectal subperitoneum, infiltrating beyond the muscularis*
B2.	*neoplasia extending beyond the serosa*
C1.	*metastasis to the pericolic or perirectal lymph nodes independently of the level of penetration into the intestinal wall*
C2.	*metastasis in the apical lymph nodes independently of the level of penetration into the intestinal wall*
D1.	*clinical or histological presence of tumour tissue on the margins of resection of the excised piece*
D2.	*distant metastasis*

Further attempts to correct the defects and disadvantages of the previously mentioned pathological or clinicopathological staging system [20] confer considerable complexity to the system, which ends up as being extremely difficult to apply, thus lacking one of the important requisites of the ideal staging system .
Jass identified, among the myriad parameters correlated to the prognosis of patients affected by a cancer of the large intestine, 4 independent predictive variables [21]: the number of lymph nodes with metastasis; the extent of the peri- and intratumour lymphocyte infiltration; the nature of the tumour growth; the degree of penetration of the tumour into the intestinal wall. On the basis of the characteristics of these factors, the author has attributed a points system, which allows for the subdivision of the patients into 4 groups (Jass grades I,II,III and IV) according to the progressive worsening of their prognosis. However, Jass's classification may be complicated by observer variation between pathologists, thus limiting its reproducibility [22-23], and recent evidence suggests that it offers no advantage over that of Dukes [24].

Comparison of different systems

On the eve of the year 2000, therefore, it is still not known which of the existing systems of classification is the most suitable for clinical use. Recent studies on the subject have reached completely contradictory conclusions [15,16,25]. Only those studies which analyse survival as a function of the various systems can provide precise indications as to their effective predictive capacity.

Our experience

The comparative analysis which follows regards 5 years survival, with a follow-up of at least 5 years, as a function of 4 different classifications, of the 721 patients undergoing curative surgery between 1976 and 1993 at the clinical Institutes of the University of Parma directed by Prof. A. Peracchia. A comparison was made of the 4 staging systems most commonly utilised in clinical practice: Dukes' classification of 1932 [2], its modification by Astler and Coller [6], the 4th edition of the TNM system, from which the classification in 4 stages was obtained [13] and the ACPS classification of 1976 [18]. Stage IV of the TNM system and stages D1 and D2 of the ACPS do not appear in this evaluation, since those patients with distant metastasis (stage D) or those in whom local diffusion did not allow for curative resection, were excluded from the study. It is, however, to be noted that for this category of patient, specific classification systems have recently been established [26].
Figure 1 shows the correlation between the 4 staging systems under examination. Figures 2,3,4 and 5 show survival at 5 years in relation to the 4 staging systems.

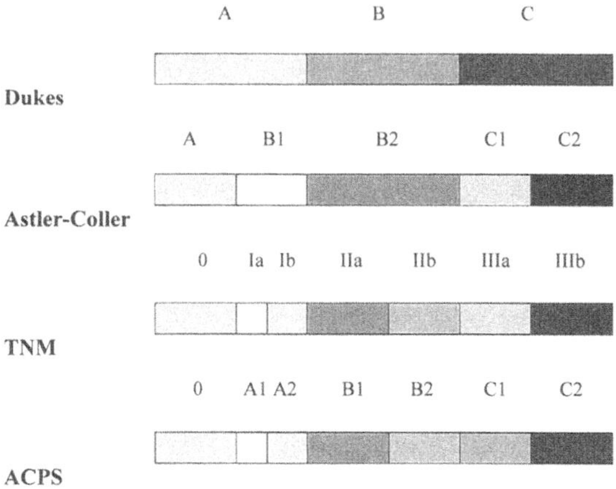

Figure 1. correlations between the 4 classifications under examination.

Figure 2. Five years survival of the 721 patients undergoing curative surgery in the period 1976-1993, at the surgical Institutes of Parma University, directed by Prof. A. Peracchia, as a function of stage according to ***Dukes' system*** of 1932.
The differences between the curves are statistically significant: A versus B $p<0.01$, B versus C $p<0.074$.

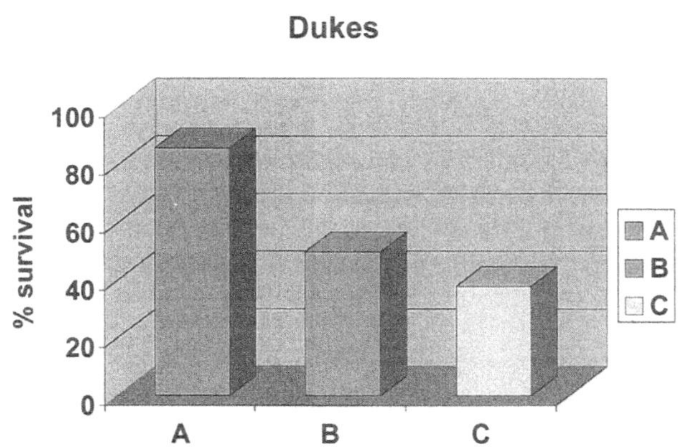

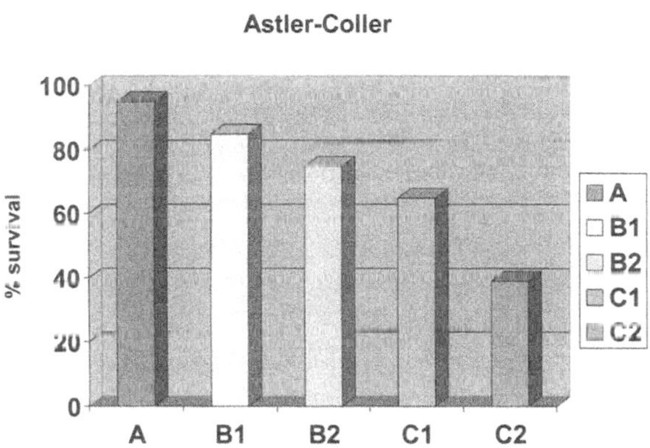

Figure 3. Five years survival of the 721 patients under examination, as a function of stage according to the classification of ***Astler and Coller***: The differences between groups A and B2 ($p<0.03$) and between groups B2 and C1 ($p<0.009$) are statistically significant.

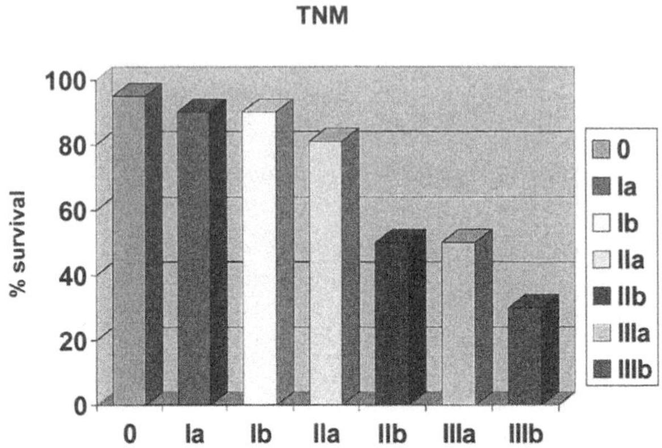

Figure 4. Five years survival of the 721 patients undergoing curative surgery as a function of stages according to the ***TNM system***. The differences between groups IIa and IIb ($p<0.01$) and between groups IIIa and IIIb ($p<0.0001$) are statistically significant.

The survival percentages decrease as the stages proceed in all the classifications, although the differences are not always significant (*Figs. 2-5*).

These results allow for a critical analysis of the classifications utilised in the study. The main objection that has been made to Dukes' system is the absence of information as to the level of penetration of the tumour into the intestinal wall (stage A in all cases of tumours not going beyond the serosa) [27]. However, when systems are utilised which break down Dukes' stage A on the basis of the level of parietal infiltration (stages 0, Ia, Ib and IIa of TNM and their equivalents 0, A1, A2 and B1 of ACPS), the survival rates observed do not statistically differ from each

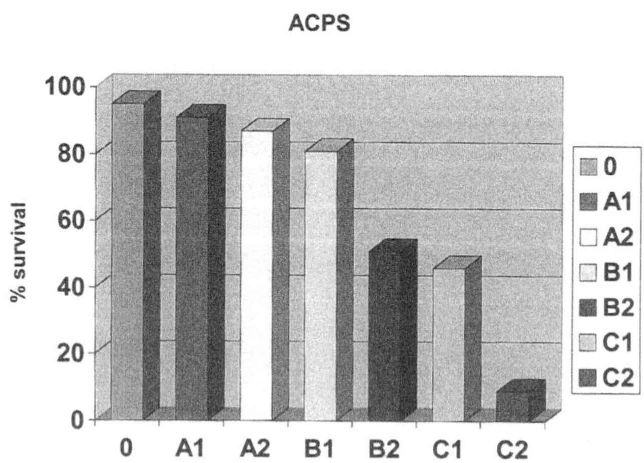

Figure 5. Five years survival of the 721 patients undergoing curative surgery asa function of the stage according to the ***ACPS system***. The differences between groups B1 and B2 ($p<0.1$) and between groups C1 and C2 ($p<0.0001$) are statistically significant

other (*Figs. 4-5*) and are comparable to those of Dukes' class A (*Fig. 1*). A higher survival rate can be observed only for stage 0 of TNM and ACPS, equivalent to stage A of Astler and Coller (*Fig. 2*), compared to the immediately subsequent stages. This difference, although of no statistical significance (*Figs. 2,3,4 and 5*), identifies a category of patients having a better prognosis. In our experience, in fact, none of the patients belonging to this class died of causes linked to the tumour. Thus, although recent studies propose detailed classification systems for early colorectal cancer [28], we maintain that the prognosis of patients with a tumour limited to the mucosa may be interpreted as being equivalent to that relating to a population not affected by cancer.

A second criticism aimed at Dukes' system concerns the absence of information regarding the degree of extraparietal infiltration (stage B in all cases of penetration beyond the serosa) [17]. On the basis of our data, however, more information in this sense does not seem to be necessary. The survival rate in patients placed in this stage and in the equivalent ones (IIb of TNM and B2 of ACPS) (*Figs. 2,4 and 5*) results in fact as being statistically worse than that of the immediately preceding stages, thus showing that the extension of the tumour beyond the colorectal wall gives rise in any case to a definite worsening of the prognosis.

Dukes' staging does not involve groups in which lymph node metastasis is combined with an incomplete penetration of the intestinal wall [17]. This is undoubtedly a serious limit if we consider that the survival rate of patients with an Astler and Coller stage C1 tumour (lymph node metastasis and parietal infiltration not going beyond the muscularis) results as being better than that of the patients in stage C2 (lymph node metastasis and infiltration beyond the muscularis) (*Fig. 3*). In our experience, in any case, the difference does not reach statistical significance.

A third criticism regards the absence of information as to the number and site of the lymph nodes involved (stage C in all cases in Dukes' staging). In effect, it is precisely the grouping in a single stage of all the patients with lymph node metastasis which constitutes, in our opinion, the most serious drawback to Dukes' system. It has been shown that the prognosis of patients with only one to four positive nodes is significantly better than that of patients with more than 4 positive nodes [29]. The survival rates relating to stages IIIb of TNM (more than 4 lymph nodes involved) and C2 of ACPS (the involvement of the apical lymph nodes) result as being significantly lower than those of the immediately preceding stages (*Figs. 4 and 5*), while those relating to Dukes' stage C, IIIa of TNM and C1 of ACPS do not differ greatly from each other (*Figs. 2,4 and 5*). It can be deduced that, although when the tumour has gone beyond the intestinal wall, the involvement of a few proximal lymph nodes does not significantly worsen the prognosis, when more than 4 lymph nodes are involved, or else the apical lymph nodes, the risk of tumour recurrence is considerably high. The survival rates in patients with metastasis in more than 4 lymph nodes (IIIb TNM) and that of patients with metastasis in the apical lymph nodes (C2 ACPS) are similar (*Figs. 4 and 5*). Indeed, it can be presumed that if there are metastases in numerous proximal lymph nodes, the tumour already involves the most distal areas [18].

All the conventional staging systems we analysed fail to take the skill of the surgeon into account when determining outcome [17]; it is therefore difficult to decide which of the classification systems examined is preferable. On the basis of our results it seems that the ease of use and high prognostic power of Astler and Coller's modification of Dukes' classification ensure that it is still a good model, against which all other classifications of colorectal cancer should be assessed. This classification in fact involves a class of patients at practically no risk, and is the only one of all the systems analysed which takes into consideration the possibility of lymph node metastasis also in the case of limited parietal infiltration.

Proposal for a new classification

On the basis of what has emerged, however, we attempted to improve the predictive value of Astler and Coller's classification system, by means of the introduction of a subclassification of stage C as a function of the number and site of the lymph nodes affected by deposits. The actuarial survival curves at 10 years obtained with this variant to the classification are shown in Figure 6; observation

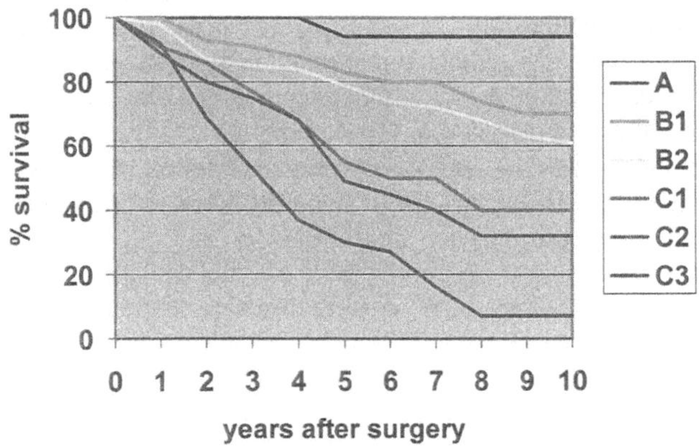

Figure 6. Actuarial survival curves of the 721 patients under examination obtained by modifying Astler and Coller's system as follows:

A. lesion limited to the mucosa

B1.lesion infiltrating the muscularis

B2.lesion extending beyond the muscularis

C1.lesion not completely penetrating the intestinal wall with metastasis in fewer than 4 pericolic or perirectal lymph nodes

C2.lesion completely penetrating the intestinal wall with metastasis in fewer than 4 pericolic or perirectal lymph nodes

C3. every degree of parietal invasion with metastasis in 4 or more pericolic or perirectal lymph nodes or in the apical lymph nodes.

The differences between groups A and B2 ($p<0.03$), between groups B2 and C2 ($p<0.009$), and between groups C1 and C3 ($p<0.009$) are statistically significant.

of this revealed the possibility of simplifying the system. The prognosis of stages B1 (infiltration limited to the muscularis without lymph nodes) and B2 (infiltration beyond the muscularis without lymph nodes) results, in fact, as being thus similar to that of stages C1 (infiltration as far as the muscularis with the involvement of fewer than 4 proximal lymph nodes) and C2 (infiltration beyond the muscularis with less than 4 lymph nodes involved). It is thus possible to formulate a really simple proximal staging system involving the merging of stages B1 and B2 into a single stage B (each degree of parietal invasion beyond the mucosa in the absence of lymph node metastasis) and of stages C1 and C2 into a single stage C1 (each degree of parietal invasion with metastasis in fewer than 4 proximal lymph nodes) (*Fig. 7*). This system, in which significance is attached to the level of lymph node

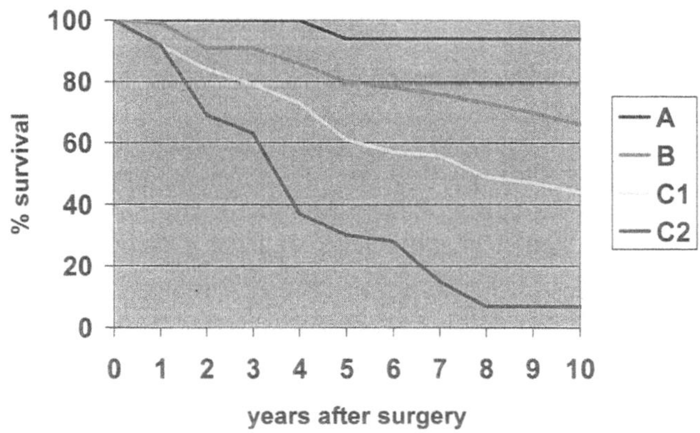

Figure 7. Actuarial survival curves of the 721 patients under examination obtained by further modification of Astler and Coller's system as follows:

A. lesion limited to the mucosa

B. each degree of parietal invasion in the absence of lymph node metastasis

C1. each degree of parietal invasion with metastasis in fewer than 4 pericolic or perirectal lymph nodes

C2. each degree of parietal invasion with metastasis in 4 or more pericolic or perirectal lymph nodes or in the apical lymph nodes.

The differences between groups A and B ($p<0.03$), between groups B and C1 ($p<0.009$) and between groups C1 and C2 ($p<0.009$) are statistically significant.

involvement rather than to the degree of parietal infiltration, would have the advantage of being able to identify, among those patients undergoing curative surgery, a class at practically no risk (class A) and a class with a poor prognosis (class C2). For the two intermediate classes, in any case with statistically different prognoses, further variables should be referred to for a better prognostic definition, since these categories are poor predictors of final outcome.

New trends

In recent years, many attempts have been made to improve the prediction of final outcome precisely in these intermediate categories. Many parameters have been studied, but, although some of these have significant predictive value, in multivariate analyses most appear to have limited independent value. In accordance with other authors [30], in a multivariate analysis carried out by us, DNA ploidy [31] and Labelling Index [23] resulted as being essential factors that could be combined with pathological staging for a better and easier definition of prognosis. Even tumour-infiltrating lymphocytes independently predict recurrence-free survival rate [32], as does the Doppler perfusion index [33]. Recent studies indicate that nuclear morphometry [34] and genetic abnormalities might be important new prognostic indicators [35,36]. One of the most promising findings in this area is an allelic loss of chromosome 18q, which allows the division of Dukes' B patients into subgroups at low or high risk for recurrent disease [37].

Finally, we deem it necessary to consider that not all the limits of predictability are to be attributed directly to the classification criteria. An important reason for lack of progress in the prognostic power of classification systems is that, on removal of the primary tumour, a significant proportion of those patients with seemingly localised disease already had undetectable micrometastases, mostly in the liver . An estimate of the risk of micrometastasis requires a prognostic classification utilising independent pathobiological variables not yet known [38].

Another factor affecting the accuracy of staging is the variability in quality of anatomopathological evaluation [39]. Histological examination is in fact not always able to provide precise information as to the number and site of the lymph nodes with metastasis [40], the involvement of the outside surface of the serosa, and the infiltration of the distal and lateral lines of resection [41]. Imprecise information leads inevitably to errors in classification and thus to inaccurate prognostic evaluation. The Cancer Committee of the College of American Pathologists has developed a protocol for the pathological examination and reporting of specimens from patients with colorectal carcinoma [42].

Conclusions

In conclusion, we maintain that of the commonly-used staging systems adopted for patients affected by colorectal cancer, Dukes' system modified by Astler and Coller is today the best reference model. The system can be fine-tuned to a certain extent, in order to improve its predictive value, by taking into account the number of lymph nodes affected by the tumour, and further improvements are foreseeable, above all by using genetic variables. However, no system of classification will be correct unless it is supported by an extremely accurate pre-operative diagnosis and post-operative histological study.

References

1. Lockhart-Mummery JP. Two hundred cases of cancer of the rectum treated by perineal excision. *Br J Surg* 1926; 14: 110-7.
2. Dukes C. The classification of cancer of the rectum. *Pathol Bacteriol* 1932; 35: 323-37.
3. Deans GT, Patterson CC, Parks TG, Spence RA, Heatley M, Moorehead RJ, Rowlands BJ. Colorectal carcinoma: importance of clinical and pathological factors in survival. *Ann R Coll Surg Engl* 1994; 76: 59-64.
4. Ropponen K, Eskelinen M, Kosma VM, Lipponen P, Paakkinen P, Alhava E. Comparison of classic and quantitative prognostic factors in colorectal cancer. *Anticancer Res* 1996; 16: 3875-82.
5. Hannisdal E, Thorsen G. Regression analysis of prognostic factors in colorectal cancer. *J Surg Oncol* 1988; 37: 109-12.
6. Astler WB, Coller FA. The prognostic significance of direct extension of carcinoma of the colon and rectum. *Ann Surg* 1954; 139: 846-52.
7. Jass JR. Future role of the pathologist in reporting colorectal cancer. *World J Surg* 1997; 21: 688-93.
8. Nathanson SD. Is there a role for clinical prognostic factors in staging patients with colorectal cancer?. *Semin Surg Oncol* 1994; 10: 176-82.
9. Crucitti F, Sofo L, Doglietto GB, Bellantone R, Ratto C, Bossola M, Crucitti. A Prognostic factors in colorectal cancer: current status and new trends. *J Surg Oncol* (suppl) 1991; 2: 76-82.
10. Turnbull RB jr. The no touch isolation technique of resection. *JAMA* 1975; 231: 1181-7.
11. Turnbull RB jr, Kyle K, Watson FR, Spratt J. Cancer of the colon: the influence of the no touch isolation technique on survival rates. *Ann Surg* 1967; 166: 420-5.
12. International Union Against Cancer. TNM: Illustrated guide to the classification of malignant tumors. Geneva, 1978.
13. American Joint Committee for Cancer Staging and End-Results Reporting : Manual for staging of cancer. Chicago, 1978.
14. D'eredita G, Serio G, Neri V, Polizzzi RA, Barberio G, Losacco T. A survival regression analysis of prognostic factors in colorectal cancer. *Aust N Z J Surg* 1996 ; 66: 445-51.
15. Gasser A, Isaak B, Maibach R, Ruchti C, Wagner HE, Nothiger F. Staging and prognosis of colorectal carcinoma. *Schweiz Med Wochenschr* 1992; 122: 1356-62.
16. Williams ST, Beart RW Jr. Staging of colorectal cancer. *Semin Surg Oncol* 1992; 8: 89-93
17. Jass JR. Staging of colorectal cancer (symposium). *Int J Colorectal Dis* 1987; 2: 123- 8.
18. Newland RC, Chapuis PH, Pheils MT, McPherson JG. The relationship of survival to staging and grading of colorectal carcinoma: a prospective study of 503 cases. *Cancer* 1981; 47: 1424-9.
19 Davis NC, Newland RC. Terminology and classification of colorectal adenocarcinoma: The Australian Clinico-Pathologic System. *Aust NZ J Surg* 1983; 53: 211-5.
20. Payne JE. International colorectal carcinoma staging and grading. *Dis Colon Rectum* 1989; 32: 282-6.
21. Jass JR, Love SB, Northover JMA. A new prognostic classification of rectal cancer. *Lancet* 1987; 1: 1303-5.
22. Secco GB, Fardelli R, La Pertosa G. Valore prognostico della classificazione di Jass nel cancro del colon sinistro e del retto. *Minerva Chir* 1990; 45: 1347-54.
23. Pietra N, Sarli L, Thenasseril B, Costi R, Cattaneo G, Gobbi S, Peracchia A. Risk factors for local recurrence of colorectal cancer: a multivariate study. *Br J Surg* 1997; 84: 63 (abstr.).
24. Deans GT, Parks TG, Rowlands BJ, Spence RA. Prognostic factors in colorectal cancer. *Br J Surg* 1992, 79. 608-13.
25. Chapui PH, Fisher R, Dent OF, Newland RC, Pheil MT. The relationship between different staging methods and survival in colorectal carcinoma. *Dis Colon Rectum* 1985; 28: 158-61.
26. Yasui K, Hirai T, Kato T, Torii A, Uesaka K, Morimoto T, Kodera Y, Yamamura Y, Kito T, Hamajima N. A new macroscopic classification predicts prognosis for patients with liver metastases

from colorectal cancer. *Ann Surg* 1997; 226: 582-6.
27. Gabriel WB, Dukes C, Bussey H. Lymphatic spread in cancer of the rectum. *Br J Surg* 1935; 23: 395-400.
28. Mainprize KS, McC Mortensen NJ,Warren BF. Early colorectal cancer: recognition, classification and treatment. *Br J Surg* 1998; 85: 469-76.
29. Hyder JW, Talbott TM, Maycroft TC. A Critical review of chemical lymph node clearance and staging of colon and rectal cancer at Ferguson Hospital, 1977 to 1982. *Dis Colon Rectum* 1990;33:923-5.
30. Pinto AE, Chaves P, Fidalgo P, Oliveira AG, Leitao CN, Soares J. Flow cytometric DNA ploidy and S-phase fraction correlate with histopathologic indicators of tumor behavior in colorectal carcinoma. *Dis Colon Rectum* 1997; 40: 411-9.
31. Pietra N, Sarli L, Sansebastiano G, Saccani Jotti G, Peracchia A. Prognostic value of ploidy, cell proliferation kinetics, and conventional clinicopathologic criteria in patients with colorectal carcinoma. A prospective study. *Dis Colon Rectum* 1996; 39:494-503.
32. Ropponen KM, Eskelinen MJ, Lipponen PK, Alhava E, Kosma VM. Prognostic value of tumour-infiltrating lymphocytes (TILs) in colorectal cancer. *J Pathol* 1997;182: 318-24.
33. Leen E, Angerson WG, Cooke TG, McArdle CS. Prognostic power of Doppler perfusion index in colorectal cancer. Correlation with survival. *Ann Surg* 1996; 223: 199-203.
34. Ropponen K, Eskelinen M, Kosma VM, Lipponen P, Paakkinen P, Alhava E. Comparison of classic and quantitative prognostic factors in colorectal cancer. *Anticancer Res* 1996; 16: 3875-82.
35. Senagore AJ, Biener JT. A newly identified pattern of K-ras mutations at codons 12 and 13 is associated with long-term survival in colorectal cancer. *Surgery* 1997; 122: 765-70.
36. Kapitanovic S, Radosevic S, Kapitanovic M, Andelinovic S, Ferencic Z, Tavassoli M, Primorac D, Sonicki Z, Spaenti S, Pavelic K, Spaventi R. The expression of p185 (HER-2/neu) correlates with the stage of disease and survival in colorectal cancer. *Gastroenterology* 1997;21: 1103-13.
37. Bosman FT. Prognostic value of pathological characteristics of colorectal cancer. *Eur J Cancer* 1995; 31: 1216-21.
38. Jass JR. Future role of the pathologist in reporting colorectal cancer. *World J Surg* 1997; 21: 688-93.
39. Sarli L, Pietra N, Carreras F, Longinotti M, Gafà M, Peracchia A. Metastasi epatiche occulte da carcinoma colo-rettale: considerazioni diagnostiche e prognostiche. *Giorn Chir* 1991; 12: 232-6.
40. Blenkinshop WK, Stewart-Brown S, Blesovsky L. Histopathology reporting in large bowel cancer. *J Clin Pathol* 1981; 34: 598-603.
41. Wolmark N, Fisher B, Wieand HS. The prognostic value of the modification of the Dukes' C Class of colorectal cancer. *Ann Surg* 1986; 203: 115-9.
42. Compton CC, Henson DE, Hutter RV, Sobin LH, Bowman HE. Updated protocol for the examination of specimens removed from patients with colorectal carcinoma. A basis for checklists. *Arch Pathol Lab Med* 1997; 121: 1247-54.

CHAPTER 11

STANDARD SURGERY AND ADJUVANT THERAPY FOR COLORECTAL CANCER.

DONATO NITTI, GIULIA VIECELI, ALBERTO MARCHET, and MARIO LISE

Department of Surgery and Oncology, 2nd Surgical Clinics, University of Padua, Padua, Italy.

Introduction

Colorectal cancer (CRC) is the second cause of death from malignant tumors in Western countries. In Italy, the overall annual age-adjusted incidence is 41 per 100.000 in men and 26 per 100.000 in women [1], with overall 5-year survivals of 46% for colonic and 39% for rectal carcinoma [2].

Notwithstanding progress in multimodal therapy achieved in recent years, the main approach for colorectal cancer is still surgical. Although at diagnosis radical resection is feasible in 70 to 80% of patients [3], the natural history of this tumor-type is characterized by the development of distant metastases in 40 to 50% of cases, and by the appearance of local recurrences in 10 to 40% of cases [4].

In the attempt to improve results following surgery, the effects of adjuvant chemo and/or radiotherapy have been tested in subgroups of patients at high risk of locoregional recurrence or distant metastasis. The risk of recurrence is increased by tumor invasion through the muscularis propria into the subserosa or non-peritonealized tissues, or into adjacent organs and structures (T3-T4), and the presence of lymphnode metastases [5, 6]. Other independent prognostic factors are: primary disease with complications (perforation, occlusion), vascular invasion, quality of surgery (e.g. complete removal of the mesorectum in rectal cancer), cell cycle parameters and ploidy, grade of differentiation and high mitotic index for neoplastic cells, genetic mutations in the tumor tissue (e.g. p53, DCC, kRAS, p21) and pre-operative serum CEA assay [7, 8].

We here define the general principles for colorectal resection, and report on the results of recent controlled clinical studies on adjuvant chemo-radio-immuno-therapy after radical surgery.

E. Zanella (ed.), Advances in Abdominal Surgery, 107–125.

Carcinoma of the Colon

Surgery

Considerable progress has been made in colon surgery since 1833, when Reybard performed the first resection with anastomosis. Radical resection still offers the only chance of cure for patients with CRC, quality of surgery playing a primary role in disease control.

Although the principles for colon resection have changed little in recent years, a greater oncological radicality has been achieved by surgeons, thanks to progress made in intensive care techniques, antibiotic therapy and anesthesia. This has reduced peri-operative mortality and morbidity in emergency surgery, in particular, which accounts for 20 to 30% of surgical procedures performed in patients with CRC.

Curative or palliative elective surgery is performed in 70 to 80% of colon cancer patients. In those with locally advanced or metastatic disease, palliative treatment must be considered with a view to preventing later complications, such as occlusion and perforation [9].

The principles for radical surgery, established in relation to the site of the primary tumor, include resection of the bowel, with disease-free resection margins, resection of the mesocolon and regional lymphnodes, ligation of the main vascular stump, and removal of adjacent affected organs.

Total colectomy should be considered a valid alternative in patients with multiple and synchronous tumors or hereditary non-polyposis colon carcinoma (HNPCC), who refuse to undergo close clinical and endoscopic control after conservative surgery [10].

A recently proposed alternative to traditional laparotomy, laparoscopic colon resection, can also be used for malignant tumors. At present, minimally-invasive surgery is not widely used because of technical difficulties involved (e.g. long period of training required), the higher risk of local recurrences, and doubts as to whether it allows radical lymphoadenectomy to be performed. Laparoscopy causes less blood loss, allows earlier bowel movement and a shorter hospital stay. However, the follow-ups in current studies [11] comparing traditional laparotomy with the laparoscopic technique are as yet too short to allow definite conclusions concerning survival and the real incidence of recurrences.

Overall, the guidelines for radical surgery in elderly patients are quite similar to those in younger patients. Radical surgery can be achieved in 54% of colorectal cancer patients over 75 years of age, and the peri-operative mortality and 5-year survival rates in this category are comparable to those in younger patients [12].

Twenty to thirty per cent of patients with colorectal tumors have occlusion or perforation requiring emergency surgery. The peri-operative mortality in these patients is three-times that of patients who undergo elective surgery, and the 5-

year survival is 10% less. In the presence of free peritonitis, resection with colonic anastomosis is associated with a high risk of anastomotic dehiscence, which can be fatal. In such cases, the treatment of choice is colostomy, with removal of the colon tract with the perforated tumor. In the presence of localized peritonitis and occlusion of the left colon, colostomy is reserved for selected cases [9].

The outcome following surgery is related to the disease stage. In patients without lymphnode metastases who have tumors involving the mucosa and the submucosa (T1), and those involving also the muscularis propria (T2, Dukes' stage B1), the 5-year survival is 90% and 80% respectively [6, 13]. In patients with extension to the entire organ wall (T3, Dukes' stage B2) the 5-year survival is 50 to 70% [6, 13]. In patients with metastases in the locoregional lymphnodes (Dukes' stage C), the 5-year survival is less than 40%, although important variations occur in relation to T stage and the number of lymphnodes involved [6, 13-16].

Therefore in patients with Dukes' stage B1 and in many patients with Dukes' stage B2 tumor surgery is curative. However, in the presence of lymphnode metastases (Dukes' stage C), surgery alone cannot provide cure.

Adjuvant treatments

Systemic chemotherapy

The history of adjuvant therapy for carcinoma of the colon can be subdivided into four fundamental stages, with studies on: **1)** the MOF regimen [5-Fluorouracil (5-FU)+MeCCNU+vincristine]; **2)** levamisole; **3)** combined 5-FU and folinic acid (FA); and **4)** ongoing new drugs.

Moreover, throughout the sixties, studies mainly utilizing adjuvant 5-FU after radical surgery in small patient series, demonstrated that this regimen had no therapeutic advantage over surgery alone, for survival or for disease-free interval (17).

1) The efficacy of MOF was evaluated in an NSABP study (National Surgical Adjuvant Breast and Bowel Project Protocol) on 1.166 patients. Although a significant improvement in the 5-year survival was found in patients given MOF, compared with those who underwent surgery alone, the use of this regimen was discontinued, because of its high toxicity and the leukemogenous effect of nitrosurea [18].

2) Levamisole, an antihelminthic, was found to have an antineoplastic effect in some animal models, above all in the presence of metastases [19]. On the basis of this preliminary finding, the North Central Cancer Treatment Group (NCCTG) made a study on levamisole used alone or associated with 5-FU in Dukes' stage B2 (negative lymphnodes) and C (positive lymphnodes) patients with colon cancer [20], and demonstrated that 5-FU associated with levamisole, but not levamisole alone, improved both the survival and the disease-free interval of Dukes' stage C patients, with respect to the controls (surgery alone). Comparable results were obtained in a confirmatory trial conducted on 1.296 patients [21] (Table 1). In 1990, based on the results of these two studies, in the "Consensus Conference" of the National Cancer Institute at Bethesda, the 5-FU and levamisole regimen was defined as standard treatment for patients with Dukes' stage C carcinoma [22].

3) The use of biochemical modulators of 5-FU, folinic acid in particular, was proposed with a view to improving the results obtained with 5-FU alone [23]. The efficacy of 5-FU+folinic acid (FUFA) in advanced disease was recently confirmed in a meta-analysis of ten controlled clinical studies: the response rate following FUFA regimen was found to be double that following 5-FU alone [24]. Moreover, the NSABP C-03 protocol comparing MOF chemotherapy with the FUFA regimen showed that the survival of patients treated with 5-FU+folinic acid was found to be 10% greater than that of patients treated with MOF [25]. The FUFA association was thus evaluated as adjuvant therapy, and the combined analysis (IMPACT) [17] of the results of three controlled clinical trials on 1.500 patients conducted in France, Canada and Italy demonstrated that the FUFA reduces mortality by 22% and recurrences by 35% with respect to surgery alone. The 5-FU+folinic acid regimen is less toxic and requires a shorter administration time than 5-FU+levamisole (6 *versus* 12 months) [25]. However, in a recent trial conducted by the NCCTG and the National Cancer Institute of Canada utilizing the 5-FU/levamisole association [26], the duration of therapy was reconsidered. A 12-month course of chemotherapy was found to have no advantages over a 6-month course, and results following the addition of folinic acid were no better than those achieved with associated 5-FU+levamisole alone.

While adjuvant chemotherapy is clearly effective in Dukes' stage C patients, its indications in Dukes' stage B patients are more controversial. Laurie and Moertel [20, 21] found that in stage B patients associated 5-FU and levamisole had no advantages in terms of survival or in risk of recurrences, and these findings were confirmed in subsequent controlled clinical studies [17]. Recently, however, the role of adjuvant chemotherapy in stage B patients was re-evaluated, and the data reported at the American Society of Clinical Oncology (ASCO) in 1996, suggest that Dukes' stage B patients treated with adjuvant chemotherapy have the same benefit as Dukes' stage C patients [25]. An important clarification on this issue will undoubtedly be made by the ongoing meta-analyses and by the forthcoming results of some important multicentric trials now underway in Europe and in North Amerca. It is, however, evident that not all Dukes' stage B tumors have the same biological behavior, and some subgroups of patients with unfavorable prognostic factors (vascular invasion, increased concentrations of CEA, poor differentiation, genetic mutations, etc.), are at greater risk of recurrence. If these subgroups are identified, a more selective utilization of adjuvant chemotherapy in Dukes' B stage patients will be achieved.

4) Ongoing studies aim to: **a)** compare the efficacy of the two regimens, which are considered standard (FUFA *versus* 5-FU+levamisole); **b)** identify new administration modalities for traditional drugs (e.g. continuous i.v. infusion *versus* i.v. bolus administration); and **c)** investigate the efficacy of new chemotherapeutic drugs active against advanced disease (e.g. tomudex, oxaliplatin, etc.).

a) Two recently completed studies on a total of 5.400 patients (Intergroup 0089 and NSABP C-04) [27, 28] have demonstrated that FUFA has a slight, but not statistically significant, advantage over 5-FU/levamisole for survival. The 5-FU+levamisole regimen is therefore considered a valid alternative to FUFA.

b) Recent studies conducted in USA and France have shown that in patients with advanced disease continuous 5-FU infusion increases the percentages of response with respect to i.v. bolus administration, without improving survival [29]. In other studies [30, 31], associated FA and 5-FU continuous infusion has increased the percentages of response in patients with advanced disease, and appears to improve the survival and reduce toxicity. Controlled clinical studies are now underway to evaluate the efficacy of continuous 5-FU infusion. In particular, a multicentric randomized study by the European Organization for Research and Treatment of Cancer (EORTC), the PETACC 2 (Pan European Trial in Adjuvant Colon Cancer) should compare FUFA administered in bolus with high dose continuous FUFA infusion, in Dukes' stage C carcinoma patients who undergo radical resection.

c) New chemotherapeutic agents for the treatment of colorectal cancer are being evaluated. Tomudex (raltitrexed), a direct inhibitor of timidilate-synthetaxis, is one of the first to be experimented [32, 33]. In three phase III randomized studies on patients with advanced disease, the response following Tomudex administration was comparable to that obtained with FUFA administered in bolus; its toxicity is similar, although it causes less neutropenia and mucositis [33]. In one trial, the survival of patients treated with FUFA was found to be slightly better than that of patients treated with Tomudex [33]. In the light of these favorable results, and in view of the fact that the drug doses are manageable (one i.v. administration every three weeks), Tomudex has been proposed as adjuvant treatment in an ongoing controlled clinical study (PETACC 1).

Two new cytotoxic agents, irinotecan (CPT-11) and oxaliplatin, are active in colorectal tumors resistant to 5-FU. Irinotecan, a topo-isomerase 1 inhibitor, has a response rate of 15 to 20% in first line treatment, and 11 to 16% in second line treatment on tumors resistant to 5-FU [34, 35]. Twenty-four to fifty-one per cent of the patients studied presented stable disease with CPT-11; the average duration of the response observed in the European phase II studies was 7.5 months, with an overall survival of 9.3 months [34, 35]. Oxaliplatin, which appears to be active against colorectal tumors resistant to 5-FU, was found to be effective when combined with 5-FU and FA. This regimen has a good response percentage when used as a second line treatment [36].

However, results from further trials are required to confirm whether these new drugs are effective as first line treatment and as adjuvant therapy.

Table 1. Controlled clinical trials on systemic chemotherapy for carcinoma of the colon

Study (year)	Stage (Dukes)	PatientsN.	Therapy	Disease-free interval P	5-year survival p
NSABP 1988[18]	B-C	1166	MOF Vs Controls	P=0.02	P=0.05
NCCTG 1989[20]	B-C	401	5-FU+LEV vs controls	P=0.0001	
INT 1990[21]	B-C	1296	5-FU+LEV vs controls	P=0.0001	P=0.006
IMPACT 1995[17]	B-C	1500	FUFA Vs Controls	P=0.001	P=0.035
NSABP-C04 1996[25]	B-C	2151	FUFA Vs 5-FU+LEV	P=n.s.	P=n.s.
INT 0089 1996[27]	B-C	3759	FUFA Vs 5-FU+LEV	P=n.s.	P=n.s.

NSABP=National Surgical Adjuvant Breast and Bowel Project Protocol; NCCTG=North Central Cancer Treatment Group; INT=Intergroup Protocol; IMPACT=International Multicenter Pooled Analysis of Colon Cancer Trials

5-FU=5-fluorouracil; MOF=MeCCNU+Vincristine+5-FU; LEV=levamisole; FUFA=5-FU+folinic acid ;.p = statistically significant; n.s. = not significant.

Intraportal chemotherapy

The liver is the most frequent site for metastases from colorectal cancer. When operated on for primary carcinoma, 14 to 25% of patients present synchronous hepatic metastates [37], while 8 to 25% develop metachronous hepatic metastases [37, 38]. In only 15 to 30% of patients with hepatic metastasis can curative resection be performed, with a 5-year survival ranging from 30 to 40% [39-41]; the average survival of patients with unresectable liver metastases ranges from 3 to 19 months [42-44].

Attempts have long been made to prevent hepatic metastases. With systemic chemotherapy modalities, relatively low drug concentrations reach the liver, and the preventive effect of systemic chemotherapy may therefore be reduced [45-48]. Tumoral invasion of the mesenteric vein causes malignant cells to spread to the

vena porta, thus leading to hepatic micrometastases. During the first phases of growth, metastatic vascularization originates in the portal branches, while larger liver metastases are supplied by the hepatic artery [49]. It is therefore reasonable to assume that in patients with a subclinical disease, chemotherapy infusion along the vena porta simulates the route of neoplastic emboli [50]. The rationale for continuous portal vein infusion (PVI) is, in fact, based on this observation; if utilized in the immediate post-operative period (7 days), it should increase the therapeutic efficacy of surgery.
The first randomized study on intraportal chemotherapy was made by Taylor [51] who, following 5-FU administration, observed a reduction in liver metastases, and an improvement in survival (Table 2). Throughout the eighties, however, different controlled clinical studies were conducted in USA and in Europe [52-57] to confirm Taylor's positive results, but their findings on efficacy of treatment were contradictory.
A meta-analysis was therefore undertaken to ascertain the effects of PVI on recurrences and survival after treatment with intraportal 5-FU, whether or not associated with other toxic agents. The 3.500 patients considered had undergone resection for colorectal cancer, and had been included in ten randomized trials started before 1987 [58] (Table 2).

Table 2. Controlled clinical trials on intraportal chemotherapy (PVI)

Study (year)	**Patients N.**	**Therapy**	**5-year survival (%) (p)**		**Reduction in hepatic recurr.**
			PVI	**Controls**	**p**
Taylor 1985[51]	277	5-FU	57.8 41.5 (p=0.008)		p=0.0001
LIMG 1997[58]	3222	5-FU+heparin ± MMC,FUDR	61.8 57.1 (p=0.006)		n.s.
EORTC 1998[59]	1235	5-FU+heparin	73 72 n.s.		n.s.

LIMG=Liver Infusion Meta-Analysis Group; EORTC=European Organization for Research and Treatment of Cancer; 5 FU=5 fluorouracil; MMC=Mitomycin C; FUDR=floxuridin; n.s.=not significant.

The two-year survival of patients treated with PVI was found to be the same as that of controls without PVI. At five years, however, a significant difference was observed, with a 4.7% increase in the PVI- treated patients (61.8% of survivors in the group treated with PVI against 57.1% in the control group), without significant differences between Dukes' stage A, B and C patients. However, the meta-analysis did not demonstrate that PVI significantly reduced the incidence of hepatic metastases. It has been suggested that the improvement in survival reported following PVI may depend on the peri-operative infusion of 5-FU, and on its systemic effect [58]. The results of this meta-analysis should be reconsidered in the light of the data obtained in two controlled clinical studies recently concluded by the EORTC [57, 59].

The first phase III controlled clinical trial, concluded by the EORTC in 1987 and included in the meta-analysis [57], evaluated the effect of adjuvant treatment with intraportal infusion of heparin and 5-FU on overall survival and the disease-free interval, in 235 patients with resectable colon cancer. No differences were found between the control group and the treated groups, for complications and hospital stay. Nor, after an average follow-up of 9 years, were any statistically significant differences found between the three groups (surgery alone, PVI with heparin and PVI with heparin+5-FU) for 5-year survival and disease-free interval.

In the second trial, conducted by the EORTC from 1987 to 1993 [59], 1.235 patients who underwent curative surgery were randomized to the control group, which had surgery only, or to a group receiving PVI with heparin (5000 UI) + 5-FU (500mg/m^2/die) for 7 post-operative days. This study confirmed that 7 days' PVI infusion alone does not improve survival or reduce the incidence of liver metastases [59] (Table 2). Therefore, although intraportal 5-FU infusion is a reliable method in expert hands and has an acceptable toxicity, it cannot be considered standard treatment for patients with resectable colon cancer.

Some clinical studies on adjuvant therapy for colorectal carcinoma, which are now being concluded, should establish whether PVI in association with systemic chemotherapy with FUFA or with 5-FU+levamisole improves the results of systemic chemotherapy alone.

Immunotherapy

Recent studies have shown that interferon α, monoclonal antibodies and active immunization are effective against colorectal cancer.

Interactions between interferon α and 5-FU [60,62] have been described in experimental studies. Interferon α can contribute to cellular necrosis from fluoropyrimidine exposure, and can increase the cytotoxicity of Natural Killer cells. In a phase I trial [61] on patients with advanced colorectal cancer, a 40 to 50% response rate was achieved. Phase II studies have confirmed these results [60, 62]. Even greater response percentages have been obtained by adding 5-FU and folinic acid to interferon α-2a [60]. This association causes a significant non-hematological toxicity (severe mucositis and diarrhea), but a negligible hematological toxicity. In the light of these results, phase III clinical studies have been initiated, some of which are also on adjuvant therapy, to evaluate the therapeutic efficacy of interferon associated mainly with 5-FU and folinic acid [63].The possibility of marking cancer cells with antibodies, especially in the early post-operative period, prompted the German Cancer Society Group [64] to use the

monocloncal antibody 17-1A as adjuvant treatment for patients with Stage III colon carcinoma. With respect to surgery alone, this immunotherapy, which does not cause important toxicity, reduces the overall mortality by 30% and the recurrence rate by 27%, and gives results comparable to those obtained with combined 5-FU+levamisole [64]. One international trial (the PANOREX Study) is now evaluating the efficacy of the 17-1A monoclonal antibody in adjuvant therapy in patients with Dukes' stage C colorectal tumors [63].
Several trials have focused on the use of an antitumoral vaccine, the Bacillus of Calmette-Guérin (BCG), as adjuvant therapy. Studies conducted utilizing BCG in association with 5-FU and nitrosurea [Gastrointestinal Tumor Study Group (GITSG) and NSABP C-01] [8, 18] showed no significant advantages in groups treated with immunotherapy, with respect to patients treated with chemotherapy, or to the control patients, who underwent surgery only. However, the unsatisfactory results obtained may have depended on the therapeutic regimens utilized. A prospective study is now underway to investigate the effects of this vaccine in association with 5-FU and levamisole [63].

Carcinoma of the rectum

It has been predicted that in 1998 there will be 37 000 new cases of rectal cancer in the USA. Even in cases in which "curative" resection is undertaken, the 5-year survival rate does not exceed 50% [65]. There are two types of recurrence after surgery: 1) distant metastases and 2) local pelvic recurrence, which is the more problematic aspect. The estimated risk of local recurrence is 20 to 50% in patients with transmural tumors or positive lymphnodes [66].

Surgery

Most patients with rectal carcinoma have regional disease through the muscularis propria into the subserosa or perirectal tissues, organs or structures (T3, T4), or diffusion to the lymphnodes of the mesorectum (which extends from the mesosigma and surrounds three quarters of the circumference of the distal rectum, and contains haemorrhoidal vessels and lymphatics).
In view of these characteristics, surgeons treating rectal carcinoma once tended to perform demolitive rather than conservative surgery in order to achieve local disease control, whatever the technique utilized and the functional results [67, 68]. Currently, the aim is to standardize a surgical technique that achieves radical resection while allowing good functional results [69].
Surgery for rectal cancer has the following objectives.
1) cure (i.e. prevention of systemic disease); 2) local control (i.e. prevention of pelvic recurrence) ; 3) preservation of the sphincters (i.e. ensuring intestinal

continuity and maintaining anorectal function); 4) preservation of sexual and urinary functions (i.e. keeping the pelvic autonomous nervous system intact).
Conventional surgery has only partly achieved these objectives [70]. In particular, in 1986 Quirke et al. [71] observed that local recurrence depends on positive resection margins and the partial excision of the mesorectum during conventional surgical procedures, that are wrongly considered curative. Fragments of adipose mesorectal tissue, including incompletely resected metastatic lymphnodes, adhere to the posterior pelvic wall, causing recurrences that appear within the following 18 months. In the presence of microscopically disease-free section margins, the incidence of recurrences is 10% or less, while in the presence of positive margins it is 85 to 90% [70].
The new surgical technique known as total mesorectal excision (TME), with autonomous nerve preservation (ANP) [72,74], is based on the possibility of completely removing the mesorectum by identifying and separating the portion of the rectum from the pelvic wall. Retrospective studies have demonstrated that the standardized use of TME reduces the percentage of local recurrences by 5-6% [69, 70], and it appears to significantly improve overall survival [69, 70, 75]. It is therefore reasonable to consider TME with ANP the new "gold standard" in surgery for rectal carcinoma.
Moreover, in patients with cancer of the lower rectum, sphincter-preserving surgery should be considered an alternative to abdomino-perineal rectal resection with colostomy, which is performed less and less frequently, being reserved for patients with rectal tumors located less than 5 cm from the anal margin. Low colorectal or coloanal anastomosis, with or without a "colon reservoir", in association with TME allows optimal local disease-control and satisfactory preservation of sphincter function. The results of conservative surgery in early stage rectal carcinomas appear identical to those obtained with abdomino-perineal resection, which has a higher mortality rate (1 to 5%) and a significant morbidity rate (e.g. genitourinary function impairment and impotence in males, psycho-social problems and difficulties related to colostomy management). Several retrospective and prospective studies have focused on improvement of quality of life, without compromising local control and survival [76].
Local excision, which can be achieved endoscopically or with a transanal, transphincteric, transcoccygeal or trans-sacral approach, guarantees satisfactory results in terms of survival, with a 10% incidence of local recurrence in over 90% of cases [77]. However, it is indicated only in patients with rectal T1 carcinoma, for whom negative resection margins have been obtained, and favorable prognostic factors identified (high or moderate grade of differentiation, absence of lymphatic and vascular invasion). Radiotherapy associated with local excision can provide excellent results in patients with a T1 tumor, but unfavorable clinical and histopathological prognostic factors, and in those with a T2 tumor [78]. A local

recurrence rate of 30 to 40% has been achieved with the same approach in patients with stage T3 tumors, and for whom therefore local therapy is contraindicated [79].
The results of surgery alone for rectal cancer depend on the extent of locoregional diffusion at diagnosis. In patients without regional lymphnode metastasis, the 5-year survival is 70 to 80% [80,82], while it does not exceed 40% in those with positive lymphnodes or tumors with extensive spread to the perirectal tissue [80,82].
Different adjuvant treatments have been proposed in recent years for rectal cancer, and among them radiotherapy has been the most widely-tested in controlled clinical trials.

Adjuvant treatments

Radiotherapy
Over the last 20 years, radiotherapy has become an integral part of the multidisciplinary approach to rectal tumors. In the light of results following radiotherapy used for advanced disease and local recurrences, it has been proposed also in adjuvant and in pre and post-operative therapy, and numerous randomized trials have been conducted to evaluate its efficacy in this setting. Most studies have demonstrated that radiotherapy significantly reduces local recurrences with respect to resection alone, while its effect on overall survival is still a matter of controversy.
The rationale for proposing pre-operative radiotherapy [83] is based on potential tumor reduction with a consequent improvement in resectability, and a minor risk of intra-operative haemorrhage, and reduced risk of neoplastic cells migrating during surgery. This technique, moreover, facilitates conservative surgery, by keeping the sphincters intact, and is associated with a smaller percentage of cases of enteritis, due to the fact that the small intestine is not dislocated into the pelvis. Post-operative radiotherapy, on the other hand, can be used to treat only patients at high risk of recurrences, and for those with residual disease [84]. It has also been demonstrated that compliance is greater for pre-operative radiotherapy than for post-operative radiotherapy (about 90% *versus* 60%) [85].
The first type of post-operative radiotherapy to be proposed was adjuvant therapy: some non-randomized clinical studies [86,87] reported a reduction in recurrences and an improved survival in patients treated with post-operative radiotherapy, with respect to patients treated with resection alone (historical control).
More recently, in three controlled clinical trials (GITSG, NSABP and Odense University Study) [88,90], two of which (GITSG and NSABP) [88, 89] included

chemotherapy arms, results reported for post-operative radiotherapy *versus* surgery alone were contradictory (Table 3).

Table 3. Controlled clinical trials on post-operative radiotherapy for rectal carcinoma

Study (year)	PatientsN.	Dose (Gy)	Local recurrence % RT+S	S	5-year survival % RT+S	S
GITSG 1988[88]	108	40-48	20	24	43	27
NSABP 1988[89]	368	46-47	16*	25*	41	43
OUS 1986[90]	494	45-50	6	8	82	67

RT=radiotherapy; S=surgery; GITSG=Gastrointestinal Tumor Study Group; NSABP=National Surgical Adjuvant Breast and Bowel Project; OUS=Odense University Study; * p=0.06.

For patients treated with post-operative radiotherapy, only the NSABP study confirmed that radiotherapy reduced local recurrences, but did not find that it improved overall survival [89]. Moreover, adequate doses and appropriate x-ray fields were utilized only by the NSABP.

Multicentric studies by the International Cancer Research Fund Trial [91], the Northwest Region Rectal Cancer Group [92], the Stockholm Rectal Cancer Study Group [93] and the EORTC [94] have demonstrated that the incidence of local recurrences significantly diminishes following pre-operative irradiation, while the survival of patients is not significantly changed (Table 4).

In a recently concluded randomized trial in Sweden [95] on 1.168 patients with Stage II or III rectal disease, who underwent surgery associated with pre-operative radiotherapy, a reduction in local recurrences was found, and there was an increase in the overall survival of the group treated with radiotherapy, with respect to the control group, which underwent surgery alone.

A study on the efficacy of pre- *versus* post-operative radiotherapy was evaluated in a randomized trial conducted in Sweden on 471 patients with Stage II or III rectal tumors [96]. It was found that pre-operative, short-term high dose radiotherapy significantly reduced the rate of local recurrences, with respect to post-operative radiotherapy, without, however, affecting survival or the incidence of distant metastases.

Results obtained so far demonstrate that pre-operative radiotherapy is more advantageous than post-operative radiotherapy for percentages of response and for complications from treatment itself. It has yet to be ascertained whether an improved standardization of surgical techniques, with the introduction of TME, can provide the same results as radiotherapy, in terms of local disease control. Randomized studies now underway may answer this question.

Table 4. Controlled clinical trials on pre-operative radiotherapy for rectal carcinoma

Study (year)	Patients N.	Dose (Gy)	Local recurrence %		5-year survival %	
			RT+S	S	RT+S	S
ICRFT 1994[91]	468	15	17	24	39	40
NRRCG 1994[92]	284	20	13	37	70	70
SRCSG 1990[93]	679	25	11	25	55	50
EORTC 1988[94]	341	34.5	15	35	69	59
SRCT 1996[95]	1168	25.5	10 ($p<0.01$)	26	60 ($p<0.01$)	46

RT=radiotherapy; S=surgery; ICRFT=Imperial Cancer Research Fund Trial; NRRCG=Northwest Region Rectal Cancer Group; SRCSG=Stockholm Rectal Cancer Study Group; EORTC=European Organization for Research and Treatment of Cancer; SRCT=Swedish Rectal Cancer Trial.

Chemotherapy

The efficacy of chemotherapy in adjuvant treatment for rectal carcinoma is not easy to evaluate, because many of the studies conducted so far have used associated radio and chemotherapy rather than chemotherapy alone.

In the NSABP study (protocol R-01) [8], which had three treatment groups, surgery alone was compared with both radio- and chemotherapy (Me-CCNU+5-FU+Vincristine). Significantly improved results, both in terms of survival and disease-free interval, were observed in the chemotherapy group. The GITSG study [88], which had one group with chemo-radiotherapy, one with surgery alone, one with radiotherapy alone and another with chemotherapy (5-FU and Nitrosurea), reports advantages only in patients who underwent combined chemo-radiotherapy. This suggests the efficacy of chemotherapy in patients who undergo "curative" resection for rectal carcinoma. However, both studies used Nitrosurea, which is considered a chemotherapeutic agent with a high myelosuppressive and leukemogenic activity.

Radio-chemotherapy

The rationale for combining radio and chemotherapy (utilizing 5-FU alone or in association) is based both on the fact that Fluorouracil has a radiosensitizing effect, and on the combined action of radio- and chemotherapy: one can contribute to the local control of the disease, while the other has a systemic activity and can therefore control distant metastases [66].

As well as the favorable results of the GITSG study [88], other studies have confirmed the advantages of combined radio-chemotherapy. In the NCCTG study [97], patients who received prolonged infusion with 5-FU during radiotherapy had a longer disease-free interval and survival and a lower incidence of distant metastases, than patients treated with 5-FU+MeCCNU or with 5-FU in bolus. An intergroup protocol (N. 0144) is now underway, to compare the efficacy of 5-FU as a single therapy in bolus, with prolonged continuous infusion in patients with Stage II and III rectal carcinoma [63, 66]. Each treatment also includes pre- and post-operative radiotherapy ("sandwich" protocol).

Finally, the favorable results obtained with pre-operative radiotherapy suggest that it is opportune to use pre-operative combined chemotherapy. Moreover, controlled clinical studies now underway aim to verify whether in high risk patients (T3-T4) pre-operative radio-chemotherapy should or should not be associated with post-operative chemotherapy [63, 66].

The following have yet to be established for carcinoma of the rectum:

1) optimal modality for administration of combined chemo-radiotherapy (concomitant, one or two cycles, sequential, bolus, continuous infusion);
2) whether, as for colon cancer, the addition of folates is more effective than 5-FU alone;
3) whether there are drugs that are more active than 5-FU;
4) whether chemotherapy associated with radiotherapy is advantageous also with respect to the cost/benefit ratio in terms of morbidity;
5) the role of TME in combined treatments.

Conclusions

The "curability" of colorectal carcinoma depends on achieving "radical" resection that fulfils standardized criteria for adequacy of surgery. New surgical approaches allow better local tumor control, while maintaining sphincteric function. Currently, abdomino-perineal rectal excision with colostomy is reserved for selected cases. The validity of laparoscopic colon resection has yet to be confirmed in larger series with longer follow-ups. Adjuvant 5-FU+folinic acid or 5-FU+levamisole reduces recurrences and markedly improves survival, in patients with colon carcinoma and lymphnode metastases. Systemic treatment is also indicated for some subgroups of Dukes' B stage patients with unfavorable prognostic factors.

Adjuvant radiotherapy undoubtedly reduces the risk of local recurrences of carcinoma of the rectum. Pre-operative radiotherapy, which is tolerated better than post-operative radiotherapy, is accompanied by a lower incidence of complications. Associated radio- and chemotherapy for carcinomas of the rectum was recently found to be effective, not only in reducing local recurrences, but also in prolonging survival.

Above all, colorectal carcinomas require "good" surgery. However, we can no longer assume that all these tumors can be controlled by surgery alone.

References

1. Registro Tumori del Veneto. Incidenza dei tumori nella regione Veneto 1990-94. CLEUP, Padova 1996.

2. Verdecchia A. Survival in adult italian cancer patients, 1978-89. *Tumori* 1997 ; 83: 39-425

3. August DA, Ottow RT, Sugarbaker PH. Clinical prospectives on human colorectal cancer metastases. *Cancer Metastases Rev* 1984 ; 3: 303-24.

4. Boring CC, Squires TS, Tong T. Cancer statistics. *Cancer J Clin* 1993; 43: 7-10.

5. Astler VA, Coller FA. The prognostic significance of direct extension of carcinoma of the colon and rectum. *Ann Surg* 1954; 139: 846-52.

6. Willett CG, Tepper JE, Cohen AM.. Failure patterns following curative resection of colonic carcinoma. *Ann Surg* 1984; 200: 685-90.

7. Hermanek P. Pathology of colorectal cancer. In : Bleiberg H, Rougier Ph, Wilke H (Eds.) Managment of colorectal cancer. Dunitz M, London 1998, pp 35-54.

8. Gastrointestinal Tumor Study Group. Adjuvant therapy of colon cancer: results of a prospectively randomized trial. *N Engl J Med* 1984; 310: 737-41.

9. Morton D, Fielding J. Surgery for colonic cancer. Colorectal cancer. In : Bleiberg H, Rougier Ph, Wilke H (Eds.) Managment of colorectal cancer, Dunitz M, London 1998, pp 79-92.

10. Lynch HT. Is there a role for prophilactic subtotal colectomy among hereditary non-polyposis colorectal cancer germline mutation carriers ? *Dis Colon Rectum* 1996 ; 39: 109-10.

11. Wexner SD, Cohen SM. Port site metastases after laparoscopic colorectal surgery for cure of malignancy. *Br J Surg* 1995; 82: 295-8.

12. Samet J, Hunt WC, Key C, et al. Choice of cancer therapy varies with age of patient. *J Am Med Assoc* 1986; 255: 3385-90.

13. Eisenberg B, DeCosse JJ, Harford F, Mickalek J. Carcinoma of the colon and rectum : the natural history reviewed in 1704 patients. *Cancer* 1982 ; 49 : 1131.

14. Cohen AM, Tremittera S, Candela F, Thaler JT, Sigurdson ER. Prognosis of node- positive colon cancer. *Cancer* 1991 ; 67 : 1859-67.

15. Wolmark N, Fisher B, Wieand HS. The prognosis value of the modifications of the Dukes'C class of colorectal cancer. *Ann Surg* 1986 ; 203 : 115-23.

16. Philips RKS, Hittinger R, Blesowsky L, Fry JS, Fielding LP. Large bowel cancer : surgical pathology and its relationship to survival. *Br J Surg* 1984 ; 71 : 604-9.

17. International Multicenter Pooled Analysis of Colon Cancer Trials (IMPACT) Investigators. Efficacy of adjuvant fluorouracil and folinic acid in colon cancer. *Lancet* 1995, 345. 939-44.

18. Wolmark N, Fisher R, Rockette H, et al. Postoperative adjuvant chemotherapy or BCG for colon cancer: results from NSABP protocol C-01. *J Natl Cancer Inst* 1988; 80: 30-6.

19. Verehaegen H, DeCree J, DeCock W, et al. Levamisole therapy in patients with colorectal cancer. In :Terry VD, Rosemberg SA (Ed) Immunotherapy of human cancer. Elsevier, New York, 1982, pp 225-9.

20. Laurie JA, Moertel CG, Fleming TR, et al. Surgical adjuvant therapy of large bowel carcinoma: an evaluation of levamisole and the combination of levamisole and fluorouracil. *J Clin Oncol* 1989; 7: 1447-56.

21. Moertel CG, Fleming TR, Mac Donald JS, et al. Levamisole and Florouracil for adjuvant therapy of resected colon carcinoma. *N Engl J Med* 1990; 322: 352-8.

22. NIH Consensus Conference. Adjuvant Therapy for patients with colon and rectal cancer. *JAMA* 1990; 264: 1444-50.

23. Glem GL, Hoth DL, Hamilton JM, King SA, Leyland-Jones B. Overwiew of current status and future directions of clinical trials with 5-FU in conbination with folinic acid. *Cancer Treat Rep* 1987; 71: 1249-64.

24. Advanced Colorectal Cancer Meta-analysis Project. Modulation of fluorouracil by leucovorin in patients with advanced colorectal cancer: evidence in terms of responsored . *J Clin Oncol* 1992; 10: 896-903.

25. Mamounas EP, Rockette H, Jones J, et al. Comparative efficacy of adjuvant chemotherapy in patients with Dukes B versus Dukes C colon cancer: results from four NSABP Adjuvant Studies. *Proc Am Soc Clin Oncol* 1996; 15: 205 (abst).

26. O'Connell MJ, Laurie JA, Shepard L, et al. A prospective evaluation of chemotherapy duration and regimen as surgical adjuvant treatment for high-risk colon cancer: a collaborative trial of the North Central cancer treatment group and the National cancer Institute of Canada clinical Trials group. *Proc Am Soc Clin Oncol* 1996 ; 15: 211 (abst).

27. Haller DG, Catalano PJ, MacDonald JS, Mayer RJ. Fluorouracil, leucovorin and levamisole. Adjuvant treatment for colon cancer: preliminary results of INT 0089. *Proc Am Soc Clin Oncol* 1996; 15: 211 (abst).

28. Wolmark N, Rockette H, Manounas EP, et al. The relative efficacy of 5-FU+Leucovorin (FU-LV), 5-FU+levamisole (FU-Lev), and 5-FU+Leucovorin+Levamisole (FU-LV-Lev) in patients with Dukes B and C carcinoma of the colon: first report of NSABP C-04. *Proc Am Soc Clin Oncol* 1996; 15: 205 (abst).

29. Rougier Ph, Pailot B, Laplanche D, et al. End results of a multicentric randomised trial comparing 5-fluorouracil in continous systemic infusion (CI) to bolus administration (B) in measurable metastatic colorectal cancer (MCC). *Proc Am Soc Clin Oncol* 1992; 11: 163 (abst).

30. De Grammont A, Bosset JF, Milan C, et al. A prospectively randomised trial comparing 5-fluorouracil bolus with low-dose folinic acid and 5-fluorouracil bolus plus continous infusion with high-dose folinic acid for advanced colorectal cancer. *Proc Am Soc Clin Oncol* 1995; 14: 194 (abst).

31. Leichman CG, Fleming TR, Muggia FM. A phase II study of 5-fluorouracil and its modulation in advanced colorectal cancer: a Southwest Oncology Group Study. *J Clin Oncol* 1995; 13: 1303-11.

32. Zalkberg JR, Cunningham D, Van Cutsem E et al. Tomudex (ZD1694), a novel thimidylate synthase inhibitor has a substantial activity in the treatment of patients with advanced colorectal cancer. *J Clin Oncol* 1996; 14: 716-21.

33. Cunningham D, Zalkberg JR, Rath U, et al. Tomudex (ZD1694): results of a randomised trial in advanced colorectal cancer demonstrate efficacy and reduced mucositis and leucopenia. *Eur J Cancer* 1995; 31: 1945-54.

34. Van Cutsem E, Rougier Ph, Droz JP, et al. Clinical benefit of irinotecan (CPT-11) in metastatic colorectal cancer resistant to 5-FU. *Proc Am Soc Clin Oncol* 1997; 16: 268 (abst).

35. Rougier P, Bugat R, Duoillard JY, et al. Phase II study of Irinotecan in the treatment of advanced colorectal cancer in chemotherapy-naive patients and patients pretreated with fluorouracil-based chemotherapy. *J Clin Oncol* 1997; 15: 251-60.

36. De Grammont A, Vignoud J, Tournigand C, et al. Oxaliplatin and high-dose leucovorin and 5-FU 48-hour continous infusion in pretreated metastatic colorectal cancer. *Eur J Cancer* 1997; 33: 214-9.

37. Finlay IG, Meek DR, Gray HW, et al. Incidence and detection of occult hepatic metastases in colorectal carcinoma. *Br Med J* 1982; 284:803-805.

38. Bengtsson G, Carlsson G, Fafstrom L, et al . Natural history of patients with untreated liver metastases from colorectal cancer. *Am J Surg* 1981; 141:586-9.

39. August D, Sugarbaker P, Ottow R, Gianola F, Schneider Ph. Hepatic resection of colorectal metastases. Influence of clinical factors and adjuvant intraperitoneal 5-Fluorouracil via Tenckhoff catheter on survival. *Ann Surg* 1985; 201:210-8.

40. Fortner JG. Recurrence of colorectal cancer after hepatic resection. *Am J Surg* 1988; 155:378-82.

41. Wagner JS, Adson MA, van Heerden JA, et al. The natural history of hepatic metastases from colorectal cancer. *Ann Surg* 1984; 199:502-8.

42. Bengmark S, Halfstrom L. The natural history of primary and secondary malignant tumors of the liver. The prognosis of patients with hepatic metastases from colon and rectal carcinoma verified by laparotomy. *Cancer* 1969; 23:198:202.

43. Nielsen J, Balslev I, Jensen HE. Carcinoma of the colon with liver metastases. *Acta Chir Scand* 1971; 137:463-5.
44. Cady B, McDermott WV. Major hepatic resection for metachronous metastases from colon cancer. *Ann Surg* 1985; 201:204-9.
45. Buyse M, Zeleniuch-Jacquotte A, Chalmers TC. Adjuvant therapy of colorectal cancer. Why we still don't know. *JAMA* 1988; 259: 3571-8.
46. Gray R, James R, Mossman J, Stenning S. AXIS-A suitable case for treatment. UK Coordinating Committee on Cancer Research (UKCCCR) Colorectal Cancer Subcommettee. *Br J Cancer* 1991; 63: 841-5.
47. Cedarmark BJ, Blumenson LE, Pickren JW, Holyoke DE, Elias EG. The significance of metastases to the adrenal glands in adenocarcinoma of the colon and the rectum. *Surg Gynecol Obstet* 1977; 144: 537-46.
48. Goslin R, Steele G Jr, Zamcheck N, Mayer R, Macintyre I. Factors influencing survival in patients with hepatic metastases from adenocarcinoma of the colon or rectum. *Dis Colon Rectum* 1982; 25: 749-54.
49. Storer EH, Akin TJ. Chemotherapy of hepatic neoplasm on the umbelical portal vein. *Am J Surg* 1966; 11: 56-8.
50. Nitti D, Marchet A, Da Pian PP, Pilati PL, Lise M. Adjuvant treatment following curative resection of liver metastasis from colorectal carcinoma. In : Bleiberg H, Rougier Ph, Wilke H (Eds.) Management of colorectal cancer, Dunitz M, London 1998, pp 185-92.
51. Taylor I, Machin D, Mullee M, Trotter G, Cooke T, West C. A randomized controlled trial of adjuvant portal vein cytotoxic perfusion in colorectal cancer. *Br J Surg* 1985; 72: 359-63.
52. Beart RW Jr, Moertel CG, Wieand HS, Leigh JE, Windschitl HE, van Heerden JA, et al. Adjuvant therapy for resectable colorectal carcinoma with fluorouracil administred by portal infusion. A study of the Mayo Clinic and the North Central Cancer Treatment Group. *Arch Surg* 1990; 125 : 897-901.
53. Fielding LP, Hittinger R, Grace RH, Fry JS. Randomised controlled trial of adjuvant chemotherapy by portal-vein infusion after curative resection for colorectal adenocarcinoma. *Lancet* 1992 ; 340 :502-6.
54. Long-term results of single course of adjuvant intraportal chemotherapy for colorectal cancer. Swiss Group for Clinica Cancer Research (SAKK). *Lancet* 1995 ; 345 : 349-53.
55. Wereldsma JC, Bruggink ED, Meijer WS, Roukema JA, van Putten WL. Adjuvant portal liver infusion in colorectal cancer with 5-fluorouracil/heparin versus urokinase versus control. Results of a prospective randomised clinical trial (colorectal Adenocarcinoma Trial I). *Cancer* 1990 ; 65 : 425-32.
56. Wolmark N, Rockette H wickerham DL, Fisher B, Redmond C, Fisher ER, et al. Adjuvant therapy od Dukes' A, B, and C adenocarcinoma of the colon with portal-vein fluorouracil hepatic infusion : preliminary results of National Surgical Adjuvant Breast and Bowel Project Protocol C-02. *J Clin Oncol* 1990 ; 8 :1466-5.
57. Nitti D, Wils J, Sahmoud, Curran D, Couvreur ML, Lise M, et al. Final results of a Phase III Clinical Trial on Adjuvant Intraportal Infusion with Heparin and 5-FU in resectable colon cancer (EORTC GITCCG 1983-1987). *Eur J of Cancer* 1997; 33: 1209-15.
58. Liver Infusion Meta-analysis Group. Portal Vein Chemotherapy for Colorectal Cancer: a Meta-analysis of 4000 Patients in 10 Studies. *J Nat Cancer Inst* 1997; 89: 497-505.
59. Rougier P, Sahmud T, Nitti D, et al. Adjuvant portal vein infusion of 5 FU and Heparin in colorectal cancer: An Inter-group phase III Trial. *Lancet* 1998. In press.
60. Grem JL, Jordan E, Robson ME, et al. Phase II study of fluorouracil, leucovorin and interferon α-2a in metastatic colorectal carcinoma. *J Clin Oncol* 1993; 11. 1737-45.
61. Pazdur R, Ajani JA, Patt YZ, et al. Phase II study of fluorouracil and recombinant interferon α-2a in previously untreated advanced colorectal carcinoma. *J Clin Oncol* 1990; 8: 2027-31.
62. Wadler S, Lembersky B, Atkins M, Kirkwood J, Petrelli N. Phase II trial of fluorouracil and recombinant inerferon α 2a in patients with advanced colorectal carcinoma : an Eastern Cooperative Oncology Group study. *J Clin Oncol* 1991; 9: 1806-10.
63. Casillas S, Pelley RJ, Milsom JW. Adjuvant therapy for colorectal cancer. Present and future prospectives. *Dis Colon Rectum* 1997; 40: 977-92.
64. Reithmuller G, Schneider-Gadicke E, Schlimok G, et al. Randomized trial of monoclonal antibody for adjuvant therapy of resected Dukes C colorectal carcinoma. *Lancet* 1994; 343: 1177-83.

65. Parker SL, Tong T, Bolden S, Wingo PA. Cancer statistics 1997. *CA Cancer J Clin* 1997; 47: 5-27.
66. Labianca R, Pessi MA, Zamparelli G. Treatment of Colorectal Cancer: Current guidelines and future prospects for drug therapy. *Drugs* 1997; 53: 593-607.
67. Enker WE, Laffer UT, Block GE. Enhanced survival of patients with colon and rectal cancer is based upon wide anatomic resection. *Ann Surg* 1979; 190: 350-60.
68. Heald RJ. A new approach to rectal cancer. *Br J Hosp Med* 1979; 277-83.
69. Sugihara K, Moriya Y, Akasu T, Fujita S. Pelvic autonomic nerve preservation for patients with rectal carcinoma: oncologic and functional outcome. *Cancer* 1996; 78: 1871-80.
70. Enker WE. Designing the optimal surgery for rectal carcinoma. *Cancer* 1996; 78: 1847-50.
71. Quirke P, Durdey P, Dixon MF, Williams NS. Local recurrence of rectal adenocarcinoma due to inadequate surgical resection. Histopatological study of lateral tumor spread and surgical excision. *Lancet* 1986; 1: 996-9.
72. Enker WE. Potency, cure, and local control in the operative treatment of rectal cancer. *Arch Surg* 1992; 127: 1396-402.
73. Havenga K, Enker WE, McDermott K, Cohen AM, Minsky BD, Guillem J. Male and female sexual and urinary function after total mesorectal excision with autonomic nerve preservation for carcinoma of the rectum. *J Am Coll Surg* 1996; 182: 495-502.
74. Arbman G, Nilsson E, Hallbook O, Sjodahl R. Local recurrence following total mesorectal excision for rectal cancer. *Br J Surg* 1996; 83: 375-9.
75. Mac Farlane J, Ryall RDH, Heald RJ. Mesorectal excision for rectal cancer. *Lancet* 1993; 341: 457-60.
76. Ng AK, Recht A, Busse P. Sphincter preservation therapy for distal rectal carcinoma. A Review. *Cancer* 1997; 79: 671-83.
77. Graham RA, Garnsey L, Jessup JM. Local excision of rectal carcinoma. *Am J Surg* 1990; 160: 306-12.
78. Willet CG, Compton CC, Shellito PC, Efird JT. Selection factors for local excision or abdominoperineal resection of early stage rectal cancer. *Cancer* 1994; 73: 2716-20.
79. Hager TH, Gall FP, Hermanek P. Local excision of cancer of the rectum. *Dis Colon Rectum* 1983; 26: 149-51.
80. Rich T, Gunderson LL, Lew R, Galdibini JJ, Cohen AM, Donaldson G. Patterns of recurrence of rectal cancer after potentially curative surgery. *Cancer* 1983 ; 52 : 1317-26.
81. Philipshen SJ, Heilweil M, Quan SHQ, Sternberg SS. Enker WE. Patterns of pelvic recurrence following definitive resections of rectal cancer. *Cancer* 1984 ; 53 :1354-62.
82. Minsky BD, Mies C, Recht A, Rich TA, Chaffey JT. Resectable adenocarcinoma of the rectosigmoid and rectum. Patterns of failure and survival. *Cancer* 1988 ; 61 :1408-16.
83. Minsky BD. Preoperative combined modality treatment for rectal cancer. *Oncology* 1994; 8: 53-68.
84. Minsky BD, Cohen AM, Enker WE, Kelsen DP, Kemeny N, Frankel J. Efficacy of postoperative 5-FU, high.dose leucovorin, and sequential radiation therapy for clinically resectable rectal cancer. *Cancer Invest* 1995; 13: 1-7.
85. Pahlman L. Preoperative treatment of rectal cancer. In: Bleiberg H, Rougier Ph, Wilke H (Eds.) Management of colorectal cancer, Dunitz M, London 1998, pp 153-66.
86. Tepper JE, Cohen AM, Wood WC, Orlow EL, Hedberg SE. Postoperative radiation therapy of rectal cancer. *Int J Radiat Oncol Biol Phys* 1987 ; 13 : 5-12.
87. Vigliotti A, Rich TA, Romsdahl MM, Withers HR, Oswald MG. Postoperative adjuvant radiotherapy for adenocarcinoma of the rectum and rectosigmoid. *Int J Radiat Oncol Biol Phys* 1987 ; 13 : 999-1005.
88. Thomas PRM, Lindblad AS. Adjuvant postoperative radiotherapy and chemotherapy in rectal carcinoma : a rewiew of the Gastrointestinal Tumor Study Group experience. *Radiother Oncol* 1988; 13: 245-52.
89. Fisher B, Wolmark N, Rockette H, et al. Postoperative adjuvant chemotherapy or radiation therapy for rectal cancer : results fron NSABP protocol R-01. *J Natl Cancer Inst* 1988; 80: 21-9.
90. Balslev I, Pedersen M, Teglbjaerg PS, et al. Postoperative radiotherapy in Dukes'B and C carcinoma of the rectum and rectosigmoid : a randomized multicenter study. *Cancer* 1986 ; 58 : 22.

91. Goldberg P, Nicholls R, Porter N, et al. Long-term results of a randomised trial of short-course low-dose adjuvant preoperative radiotherapy for rectal cancer: reduction in local treatment failure. *Eur J Cancer* 1994; 30: 1602-6.
92. Marsh PJ, James RD, Schfield PF. Adjuvant preoperative radiotherapy for locally advanced rectal carcinoma : results of a prospective randomised trial. *Dis Colon Rectum* 1994; 37: 1205-14.
93. Cedermark B, Johansson H, Rutqvist L, Wilking N. The Stockholm I trial of preoperative short term radiotherapy in operable rectal carcinoma. *Cancer* 1995; 75: 2269-75.
94. Gerard A, Buyse M, Nordlinger M et al. Preoperative radiotherapy as adjuvant treatment in rectal cancer: final results of a randomized study of the EORTC. *Ann Surg* 1988; 208: 606-14.
95. Swedish Rectal Cancer Trial. Five-year survival after preoperative radiation in rectal cancer. *Int J Colorectal Dis* 1996; 11: 198 (abst).
96. Pahlman L,Glimelius B. Pre- or postoperative radiotherapy in rectal and rectosigmoid carcinoma: report from a randomized multicenter trial. *Ann Surg* 1990; 211: 187-95.
97. O'Connell MJ, Martenson JA, Wieand HS, et al. Improving adjuvant therapy for rectal cancer by combining protracted-infusion fluorouracil with radiation therapy after curative surgery. *N Engl J Med* 1994; 331: 502-7.

CHAPTER 12

THE FOLLOW-UP IN COLORECTAL CANCER.

ANACLETO PERACCHIA, NICOLA PIETRA, and LEOPOLDO SARLI

Institute of Surgical Clinics, University of Parma, Parma , Italy

Summary

After an overview of the various procedures best able to achieve early diagnosis of recurrence of colorectal cancer, two different follow-up plans were compared in 207 consecutive patients, who had undergone curative resections for primary untreated large bowel carcinoma, at Parma University's Istituto di Clinica Chirurgica Generale e Terapia Chirurgica. The intense follow-up led to more frequent identification of local recurrences without distant metastases, and to the detection of local recurrences in a high percentage of cases with as yet no manifestation of symptoms clearly indicative of recurrence. The intense follow-up led to a greater number of re-resections for local recurrences than those performed in the control group submitted to conventional follow-up (17 versus 2; $p<0.01$), and we observed an improved 5-year survival in patients undergoing intense follow-up (73.1% versus 58.3%; $p<0.02$).

Our data support use of an intense follow-up plan after primary resection of large bowel cancer, at least in rectal cancer patients.

Introduction

The necessity of carrying out periodical clinical and instrumental checks after curative resection of a colorectal cancer, is motivated by the observation that about around half those patients face local or distant recurrence, with consequent negative effects on the survival rate [1,2]. The follow-up of these patients should thus allow *early diagnosis of recurrence*, and the application of a surgical, radiological or pharmacological therapy from which the patient can benefit in terms of quality of life and survival [3-9]. Another aim of the follow-up should be the *early diagnosis of metachronous colorectal neoplasia*, because of which these patients are at high risk.

Follow-up procedures depend on knowledge of the natural history of colorectal cancer. An ideal procedure must always take into account the following biological indices [10]:

Site of recurrence probability;

Time of recurrence probability;

Higher risk patients.

As regards possible sites of recurrence, Sugarbaker et al. calculated that recurrence

E. Zanella (ed.), Advances in Abdominal Surgery, 127–141.

in 63% of cases is exclusively endoperitoneal and in 21% of cases involves both the peritoneal cavity and other sites: in all, recurrence affects the abdominal cavity in 84% of cases [11].

Locoregional recurrences are the most frequent (30-40%), while the liver is the most common site of distant metastasis, being affected in 50% of patients with disseminated disease [12,13]. Lung metastasis occurs in around 11% of patients who undergo resection of the rectum, and in 3.5% of those undergoing resection of the colon [14]. Recurrence can also be observed, more rarely, in other sites, such as the bone and the central nervous system (4-7%), generally in association with liver and/or lung metastasis (Fig. 1) [15].

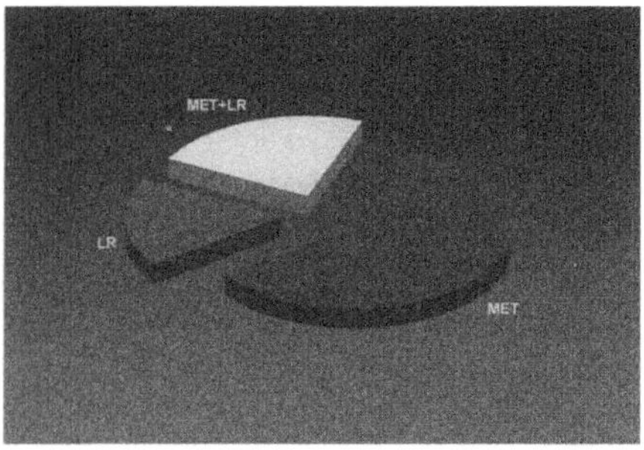

Figure 1. 791 patients underwent curative exeresis for colorectal cancer and 721 were subjected to subsequent regular follow-up at the clinical Institutes of the University of Parma, directed by Prof. A. Peracchia, in the period between 1976 and 1993. A recurrence was detected in 198 of them (27.5%). In 81 cases (11.2%) an LR was found, isolated in 36 cases and associated with distant metastasis in 45. In 117 cases (16.2%), distant metastases were found not associated with LR.

The study of the time of recurrence has shown that it mostly (80%) appears within the first 24 months after surgery, rarely appearing after 5 years (Figs. 2,3) [16,17].

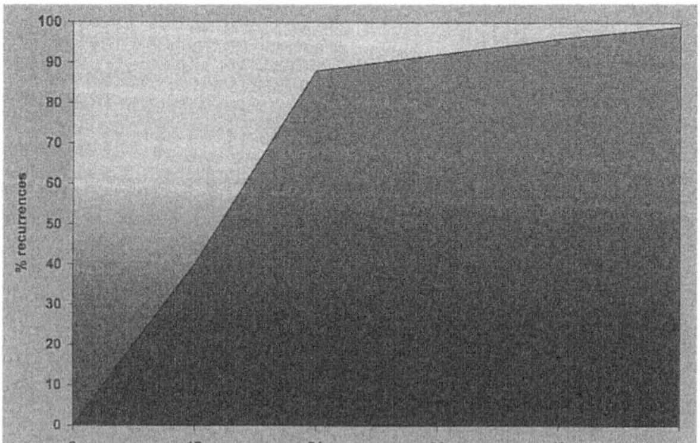

Figure 2. In the personal series of 721 patients subjected to radical resection of colorectal cancer and subsequent regular follow-up in the period between 1976 and 1993, local recurrences and/or distant metastases were found in 198 cases (27.5%). Most of the recurrences were observed within the first 2 years of follow-up, after a mean disease-free interval of 17 months. Only in 2 cases (1%) did a recurrence show up after the fifth year of observation.

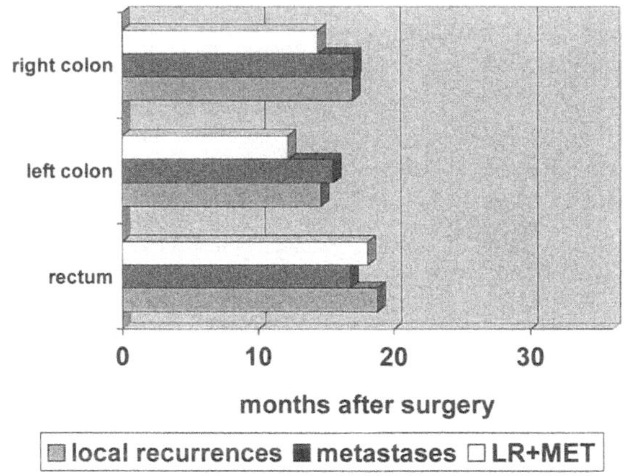

Figure 3. Mean duration of the disease-free interval in relation to the site of the primary tumour in our experience (198 recurrences in 721 patients).

Despite the considerable number of contributions to the literature regarding the analysis of clinical and anatomopathological variables which are useful in identifying higher risk patients, it is not easy to shed light on the subject [18,19], and the anatomopathological stage is still the single factor considered as being of the greatest predictive value [20].

Multivariate statistical analysis of the data relating to 721 patients undergoing radical surgery at the surgical institutes of the University of Parma, directed by Prof. A. Peracchia, in the period between 1976 and 1993, and subjected to subsequent regular follow-up, showed that the two factors which most increased the risk of recurrence were *tumour stage* (Risk Ratio [RR]: 1.98; Confidence Interval [CI]: 1.45-2.69; $p<0.0001$) and *tumour perforation* (RR 2.69; CI 1.81-3.99; $p<0.0001$) (Figs. 4,5) [20]. It would thus be logical to expect follow-up

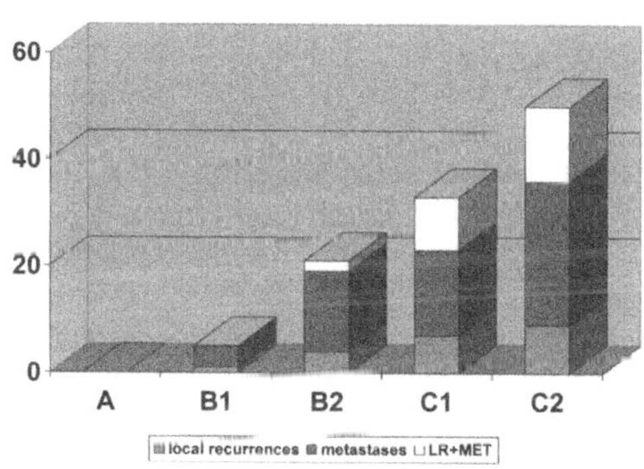

Figure 4: Incidence of recurrences and anatomopathological stage (Dukes' classification modified by Astler and Coller) in the personal series of 721 patients submitted to radical exeresis of colorectal cancer and subsequent regular follow-up. The differences between the frequencies are significant, with $P<0.0001$.

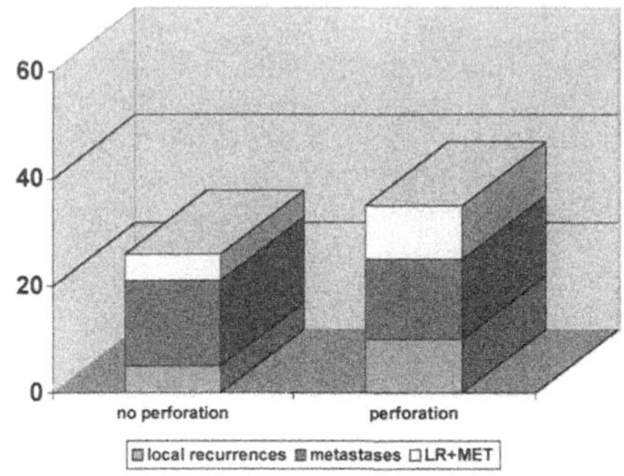

Figure 5. Incidence of recurrences and presence of perforative complications of the primary tumour in the personal series of 721 patients submitted to radical exeresis of colorectal cancer and subsequent regular follow-up. The difference between the frequencies is significant, with P<0.0001.

procedures to involve differing examinations according to the tumour stage; however, debate on the subject is still under way [21,22].

Diagnosis of locoregional recurrence

LOCOREGIONAL RECURRENCES (LR) can appear at the site of the primary tumour, on the laparotomic or perineal scar, at the pericolostomic level or along the pathway of a drain, in correspondence with the regional lymph nodes, or at the level of the intestinal anastomosis [20]. The anastomosis may be the only site of an LR, which in this case is defined as primary anastomotic, but the patient is more often affected by a contiguous, perianastomotic LR, which projects into the intestinal lumen, configuring the so-called "iceberg" recurrence.

Surgery is the only option for curative therapy for these recurrences. However, radical surgery for LR, when these are already symptomatic, is possible only in selected cases: in our experience, LR resulted as being suitable for radical exeresis in only 22.9% of the cases [23]. The only LR which lend themselves to satisfactoy radical exeresis are primary anastomotic recurrences, which are, however, not at all frequent (5% in our experience, 4-20% in the series in the literature).

These considerations justify the need to establish the nature and frequency of the follow-up procedures best able to achieve early diagnosis of LR, in the hope that this will lead to greater possibilities of cure.

Clinical examination is indispensable and must be carried out every time the patient is seen. Although prospective studies have shown that physical examination is the first indication of recurrence in 21-48% of cases [11], it must be borne in mind that this factor often contributes to the diagnosis of recurrence only when this is already symptomatic [24].

Endoscopy is the examination of choice for primary anastomotic LR. It is preferable to *double contrast enema* since it is of higher diagnostic reliability (98%), with a decidedly lower risk of false negatives than with radiological examination. Above all, thanks to histobioptic examination, it does not produce the false positives which are always possible with barium enema. The disadvantage of endoscopy, besides morbidity and mortality rates of 0.25-2% and 0.01-0.1% respectively, is its incompleteness, which in expert hands affects 2% of cases, but which reaches a mean 25% [25].

Transrectal ultrasound is today the first-choice examination for the pelvis, in the follow-up of patients undergoing resection of the left colon or of the rectum with colorectal anastomosis [26]. This examination is particularly useful for the identification of perirectal recurrences before these become a cause of endoluminal infiltration, and it permits the taking of samples aimed at the histopathological confirmation of LR, in those cases where the difference in diagnosis between recurrence and inflammatory processes is particularly difficult.

Abdominal ultrasound and *computed tomography* (CT) can be utilised for the study of the peritoneal cavity, although it must be remembered that the involvement of the peritoneum in cases of peritoneal carcinosis is still difficult to identify, even by the most expert examiners. The sensitivity of ultrasound in the identification of LR depends largely on the dimensions of the lesions. However, it remains an easily-applied, non-invasive, low-cost examination which is routinely used in the procedures of most European schools. On a systematic basis CT does not seem to be useful, above all because of the high frequency of false positives and the considerable costs [11,24]. Its use is advisable whenever other examinations reveal a suspect of recurrence [27]. Its sensitivity in the follow-up for the detection of a suspected recurrence results as being 85%.

Among serological examinations, measurement of the serum concentration of *carcinoembryonic antigen* (CEA) [28], a glycoprotein produced by over 90% of colorectal adenocarcinomas, achieves major consensus and is generally deemed to be a necessary feature of any post-operative follow-up plan [29,32]. High serum levels of this antigen lead to the indication of a suspected recurrence before any other serological or instrumental examination, with the exception of poorly-differentiated neoplasms [33]. Sugarbaker et al., on the basis of a prospective study, show that its increase constitutes, in 60-70% of cases, the first indicator of a recurrence and must always lead to further diagnostic investigation [11]. The usefulness of serum concentration measurement of other tumour markers, such as *membrane-associated glycoproteins CA19 9, CA-242, CA125, CA15-3* and *CA72-4, Tissue Polypeptide Antigen, Tissue Polypeptide-Specific antigen* and *Tissue Polypeptide Monoclonal antigen,* has not yet won complete agreement, and thus the most commonly-used follow-up plans do not include these markers [34,35].

Diagnosis of distant recurrence

As regards the DISTANT RECURRENCE of a colorectal carcinoma, the removal of the liver metastases is solely a curative indication, and is thus acceptable only if the involvement of the liver is the sole manifestation of recurrence. The infiltration of an extrahepatic structure, or the presence of lymph node metastases on the hepatic pedicle or at the coeliac tripod, are elements which, when present, are a contraindication for exeresis [36]. The only exception is the coexistence of lung metastases, a situation which does not absolutely exclude a double exeresis, although its significance is negative, since it testifies to the probable generalisation of the disease. The presence of lung metastases may be an indication for exeresis in selected patients. Some authors report not-inconsiderable survival rate [20], in these cases.

First choice for the examination of the liver is *ultrasound*. The sensitivity of this examination depends on the experience of the examiner, on the quality of the instrument and on the dimensions and site of the metastases. Under optimal conditions, it is equal to, if not greater than, that of more sophisticated examination procedures such as *angio CT* or *magnetic resonance*.

Chest X-ray allows the diagnosis of lung metastases. No randomised studies exist to establish whether this examination makes for better results when carried out at very close intervals. *Thoracic CT* may also be usefully applied in cases in which standard chest X-ray reveals suspected lung metastases.

Diagnosis of Metachronous tumours

Endoscopy is also the chosen examination in the identification of metachronous colorectal neoplasms. The mean interval between the preceding check-up and the appearance of METACHRONOUS COLORECTAL TUMOURS is 18 months for adenomas and 24 months for adenocarcinomas [37]. Sometimes, however "early" metachronous lesions are found, which must be interpreted as having been already present, but having escaped detection, at the preceding check-up (Fig. 6) [25].

Thus a complete colonoscopy must be carried out before surgery, or, in the case of obstructing lesions, in the course of surgery itself, or as soon as possible after operation, so that unidentified synchronous tumours will not subsequently be interpreted as metachronous tumours [38].

The highest incidence of metachronous tumours is observed between five and twelve years after surgery, but lesions are also detected after a longer time; it is thus necessary to continue the follow-up plan designed for their detection throughout the patient's life [39].

The diagnosis of metachronous carcinoma in the course of regular follow-up carried out along the lines proposed in Table 1, varies between 1.5% and

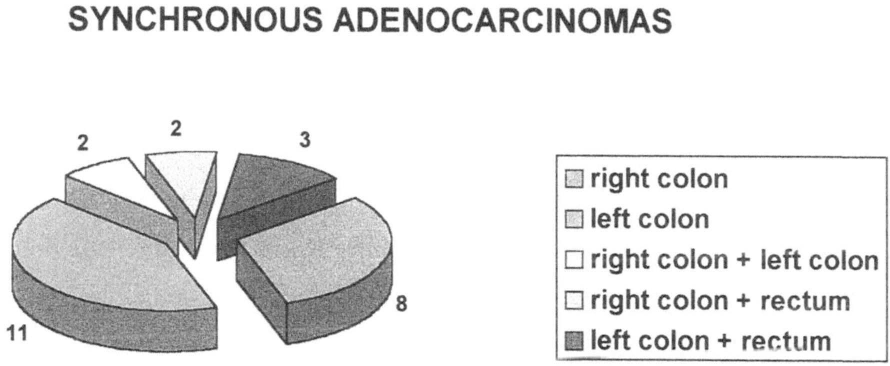

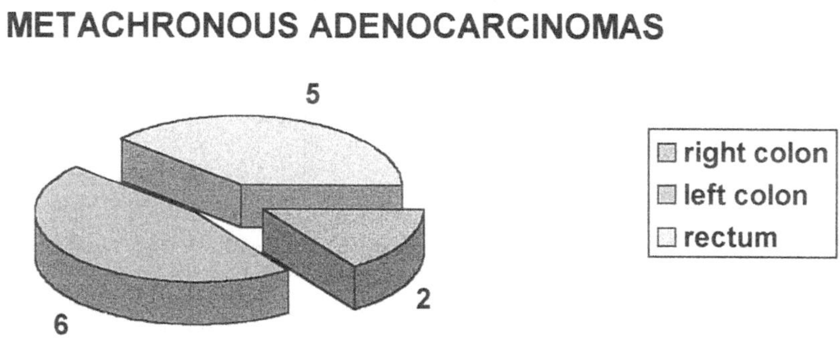

Figure 6: Frequency and site of synchronous colorectal adenocarcinomas in the personal series of 791 patients submitted to radical exeresis of colorectal tumours in the period between 1976 and 1993 and of metachronous adenocarcinomas in the series of 721 patients undergoing regular follow-up.

Table 1. Follow-up plan proposed by Ovaska et al.[48]

MONTHS AFTER SURGERY	3	6	12	18	24	36	48	60
Physical examination	X	X	X	X	X	X	X	X
Laboratory tests	X	X	X	X	X	X	X	X
CEA measurement	X	X	X	X	X	X	X	X
Occult blood test	X	X	X	X	X	X	X	X
Rectosigmoidoscopy	X	X	X	X	X	X	X	X
Barium enema		X	X		X	X	X	X
Chest X-ray		X	X		X	X	X	X

3.8% (Fig. 6) [40,43], and, although no comparative prospective studies have been reported, in these cases the follow-up proves to be extremely useful. In the experience of St Mark's Hospital, metachronous neoplasms diagnosed in the course of routine check-ups were shown to be at an earlier stage than those detected in subjects not regularly controlled [38]. During follow-up, metachronous adenomas are detected in 9-50% of cases and are generally removed in the course of endoscopy. It has not, however, been proved that their removal reduces the incidence of metachronous carcinomas [44].

Follow-up procedure

Intensive follow-up, leading to early detection and resection of recurrences, is advocated by many authors as a way of increasing the survival of these patients [45,48]. Other authors [49,52], however, criticize the use of extensive post-operative diagnostic tests, because the extra cost and time involved do not seem to lead to a better survival rate: Martin et al. [53] reported an increase in the resectability of recurrences from 27% to 60% when the CEA levels were measured every 4 to 6 weeks during the first 2 post-operative years, and Minton et al. [54] emphasized that an aggressive CEA-based follow-up can lead to a considerable cure rate. Using an intensive follow-up during the first 2 post-operative years, Reid et al. [55] found that half their patients with recurrence were asymptomatic, but were identified at scheduled visits; Ovaska et al. [48] were in agreement, reporting that 83% of recurrences in their series were detected at scheduled visits. On the other hand, Cochrane et al. [56] and Hulton and Hargreaves [57] noted that the majority of patients with LR presented themselves between routine clinic appointments; Beart and O'Connell [23] reported that 41 out of 48 patients who were being followed at intervals of 3 months had noticed symptoms suggesting recurrence since their last clinic visit. Makela et al. [49] found that earlier detection of recurrence by intensified follow-up did not lead to significantly more radical re-operations or to a better long-term survival; Kjeldsen et al. [52] reported that

patients subjected to intensive follow-up have recurrence diagnosed earlier, and have more operations for recurrence, but without any positive effect on survival. In contrast, Barillari et al. [29] found that serial tumor marker evaluation is of help in earlier diagnosis of LR and allows asymptomatic patients to undergo further curative surgery in a greater number of cases, and to have a better survival rate.
It is difficult to see why the results of these papers vary so widely, especially since the population studied and the follow-up protocols were similar.
In a study conducted by us, a comparison was made between two different follow-up plans, in 207 consecutive patients who had undergone curative resections for primary untreated large bowel carcinoma between 1987 and 1990 [58]. These patients were randomized into a conventional follow-up group (group A, N=103) and into an intense follow-up group (group B, N=104). The two groups were similar with respect to baseline clinical and pathological data. One full colonoscopy was performed 3 months after surgery to ensure a clean colon, if it had not been performed prior to operation. The protocols for conventional and intense follow-up are reported in Table 2, and the same clinical and/or instrumental tests were carried

Table 2. Intense and conventional follow-up plans applied in 207 patients of our series.

MONTHS AFTER SURGERY	3	6	9	12	15	18	21	24	30	36	42	48	54	60
CONVENTIONAL FOLLOW-UP														
Physical examination		X		X				X		X		X		X
Ultrasound		X		X				X		X		X		X
CEA measurement		X		X				X		X		X		X
Chest X-ray				X				X		X		X		X
Colonoscopy				X				X		X		X		X
INTENSE FOLLOW-UP														
Physical examination	X	X	X	X	X	X	X	X	X	X	X	X	X	X
Ultrasound	X	X	X	X	X	X	X	X	X	X	X	X	X	X
CEA measurement	X	X	X	X	X	X	X	X	X	X	X	X	X	X
Chest X-ray				X				X		X		X		X
Colonoscopy				X				X		X		X		X
Computed tomography				X				X		X		X		X

out whenever a patient of either group presented symptoms suggestive of a possible recurrence of the disease (abdominal or perineal pain, altered bowel movements, change in fecal color, weight loss). In the case of persistent increase in CEA serum level, with no evidence of tumour recurrence, a surgical second-look was performed. Patients with rectal cancer received post-operative irradiation, whereas no patient was submitted to adjuvant chemotherapy, which was introduced into our therapeutic procedure for colorectal cancer after 1991. All the patients were followed prospectively, and the outcome is known for all of them five years after. The results of our study are reported in Figures 7-10.

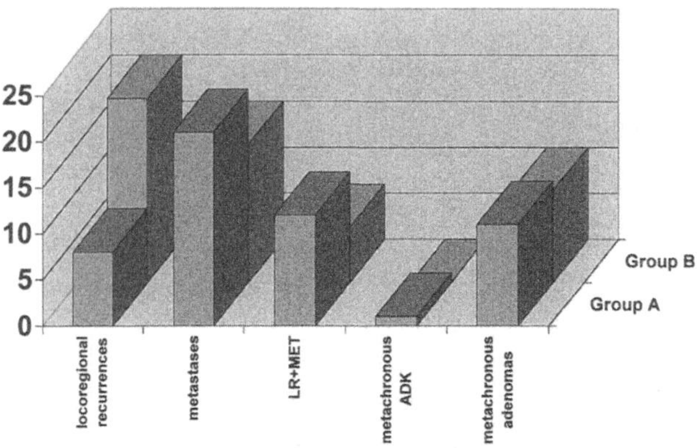

Figure 7: Results of follow-up obtained in 103 patients submitted to conventional follow-up (Group A) and 104 patients submitted to intense follow-up (Group B). The intense follow-up led to more frequent identification of LR without distant metastases (P<0.05).

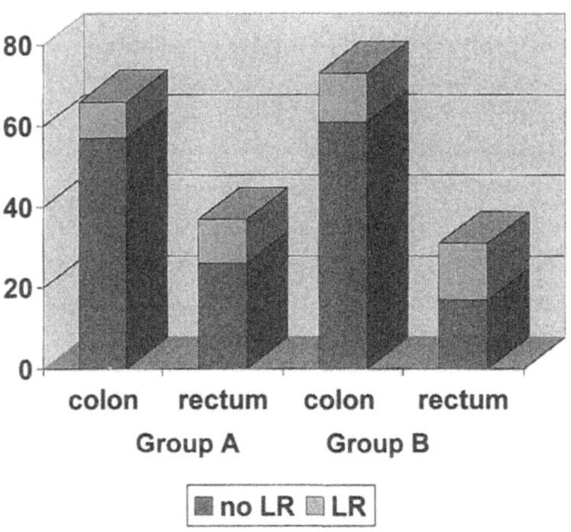

Figure 8: Site of the primary tumor and incidence of LR.

The intense follow-up led to a greater number of re-resections for LR than those performed in the control group, submitted to conventional follow-up (17 versus 2; $p<0.01$) (Fig. 9) and we observed an improved 5-year survival in patients who had undergone intense follow-up (73.1% versus 58.3%; $p<0.02$) (Fig. 10).

In particular, the intense follow-up led to more frequent identification of LR without distant metastases, and to the detection of LR in a high percentage of cases with as yet no manifestation of symptoms clearly indicative of recurrence. An important consequence of the absence of distant metastases and of early diagnosis was the possibility to carry out a greater number of re-resections. These observations confirm what has been stated in other contributions of literature, that is, if an LR is diagnosed early there is a greater probability of being able to proceed with curative re-resection [59,62]. The results listed in Figures 8 and 9 suggest that

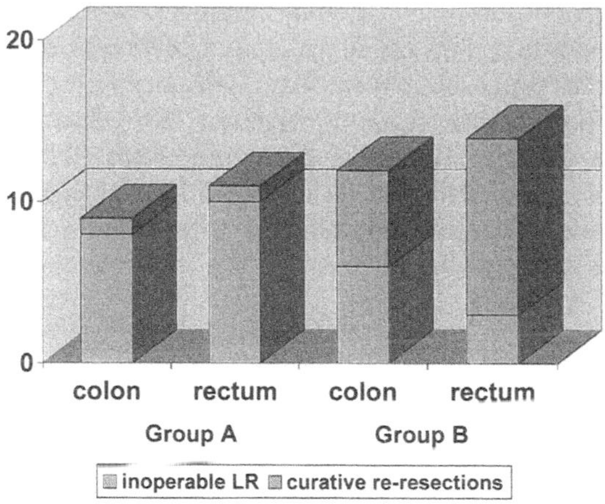

Figure 9: Site of the primary tumor and curative re-resections in patients with LR.

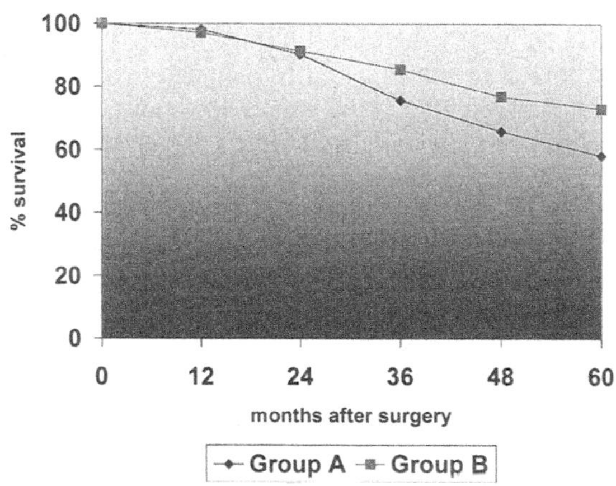

Figure 10: Cumulative five-year survival rate in patients submitted to the conventional follow-up (group A, 103 patients) and in patients submitted to the intense follow-up (group B, 104 patients). The difference between the survival curves is significant ($p<0.02$).

the significant differences in the two groups were limited to the rectal cancer patients, and that intensive follow-up may be more beneficial for rectal cancer patients than colon cancer patients. More meaningful interpretation would be helped with stratification by stage and site of the primary tumour, but the limited number of patients precludes this statistical evaluation.

The commonest sign indicating LR in both groups, when no clinical symptoms were present, was an elevation of the CEA value. None of the other clinical and/or instrumental tests, including CT, used in routine fashion, were cost-efficient in screening for LR, as has already been observed by other authors [11]. These results prompt us to state that, although the most cost-effective follow-up schedule

remains to be defined, CEA is the most effective indicator of recurrent disease and we suggest that a *simplified intense follow-up program with frequent CEA assays* is an optimal plan [11,63]. The planning of a follow-up programme must also take into account the *level of specialisation of the clinic where follow-up is conducted* [64]. In other words, highly specialised centres should be used, capable of carrying out both an accurate diagnosis of recurrences and their prompt treatment.
CEA measurement was also seen to be a useful indicator of second-look procedures [58]. Results of other studies on the subject are contradictory [65,67], although progress in radioimmuno-guided surgery, using anti-CEA antibodies or other more sensitive markers, could in the near future lead to further improvement in the results of second-look surgery in identifying and treating tumour recurrences.

Conclusion

One of our randomized trials showed that the survival of large bowel cancer patients is improved with more frequent follow-up, primarily because LR are more resectable when promptly detected. Our results suggest that an intense surveillance program using CEA assays may be more beneficial for rectal cancer patients than for colon cancer patients, but this does not necessarily include all colon cancer patients; however LR are more common after rectal cancer resections. In order to extend this policy to all colon cancer patients, a trial with a larger population is needed, since the risk of LR is lower in colon cancer patients, and the overall number of resectable LR does not appear to be cost-efficient. The most cost-effective follow-up schedule remains to be defined. In any case, follow-up must be carried out in highly specialized centres where prompt local recurrence treatment can be provided.

References

1. Peracchia A, Sarli L, Carreras F, Pietra N, Longinotti E, Gafà M. Recidive loco-regionali dopo chirurgia curativa per cancro del colon. *Ann. It Chir* 1991; 62: 37-44.
2. Peracchia A, Sarli L, Pietra N, Carreras F, Longinotti E, Gafà M. Recidive pelviche dopo chirurgia curativa per cancro del retto. *Ann It Chir* 1991; 62, 151-7.
3. Bergamaschi R, Arnaud JP. Routine compared with non-scheduled follow-up in patients with "curative" surgery for colorectal cancer. *Ann Surg Oncol* 1996; 3: 464-9.
4. Pecorella G, Bracchitta S, Petrolito E, Cacciaguerra B, Blanco F, Cirino E. Follow-up in carcinoma of the large intestine. *Ann Ital Chir* 1996; 67: 41-8.
5. Tominaga T, Sakabe T, Koyama Y, Harano K, Yasutomi M, Takahashi T, Kodaira S, Kato T, Ogawa N. Prognostic factors for patients with colon or rectal carcinoma treated with resection only. Five year-follow-up report. *Cancer* 1996; 78: 403-8.
6. Khoury DA, Opelka FG, Beck DE, Hicks TC, Timmcke AE, Gathright JB Jr. Colon surveillance after colorectal cancer surgery. *Dis Colon Rectum* 1996; 39:252-6.
7. Mella J, Datta SN, Biffin A, Radcliffe AG, Steele RJ, Stamatakis JD. Surgeons' follow-up practice after resection of colorectal cancer. *Ann R Coll Surg Engl* 1997; 79: 206-9.
8. DeSalvo L, Razzetta F, Arezzo A, Tassone U, Bogliolo G, Bruzzone D, Mattioli F. Surveillance

after colorectal cancer surgery. *Eur J Surg Oncol* 1997; 23: 522-5.
9. Stiggelbout AM, de Haes JC, Vree R, van de Velde CJ, Bruijninckx CM, van Groningen K, Kievit J. Follow-up of colorectal cancer patients: quality of life and attitudes towards follow-up. *Br J Cancer* 1997; 75: 914-20.
10. Arnaud JP, Cervi C, Bergamaschi R, Tuech JJ. Value of oncologic follow-up of patients operated for colorectal cancer. A prospective study of 1000 patients. *J Chir* 1997; 134: 45-50.
11. Sugarbaker PH, Gianola FJ, Dwyer A, Newman NR. A simplified plan for follow-up of patients with colon and rectal cancer supported by prospective studies of laboratory and radiologic test results. *Surgery* 1987; 102, 79-87.
12. Fegiz G, Indinnimeo M, Gozzo P, Brozzetti S, Ramacciato G. The basis of a comprehensive follow-up in colorectal cancer. In: Fegiz G, Ramacciato G, Vitelli C, De Angelis R, ed., Current Topics in surgical oncology. Milano: Masson; 1991: 451-64.
13. Gilbert JM, Jeffrey I, Evans M. Sites of recurrent tumor after curative colorectal surgery: implications for adjuvant therapy. *Br J Surg* 1984; 71: 203-5.
14. Pihl E, Hughes ESR, McDermott FT. Lung recurrence after curative surgery for colorectal cancer. *Dis Colon Rectum* 1987; 30: 417-9.
15. Bonnheim DC, Petrelli NJ, Herrera L, Walsh D, Mittelman A. Osseous metastasis from colorectal carcinoma. *Am J Surg* 1986; 151: 457-9.
16. Abulafi AM, Williams NS. Local recurrence of colorectal cancer: the problem, mechanisms, management and adjuvant therapy. *Br J Surg* 1994; 81: 7-19.
17. Marsh PJ, James RD, Schofield PF. Definition of local recurrence after surgery for rectal carcinoma. *Br J Surg* 1995; 82: 465-8.
18. Pietra N, Sarli L, Thenasseril BJ, Costi R, Sansebastiano G, Peracchia A. Risk factors of local recurrence of colorectal cancer. A multivariate study. *Hepato-gastroenterol* 1998; (in press).
19. Pietra N, Sarli L, Sansebastiano G, Saccani Jotti G, Peracchia A. Prognostic value of ploidy, cell proliferation kinetics, and conventional clinicopathologic criteria in patients with colorectal carcinoma: a prospective study. *Dis Colon Rectum* 1996; 39: 494-503.
20. Peracchia A, Sarli L. Il cancro del colon e del retto operato. Torino, Minerva Medica, 1996.
21. Audisio RA, Setti-Carraro P, Segala M, Capko D, Andreoni B, Tiberio G. Follow-up in colorectal cancer patients: a cost-benefit analysis. *Ann Surg Oncol* 1996; 3: 349-57.
22. Li Destri G, Rinzivillo C, Craxi G, La Greca G, Di Cataldo A, Puleo S, Licata A. Colorectal follow-up planning modified on the basis of our personal experience. *Dig Surg* 1988; 15: 64-8.
23. Peracchia A, Sarli L, Pietra N, Choua O, Maggiore SM. Chirurgia delle recidive loco-regionali del cancro del colon e del retto. *Ann. It Chir* 1995; 1: 69-83.
24. Beart RW Jr, Metzger PP, O'Connell MJ, Schutt AJ. Postoperative screening of patients with carcinoma of the colon. *Dis Colon Rectum* 1981; 24: 585-8.
25. Barlow AP, Thompson MH. Colonscopic follow-up after resection for colorectal cancer: a selective policy. *Br J Surg* 1993; 80: 781-4.
26. Longinotti E, Sarli L, Cerimele M, Miselli A, Carreras F, Pietra N, Peracchia A. Ruolo dell'endosonografia rettale nella diagnosi di recidiva anastomotica del carcinoma colo-rettale. XVI Congresso Nazionale Società Italiana Chirurgia oncologica, Trieste, 19-21 Novembre 1992, pp 93-96.
27. Shirkhoda A, Staab EV, Bunce LA, Herbst CA, McCartney WH. Computed tomography in recurrent or metastatic colon cancer: Relation to rising serum carcinoembrionic antigen. *J Comput Ass Tomogr* 1984; 8: 704-8.
28. Tartter PI, Slater G, Gelernt I, Aufses AH. Screening for liver metastases from colorectal cancer with CEA and alkaline phosphatase. *Ann Surg* 1981; 193: 357-60.
29. Barillari P, Ramacciato G, Manetti G, Bovino A, Sammartino P, Stipa V. Surveillance of colorectal cancer: Effectiveness of early detection of intraluminal recurrences on prognosis and survival of patients treated for cure. *Dis Colon Rectum* 1996; 39: 388-93.
30. Korenaga D, Saeki H, Mawatari K, Orita H, Maekawa S, Ikeda T, Sugimachi K. Serum carcinoembryonic antigen concentration doubling time correlates with tumor biology and life expectancy in patients with recurrent gastrointestinal carcinoma. *Arch Surg* 1997; 132: 188-94.

31. Tobaruela E, Enriquez JM, Diez M, Camunas J, Muguerza J, Granell J. Evaluation of serum carcinoembryonic antigen monitoring in the follow-up of colorectal cancer patients with metastatic lymph nodes and a normal preoperative serum level. *Int J Biol Markers* 1997; 12: 18-21.
32. Harrison LE, Guillem JC, Paty P, Cohen AM. Preoperative carcinoembryonic antigen predicts outcomes in node-negative colon cancer patients: a multivariate analysis. *J Am Coll Surg* 1997; 185: 55-9.
33. McCall JL, Black RB, Rich CA, Harvey JR, Baker RA, Watts JM, Toouli J. The value of serum carcinoembryonic antigen in predicting recurrent disease following curative resection of colorectal cancer. *Dis Colon Rectum* 1994; 37: 875-81
34. Plebani M, De Paoli M, Basso D, Roveroni G, Giacomini A, Galeotti F, Corsini A. Serum tumor markers in colorectal cancer staging, grading, and follow-up. *J Surg Oncol* 1996; 62: 239-44.
35. Gebauer G, Muller-Ruchholtz W. Tumor marker concentrations in normal and malignant tissues of colorectal cancer patients and their prognostic relevance. *Anticancer Res* 1997; 17: 2731-4.
36. Launois B. Métastases hépatiques des cancers colorectaux. Quels sont les éléments anatomiques hépatiques qui vous font renoncer à l'exérèse? *Ann Chir* 1990; 44: 193-6.
37. Juhl G, Larson GM, Mullins M, Bond S, Polk HC Jr. Six-year results of annual colonoscopy after resection of colorectal cancer. *World J Surg* 1990; 14: 255-60.
38. Heald RJ, Lockhart-Mummery HE. The lesion of the second cancer of the large bowel. *Br J Surg* 1972; 59: 16-9.
39. Bulow S, Svendsen LB, Mellemgaard A. Metachronous colorectal carcinoma. *Br J Surg* 1990; 77: 502-5.
40. Safi F, Link KH, Beger HG. Is follow-up of colorectal cancer patients worthwhile? *Dis Colon Rectum* 1993; 36: 636-44.
41. Welch JP. Multiple colorectal tumors. *Am J Surg* 1981; 42: 274-8.
42. Cunliffe WJ, Hasleton PS, Tweedle DE, Schofield PF. Incidence of synchronous and metachronous colorectal carcinoma. *Br J Surg* 1984; 71: 941-3.
43. Sugarbaker PH. Follow-up of colorectal cancer. *Tumori* 1995; 81: 126-34
44. Winawer S. Follow-up after polypectomy. *World J Surg* 1991; 15: 25-8.
45. Bruinvels DJ, Stiggelbouf AM, Kievit J, van Houlwelingen HC, Habbema JD, van der Velde CJ. Follow-up of patients with colorectal cancer. A meta-analysis. *Ann Surg* 1994; 219: 174-82.
46. Quentmeier A, Schlag P, Smok M, Herfarth C. Reoperation for recurrent colorectal cancer: the importance of early diagnosis for resectability and survival. *Eur J Surg Oncol* 1990; 16: 319-25.
47. Pedro de Azevedo J, Dozois RR., Gunderson LL. Locally recurrent rectal cancer: surgical strategy. *World J Surg* 1992; 16: 490-4.
48. Ovaska J, Jarvinen H, Kujari H, Pertilla I, Mecklin JP. Follow-up of patients operated on for colorectal carcinoma. *Am J Surg* 1990; 159: 593-6.
49. Makela JT, Laitinen SO, Kairaluoma MI. Five-year follow-up after radical surgery for colorectal cancer. *Arch Surg* 1995; 130: 1062-7.
50. Virgo KS, Wade TP, Longo WE, Coplin MA, Vernava AM, Johnson FE. Surveillance after curative colon cancer resection: practice patterns of surgical subspecialists. *Ann Surg Oncol* 1995; 2: 472-84.
51. Edelman MJ, Meyers FJ, Siegel D. The utility of follow-up testing after curative cancer therapy. A critical review and economic analysis. *J Gen Intern Med* 1997; 12: 318-31.
52. Kjeldsen BJ, Kronborg O, Fenger C, Jorgensen OD. A prospective randomized study of follow-up after radical surgery for colorectal cancer. *Br J Surg* 1997; 84: 666-9.
53. Launois B. Métastases hépatiques des cancers colorectaux. Quels sont les éléments anatomiques hépatiques qui vous font renoncer à l'exérèse? *Ann Chir* 1990; 44: 193-6.
54. Minton JP, Hoehn JL, Gerber DM. Results of a 400-patient carcinoembryonic antigen second-look colorectal cancer study. *Cancer* 1985; 55: 1284-90.
55. Reid JD; Robins RE, Atkinson KG. Pelvic recurrence after anteriorresection and EEA stapling anastomosis for potentially curable carcinoma of the rectum. *Am J Surg* 1984; 147: 629-32.
56. Cochrane JP, Williams JT, Faber RG, Slack WW. Value of outpatient follow-up after curative surgery for carcinoma of the large bowel. *BMJ* 1980; 280: 593-5.
57. Huton NR, Hargreaves AW. Is long-term follow-up of all colorectal cancer necessary? *J R Coll*

Surg Edinb 1989; 34: 21-5.
58. Pietra N, Sarli L, Costi R, Choua O, Grattarola M, Peracchia A. The role of follow-up in the management of local recurrences of colorectal cancer. A prospective randomized study. *Dis Colon Rectum* 1998; (in press).
59. Deveney KE, Way LW. Follow-up of patients with colorectal cancer. *Am J Surg* 1984; 148, 717-22.
60. Staab HJ, Anderer A, Stumpf E. Eighty-four potential second-look operations based on sequential carcinoembryonic antigen determination and clinical investigations in patients with recurrent gastrointestinal cancer. *Am J Surg* 1985; 149, 198-204.
61. Waldron RP, Donovan JA. Clinical follow-up and treatment of locally recurrent colorectal cancer. *Dis Colon Rectum* 1987; 30: 428-30.
62. Herfarth C, Schlag D, Hohenberger P. Surgical strategies in locoregional recurrences of gastrointestinal carcinoma. *World J Surg* 1987; 11: 504-10.
63. Fantini GA, DeCosse JJ. Surveillance strategies after resection of carcinoma of the colon and rectum. *Surg Gynecol Obstet* 1990; 171: 267-73.
64. Steele G Jr. Follow-up plans after treatment of primary colon and rectum cancer. *World J Surg* 1991; 15: 583-8.
65. Martin EW Jr, Minton JP, Carey LC. CEA directed second-look surgery in the asymptomatic patient after primary resection of colorectal carcinoma. *Ann Surg* 1985; 202, 310-7.
66. Carlsson U, Stewenius J, Ekelund G, Leandoer L, Nosslin B. Is CEA analysis of value in screening for recurrences after surgery for colorectal carcinoma? *Dis Colon Rectum* 1983; 26: 369-73.
67. Hida J, Yasutomi M, Shindoh K, et al. Second-look operation for recurrent colorectal cancer based on carynoembryonic antigen and imaging techniques. *Dis Colon Rectum* 1996; 39: 74-9.

CHAPTER 13

EFFECT OF PERI-OPERATIVE TRANSFUSION OF WHOLE BLOOD VS LEUCOCYTE-DEPLETED BLOOD ON SURVIVAL AFTER CURATIVE SURGERY FOR COLORECTAL CANCER.

MARIO RUBINO, DONATO ALTOMARE, LUIGI LUPO, ELISABETTA MARTINELLI, ORONZO C. PANNARALE, FRANCESCO PUGLISI, and * GABRIELLA SERIO

*Institute of Surgical Clinics, and * Institute of Hygene, University of Bari, Bari, Italy*

Summary

Introduction Peri-operative blood transfusion has been reported to have an adverse effect on prognosis after curative surgery for colorectal cancer, perhaps due to an immunosuppressive effect. In this multicentre randomised trial comparison was made of five-year survival of patients receiving peri-operative whole blood transfusion (WB), versus those receiving leucocyte-depleted red cells (LDB).

Patients and methods From a total of 279 patients, 80 were randomly assigned to receive WB and 67 LDB. A second group of 132 patients, considered as unlikely to need transfusion, was not randomised and served as a control group outside the trial.

Results 5-year survival was 64.4 per cent (WB) and 75.2 per cent (LDB) (P = 0.41). Cox analysis showed a slightly increased relative risk (RR) of mortality in the WB group (1. 19). Strong independent risk factors were tumour stage and grading. Plasma had no apparent influence on survival. Similar results were found in patients effectively transfused in the non-randomised group; survival was 77.9 per cent. Overall RR was slightly higher in randomised patients than in non-randomised (1.17) and in transfused than non-transfused (1.26 LDB, 1.40 WB).

Conclusions Transfusion does not adversely affect survival after curative surgery for colorectal cancer, but in view of the modest increase in RR observed in the WB group it is advisable to use LDB.

Introduction

Several studies have been aimed at verifying whether transfusion has an adverse effect on survival of patients operated on for colorectal carcinoma, since a letter by Gantt [1] published in the Lancet in 1981 first suggested this possibility. Nearly all these studies were retrospective, and contradictory results were obtained, as only about half of them supported an adverse effect on survival, attributed to impairment by allogenic transfusion of the natural immune response to the tumour. This subject has been extensively dealt with in some recently published reviews and meta-analyses [2-8]. Table 1 summarises the results of the three randomised trials so far published. In the present trial we started from the hypothesis that the immunological factors influencing survival were mainly

E. Zanella (ed.), Advances in Abdominal Surgery, 143–151.

Table 1. Previous trials on survival

1st	n.pts	endpoint	Study group(A)	Control group (B)	Diff. A-B	Diff.transf. vs non transf. (observational data)
Bush 1993-4-5	423	Tumour-free survival	Autol. Blood	Whole blood	NS	yes
Heiss 1994	120	Tumour-free survival	Autol.red cells	Homol. red cells	NS	yes
Houbiers 1994	697	Tumour-free survival	LD red cells	Buffy-coat-poor red cells	NS	yes

cellular (leukocytes and platelets). Although it would be possible for erythrocytes to have an adverse effect, as suggested by Tartter [9] and Heiss [10], this cannot be investigated in a randomised trial. We therefore compared the effect of transfusion of two different blood products, whole blood (WB) and leucocyte-depleted red cells (LDB), on 5-year survival of a group of patients judged by the surgeon prior to operation as being likely to need transfusion. These patients were randomised to receive one or other of the blood products. In another group of patients, transfusion was not deemed necessary on the basis of objective clinical data (general conditions, size and site of the tumour), and these patients were not randomised, but recorded and followed-up as a second control group outside the trial. The decision was made to assign the non-transfused patients to a separate group, to avoid including them in the randomised groups and then eliminating them as dropouts, as was done in other similar trials, so markedly reducing the real sample size.

Patients and methods

Protocol

Between January 3, 1990 and December 21, 1993, 684 patients with histologically proven colorectal cancer were operated on in 8 University surgical departments (list at the end of the article). Of candidates considered eligible for curative surgery, 331 were enrolled in the study, the remaining 353 being excluded for one or more of the following criteria: advanced local spread, distant metastases, history of previous operations (e.g. emergency colostomy), emergency presentation (obstruction, perforation of the tumour or of diverticula), second primary turnout in another organ, severe anaemia or hypoproteinaemia requiring transfusion, severe cardiovascular or respiratory pathology, history of recent transfusion, patient's refusal of transfusion or randomization, or age under 20. A further 52 patients were later excluded, 42 due to the presence at operation of advanced local disease or distant metastases, and 10 for lack of information from their centre. The study was thus conducted on 279 patients.

Operations were performed according to the usual oncological criteria and under antibiotic prophylaxis. Radiotherapy was given to 21 randomised and 13 non-randomised patients with rectal cancer. 13 patients received prophylactic adjuvant chemotherapy, four of them by cannulation of a branch of the portal vein, the others by systemic route. It should be remembered that at the start of the trial, adjuvant chemotherapy had not yet become universally accepted as a routine treatment in this country.

Blood products

Leucocyte-depleted blood was prepared in the following way: red cells separated from the plasma, were filtered through a MUGARD IG 500 filter (two centres used the PALL RC 50 filtre). The filters were then washed with 150 ml of saline to recover the residual red cells; the blood was centrifugalized for 15' at 1000 rpm and the supernatant was removed. This method prevents not only transfusion reactions, but also the production of antileucocyte antibodies. The final product contained only 2% of leucocytes and 87% of red cells, with respect to the initial values.

Outcome

The primary end result was 5-year survival, considering deaths from any cause but excluding operative mortality.

Sample size

According to the formula suggested by Pocock [11], around 200 patients in each group were calculated as being necessary, to detect an increase in survival, which at 5 years was from 60 per cent to 75 per cent ($P = 0.05$, power = 0.9) in patients transfused with LDB. We calculated an approximately equal number of non-transfused patients, making a total of 800. This number was liable to undergo further increases to compensate for any losses due to protocol deviations [12]. After three years it appeared that the actual period would have to be much longer than foreseen.

We therefore decided to stop the trial, as a change in transfusion policy was also taking place in many surgical centers, which would have further protracted such times and rendered the groups less homogeneous.

Statistical analysis

Survival was calculated by the Kaplan Meier method, and comparison between the two samples by the Mantel-Cox (log-rank) test. In view of the insufficient final size of the sample in our trial, non-significant results were to be expected, as the log-rank test is very sensitive to sample size. Under such circumstances, it was judged advisable to go beyond simple hypothesis-testing, by estimating the magnitude of the association. We therefore also adopted an alternative to significance tests, by calculating the relative risk (RR) and the confidence intervals. The point-estimates of the differences, taking into account the confounding variables, were calculated with the Cox proportional hazard model. All analyses were made according to the "intention-to-treat" principle and, when necessary, also according to the efficacy principle.

Assignment

To ensure completely unpredictable treatment simple randomization was adopted, employing a table of random digits from 0 to 9. Each centre initially received 30 sealed opaque envelopes indicating the type of blood to be transfused. The envelopes were opened after the decision to transfuse had been taken by the surgeon and the anaesthetist on the day before the operation, to allow the blood bank to prepare the filtered blood. A blind design was not considered necessary, the end-point being death. All patients gave written informed consent. Due to simple randomization the two groups resulted as slightly unbalanced and dishomogeneous.

Follow-up

The patients underwent three-monthly clinical examination and blood tests, including carcino-embryonic antigen (CEA) and six-monthly liver ultrasound (US) scan and endoscopy for the first two years, and annual controls thereafter. Survival was calculated starting from the day of operation. The last control was made on February 29, 1996. Three patients were lost at 24, 38 and 46 months. Mean patient follow-up was 48 months (range 6-73 months).

Baseline data are summarised in table 2.

Table 2. Baseline data of all patients

*Dukes A and B were grouped together because of the small number of Dukes A

	Randomised (147)		Non-randomised (132)	Total (279)
	Whole blood	LD red cells		
N	80	67	132	279
Sex M	38	36	78	152
F	42	31	54	127
Mean age (range)	67.1 (38-86)	65 (28-94)	64.3 (20-86)	65.1 (20-94)
Site of the Tumour	N (%)	N (%)	N (%)	N (%)
Right Colon	26 (32.5)	10 (14.9-P<0.02)	37 (28)	73 (26.2)
Left colon	24 (30.0)	27 (40.3)	57 (43.2)	108 (38.7)
Rectum	30 (37.5)	30 (44.8)	38 (28.8)	98 (35.1)
Dukes				
Dukes A+B*	55 (68.7)	42 (62.7)	100 (75.8)	197 (70.6)
Dukes C	25 (31.3)	25 (37.3)	32 (24.2)	82 (29.4)
Grading				
G1+G2	55 (68.7)	49 (73.1)	111 (84.0)	215 (77.1)
G3	25 (31.2)	18 (26.9)	21 (16.0)	64 (22.9)

Protocol deviation

15 randomised patients were not transfused and 8 non-randomised patients required transfusion. 19 patients in the non-randomised group were transfused

with autologous blood. 20 patients randomised to receive LDB had additional plasma transfused after operation.

Results

Randomised patients (n 147).

Data were first analysed according to the "intention-to-treat" principle. 5-year survival (Kaplan-Meter) was 64.4 per cent (CI 52-76 per cent) in patients randomised to receive WB, and 75.2 per cent (CI 64-85 per cent) in patients randomised to receive LDB (Figure 1). The difference was not significant at the log-rank test (P = 0.41).

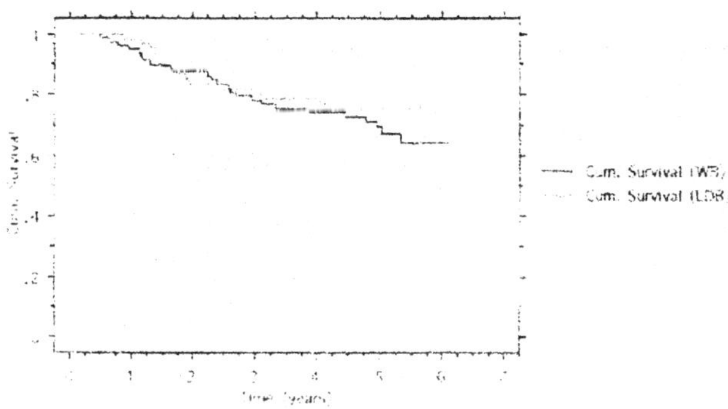

Figure 1. five-year survival (Kaplan- Meier) of randomised patients

Univariate analysis of confounding factors showed that tumour stage (Dukes), grading and age strongly influenced long term prognosis. In effectively transfused patients the results were similar but there was a modest increase in RR in those receiving more than two units of blood.The results of multivariate analyses with the Cox proportional hazard model are shown in tables 3 (intention-to treat) and 4 (efficacy).

Table 3. Cox model analysis of randomised patients

	RR	P	CI
Rand. LD	1		
Whole	1.194	0.58	0.631 – 2.260
Dukes A+B	1		
Dukes C	2.071	0.02	1.110 – 3.865
Grading G1+G2	1		
G3	2.094	0.02	1.112 3.945
Age < 70	1		
Age > 70	1.661	0,11	0.882 – 3.094
Sex F	1		
Sex M	1.174	0.62	0.0622 – 2.217

Table 4. Cox model analysis of effectively transfused patients

	RR	P	Cl
Transf. LD	1		
Whole	1.221	0.55	0.630 – 2.366
Dukes A+B	1		
Dukes C	2.119	0.02	1.121 – 4.004
Grading G1+G2	1		
G3	1.814	0.07	0.955 – 3.445
Age < 70	1		
Age > 70	1.742	0.08	0.928 – 3.272
Sex F	1		
Sex M	1.416	0.28	0.744 – 2.697
N° units <2	1		
N° units >2	1.363	0.34	0.719 – 2.584

Non-randomised patients (n 132).

5-year survival was 77.9 per cent (Kaplan-Meier), slightly better than in the LD group but again not significantly so.

Finally, all patients were analysed, comparing randomised to non-randomised and transfused to non-transfused patients. These data, all observational, are summarised in table 5. The final power of the trial, calculated retrospectively [22], was between 0. 70 and 0.75.

Table 5. Cox model analysis of 279 patients (observational data)

	RR	P	Cl
Non-rand.	1		
Rand.	1.173	0.54	0.701 – 1.960
Dukes A+B	1		
Dukes C	2.767	0.0001	1.693 – 4.522
Grading G1+G2	1		
Grading G3	1.528	0.14	0.867 – 2.693
Age < 70	1		
Age > 70	2.100	0.002	1.294 – 3.406
Sex F	1		
Sex M	1.599	0.07	0.960 – 2.665
Non Transf.	1		
Transf. LD	1.267	0.48	0.652 – 2.462
Transf whole	1.407	0.24	0.790 – 2.507
Dukes A+B	1		
Dukes C	2.799	0.0001	1.716 – 4.567
Grading G1+G2	1		
Grading G3	1.442	0.21	0.811 – 2.564
Age < 70	1		
Age > 70	2.098	0.002	1.290 – 3.412
Sex F	1		
Sex M	1.669	0.05	0.996 – 2.797

Discussion

Since the beginning of our study four randomised trials on immediate post-operative complications [13-16] and three on long term survival [17-21], but [17,18,19] describing the same trial (table 1), have been published. Jensen et al [13,15,16] found that transfusion of autologous blood is followed by a significant depression of immunocompetence and an increased number of post-operative infections, as compared with transfusion of leucocyte-depleted blood. A similar difference in infection rate was observed comparing the use of buffy-coat poor blood to leucocyte-depleted blood. Heiss et al [14] confirmed an increased infection rate after transfusion of whole blood as opposed to autologous blood.

On the contrary, no significant difference in survival rate was found in the three trials comparing autologous to homologous blood [17-19], autologous to homologous packed red cells [20] and leucocyte-depleted to buffy-coat poor red cells [21], implying that the supposed immunodepression might be more active in the short-term period. However, in the same trials a worse survival rate was observed in transfused patients as compared to non-transfused, although the latter conclusion was based only on observational data and the authors were very cautious in interpreting their results as a cause-effect relationship. In this context it must be borne in mind that randomization can be effected between different blood products, but not between transfusion and non-transfusion, for obvious ethical reasons. It is difficult to explain why Busch et al [17] found an increased number of local recurrences and Heiss et al [20] of distant metastases in transfused patients, whereas Houbiers et al [21] found no differences.

The results of our study indicate that in patients operated on for colorectal cancer, overall survival was marginally but not significantly better in those patients randomised to receive LDB than in those randomised to receive WB (RR 1.19, CI 0.631-2.260). Confidence intervals, although large, were all skewed to the right.

Comparable results were observed for patients effectively transfused. No important adverse effect of transfusion was found when comparing randomised to non-randomised and transfused to non-transfused patients (observational data). Plasma did not seem to affect prognosis; 20 patients transfused with LDB received additional plasma during the operation and then were compared to the patients transfused with LDB only (Cox model). The relative risk was 1.1 (CI 0.3-3.95).

Our data on the association between transfusion and survival are not concordant with those described by Busch, by Heiss or by Houbiers This and other differences could be explained by different patient selection and by the small sample size (in two of the published trials, and in ours).

However, some reviews and meta-analyses [2,8,9,18] have concluded that there is only a very slight or no difference in survival between transfused and

non-transfused patients. In all their papers as in ours', survival was strongly influenced by turnout stage and grading and by age.
A notable difference between our trial and the others is the presence of a separate group of non-randomised patients, which avoided the considerable number of losses reported by the other groups (44 per cent in Busch's trial), and increased the reliability of our "intention-to-treat" analysis.
Being an important confounding factor, surgical experience is difficult to assess, and even tumour staging, at present based on crude morphological data, may be misleading, because of the difficulty 9 of recognising micrometastases and sometimes advanced local extension. In our opinion, more studies are necessary to clarify the situation, with the proviso that only trials comparing different blood products can be planned, and starting from the hypothesis that leucocytes have an immune suppressive effect. To obtain a sufficient sample size [12] and to enable a reliable "intention-to-treat" analysis, losses of any kind (e.g.: dropouts) should be reduced, by randomising the patient at the moment the transfusion becomes necessary, and by using bedside filters. The problem of surgical skill could be solved by standardizing the operative technique [23] and excluding patients operated on by inexperienced surgeons.
We conclude that although no significant beneficial effect of LD blood emerges from our study, the modest decrease in RR observed in this group makes its use advisable if a transfusion is necessary, since it poses no ethical problems and involves an acceptable cost. Finally, indications for blood transfusion can and should be reduced.

List of centres and researchers participating in the trial:
Istituto di Clinica chirurgica, University of Varese (Prof R Dionigi)
Istituto di Clinica chirurgica II University of Padua (Prof M Lise)
Divisione di Chirurgia geriatrica, University of Padua (Prof O Terranova)
Istituto di Clinica chirurgica, University of Modena (Prof P Casolo)
Istituto di Clinica chirurgica I, University of Parma (Prof A Peracchia)
C!inica chirurgica VI, University "La Sapienza", Rome (Prof G Ribotta)
Istituto di Clinica chirurgica, University of Bari (prof M Rubino)
Dipartimento di Chirurgia, University of Catania (Prof S Latteri)

References

1. Gantt CL. Red blood cells for cancer patients. *Lancet* 1981; ii: 363.
2. Franci(letter to the Editor s DMA. Relationship between blood transfusion and tumour behaviour. *Br J Surg* 1991; 78: 1420- 8.
3. Nielsen HJ. Detrimental effect of perioperative blood transfusion. *Br J Surg* 1995; 82: 582-7.
4. Lont HE, Busch ORC, van Eijck CHJ, Marquet RL, Jeekel J. Blood transfusion: What does it mean to the surgeon? *Dig Surg* 1997; 14: 2-8.
5. Chung M, Steinmetz OK, Gordon PH. Perioperative blood transfusion and outcome after resection for colorectal carcinoma. *Br J Surg* 1993; 80: 427-32.

6. Amato A, Pescatori M. Perioperative blood transfusion and outcome after resection for colorectal carcinoma. *Br J Surg* 1994: 81: 313-4.
7. Vamvakas E, Moore SB. Perioperative blood transfusion and colorectal cancer recurrence: a qualitative statistical overview and meta-analysis. *Transfusion* 1993; 33: 754-65.
8. Vamvakas E. Perioperative blood transfusion and cancer recurrence: meta-analysis for explanation. *Transfusion* 1995; 35: 760-8.
9. Tartter P. Does blood transfusion predispose to cancer recurrence? *J Clin Oncol* 1989; 12: 169-72.
10. Heiss MM, Mempel W, Jauch K-W, Schildberg FW. Leucocyte-depleted or buffy-coat-depleted blood in surgery for colorectal cancer. *Lancet* 1994; 344: 1429-30.
11. Pocock SJ. The Size of a Clinical Trial. In: Pocock SJ Clinical Trials, John Wiley & Sons, Chichester 1983, pp 123-41.
12. Meinert CL. Sample size and power estimates. In: Meinert CL ClinicalTrials. Design,Conductand Analysis. Oxford University Press, New York and London 1986, pp 71-89.
13. Jensen LS, Andersen AJ, Christiansen PM, Hokland P, Juhl CO, Madsen C, Mortensen J, Maller-Nielsen C, Hanberg-Sorensen F, Hokland M. Postoperative infection and natural killer cell function following blood transfusion in patients undergoing elective colorectal surgery. *Br J Surg* 1992; 79: 513-6.
14. Heiss MM, Mempel W, Jauch K-W, Delanoff C, Mayer G, Mempel M, Eissner H-J, Schildberg FW. Beneficial effect of autologous blood transfusion on infectious complications after colorectal cancer surgery. *Lancet* 1993; 342: 1328-33.
15. Jensen LS, Hokland M, Nielsen HJ. A randomized controlled study of the effect ot bedside leucocyte depletion on the immunosuppressive effect of whole blood transfusion in patients undergoing elective colorectal surgery. *Br J Surg* 1995; 83: 973-7.
16. Jensen LS, Kissmeyer-Nielsen P, Wolff B, Qvist N. Randomised comparison of leucocytedepleted versus buffy-coat-poor blood transfusion and complications after colorectal surgery. *Lancet* 1996; 348: 841 -5
17. Busch ORC, Hop WCJ, Hoynck van Papendrecht MAW, Marquet L, Jeekel J. Blood transfusion and prognosis in colorectal cancer. *N Eng J Med* 1993; 328: 1372-6.
18. Busch OR, Hop WCJ, Marquet RL, Jeekel J. Blood transfusion andlocaltumorrecurrencein colorectal cancer. *Ann Surg* 1994 ; 220: 791-7.
19. Busch ORC, Hop WCJ, Marquet RL, Jeekel J. The effect of blood transfusions onsurvivalafter surgery for colorectalcancer. *Eur J Cancer* 1995; 31A: 1226-8.
20. Heiss MM, Mempel W, Delanoff C, Jauch K-W, Gabka C, Mempel M, Dieterich H-J, Eissner H-J, Schildberg F-W. Blood transfusion-modulated tumor recurrence: first result of a randomized study of autologous versus allogeneic blood transfusion in colorectal cancer surgery. *J Clin Oncol* 1994;12: 1859-67.
21. Houbiers JGA, Brand A, van der Vatering LMG, Hermans J, Verwey PJM, Bijnen AB, Pahiplatz P, Eeftink Schattenkerk M, Wobbes Thj de Vries JE, Klementschitsch P, van de Maas AHM, van der Velde CJH. Randomised controlled trial comparing transfusion of leucocyte-depleted or buffy-coat-depleted blood in surgery for colorectal cancer. *Lancet* 1994; 344: 573-8.
22. Benjamin IS, Boesby S. The controlledclinicaltrial. In MathieRT,TaylorKM,CalnanJS Principles of surgical research. Butterworths, London 1989, pp 43-53.
23. Cuschieri A, Fayers P, Fielding J, Craven J, Bancewicz J, Joypaul V, Cook P. Postoperative morbidity and mortality after D1 and D2 resections for gastric cancer: preliminary results of the MRC randomised controlled surgical trial. *Lancet* 1996; 347: 995-9.

CHAPTER 14

RADIOIMMUNOGUIDED SURGERY IN COLORECTAL CARCINOMA PATIENTS.

MARIO ROSELLI, ORESTE BUONOMO, and CARLO UMBERTO CASCIANI

Department of Surgery, University of Rome "Tor Vergata", Rome, Italy

Introduction

Colorectal tumour is a frequent cause of death from cancer, ranking as the third most common cause after lung cancer in men and breast cancer in the female population. There is substantial international variation in incidence with the highest occurrence found in North America, Australia, and New Zealand, and decreasing rates in western Europe, eastern Europe, Africa, Asia and Latin America [1]. To date, diagnosis and staging of colorectal cancer are achieved by means of endoscopy, liver ultrasonography, computerized tomography, as well as serum determination of carcinoembryonic antigen (CEA) and tumour associated glycoprotein-72 (TAG-72). Despite all efforts, surgical procedure can be defined as radical only in 50-70% of the cases, and locoregional recurrence can be regarded as one of the causes of major morbidity and, possibly, mortality. Indeed, ten to fifty percent of patients with colorectal cancer will develop recurrent disease following resection of their primary disease, the recurrence occurring either at the site of primary tumours or in the draining lymph-nodes. Moreover, the survival rate after 5 years is approximately 54 to 85% in Dukes stages B or C. In spite of refinements in surgical technique and diagnostic methods, and in traditional aggressive follow-up using multiple modalities, patient survival has not improved significantly over the past 15-20 years. Clearly, new approaches to diagnosis and treatment are needed.
Since current chemotherapeutic agents used in colorectal cancer have a response rate of only 10 to 20%, it would appear that the key to further improvement of the survival rate would lie in more extensive surgical excision [2,3]. Moreover, an improved knowledge of tumour biology may help to stratify patients into diagnostic subgroups, with different prognosis and therapeutic perspectives. The development and

E. Zanella (ed.), Advances in Abdominal Surgery, 153–162.

characterization of new methodologies, such as the hybridoma technique, has offered new instruments in the diagnosis and treatment of colorectal cancer. Many monoclonal antibodies (MAbs) of either human or murine origin have been developed, which recognize various specific tumour-associated antigens (TAAs). Because of their diversity, specificity and biological activity these MAbs are potentially ideal agents for a variety of applications in malignant disorders, such as: 1) early detection and staging of disease (immunoscintigraphy); 2) intra-operative estimation of tumour margins and identification of occult disease (radioimmunoguided surgery); 3) as carriers for delivering therapy (immunotherapy): several radionuclides have been coupled to MAbs to construct radioimmunoconjugates with a potential for more selective destruction of disseminated cancer. The use of radiolabeled MAbs offers obvious advantages to the various MAb-mediated modalities (drug or toxins). Many of the radionuclides being considered, in fact, can kill from 5 to 10 cell diameters, thus offering the possibility of overcoming tumour cell antigenic heterogeneity and/or phenotypic drift. Consequently, tumour cells devoid of antigen can be destroyed by radiation "cross-fire" from adjacent antibody-bearing cells. Moreover, radiolabeled MAbs do not need to be internalized to kill the tumour cell [4].

Radioimmunoguided Surgery

In an attempt to develop a more sensitive detection system which could provide immediate intra-operative definition of malignant versus normal tissues, not identified either before or during surgery , radioimmunoguided surgery was developed. With improved probe design and optimization of the radionuclide and monoclonal antibodies, radioimmunoguided surgery (RIGS) technology has evolved into a sophisticated diagnostic tool capable of finding occult disease (micrometastases or other disease-related by-products), identifying patterns of disease and metastases that are not detectable by traditional surgical and pathological examination, and providing more accurate prognostic data. RIGS is a surgical method in which a cancer-specific targeting agent, most commonly a MAb, is labeled with a radionuclide and then injected into a patient prior to surgical exploration for cancer. The targeting agent localizes the tumour and a hand-held γ-detecting probe (GDP) is then used to detect cancer during surgery, with the aim of providing a more complete resection and localizing residual unresectable disease, for future focus of additional non-surgical therapy [5-10]. RIGS information has allowed more appropriate surgical resection, better evaluation of surgical margins, and earlier and more appropriate post-surgical therapy. Certain concerns exist, however. Ongoing research is attempting to define more clearly and resolve such problems as antibody specificity, biodistribution, clearance times, antibody immunogenicity, and subsequent development of human anti-murine antibody response, as well as heterogeneity of tumour cell populations.

Clinical Trials

RIGS technique, first reported in 1985, was developed at the Ohio State University by Dr. E. Martin Jr. in collaboration with the Neoprobe Corporation, Columbus, Ohio, USA [5]. Several different carriers were employed including anti-CEA antibodies (FO23C5 and A5B7) as well as anti-TAG-72 antibodies (B72.3 and CC49) which target antigens expressed on human colon and rectal cancer cells [11,13]. The initial studies were carried out using the anti-TAG-72 MAb B72.3. The overall results demonstrated probe positivity in 70-80% of tumour lesions. Moreover, the use of RIGS technique permitted the detection of previously unrecognized tumour lesions, and the subsequent modification of surgical procedure, in approximately 25% of the cases. A strong correlation was also found between positive probe ratios and the presence of TAG-72 in tumour biopsies These findings provided evidence for the selective expression of TAG-72 by primary as well as metastatic colorectal carcinoma, and the preferential localization of 125I-B72.3 MAb [14,15].
Subsequently, the use of second generation anti-TAG-72 MAb (CC49) improved the intra-operative detection of carcinoma lesions, proving to be more specific than B72.3 especially in detecting lymph-node metastases. The first RIGS study using the second generation anti-TAG-72 antibody CC49 was reported by Arnold et al [16], as a dose-ranging study with cohort groups of 20 patients each. Doses of 2 mCi 125I radiolabeled with 0.2, 1.0, and 10.0 mg of CC49 were injected. 86% of the primary tumours were localized by CC49, the primary tumour localization was not affected by the variation of the injected dose. 97% of patients with recurrent disease were localized. RIGS findings led to 16 changes in the therapeutic plan for 12 patients (50%) including more extensive surgery, more extensive node dissection and 1 less extensive surgery, when planned placement of a hepatic artery pump was abandoned upon finding RIGS positive extra-hepatic disease. More recently, a multicenter Phase III RIGS study [17] has been carried out using 125I-CC49 MAb. Overall primary tumour localization rate was 75% in the operating room. When surgical specimens were evaluated by pathologists using the GDP, 80% were localized. Fifty five percent of patients with primary disease had additional information generated by the RIGS system, which was not recognized traditionally, resulting in changes in surgical management in 68 cases.
Arnold [18] has recently published data documenting in 31 patients with 3 years mean follow-up (range 30-54 months), that patients without any RIGS positive tissues left at

the end of surgery had a better survival rate than those with remaining RIGS positive tissues. In this study 14 patients were cleared of RIGS positive tissues, while in 17 patients RIGS positive tissues could not be removed completely because of their anatomical locations. Survival based on the TNM staging system was compared to staging by RIGS assessment. On analysis, Stage I/II patients lived longer than Stage III/IV patients. Comparing survival based on RIGS assessment at the end of surgery, approximately 93% of RIGS negative patients remain disease free, whereas 88% of patients with residual positive RIGS tissues died of their disease. In summary, the RIGS status at the end of surgery was found to be a more accurate predictor of prognosis and survival than the TNM pathological staging system. Another study by Martinez *et al.* [19] has also reported an analysis of 212 patients with primary and recurrent colorectal cancer undergoing RIGS, in which the 74 patients who were RIGS negative at the close of surgery had a significantly better 5 year survival than any other group of patients.

In studies performed at the Department of Surgery of the University of Rome "Tor Vergata", our group concentrated on the improvement of the RIGS technology to be used, in combination with the second generation MAb CC49 or anti-CEA MAbs. In particular, we focused our attention on the selection criteria for the recruitment of cancer patients suitable for the RIGS procedure. Moreover, we evaluated the possibility of improving MAb intake by the tumour, to optimize targeting and intra-operative tumour detection.

Selection Criteria

To optimize the RIGS system it is of paramount importance to correctly identify those patients who may benefit from this approach. To date, serum positivity of the antigen recognized by the MAb to be administered has been used as a predictive criterion for positive MAb tumour localization. In the case of colorectal cancer, patients with CEA serum-negative levels have been considered as inappropriate candidates for anti-CEA radiolabeled MAb administration. It should be noted that elevated serum CEA levels are shown in no more than 40% of patients in whom primary tumour has been diagnosed, while recurrent disease demonstrated an increase of CEA-positive serum levels in approximately 60% of patients [20,21]. However, the overall utility of RIGS will be limited unless the efficacy of this technique can be demonstrated also in the treatment of primary patients, who have been selected following good criteria of eligibility. In a recent study we have shown the absence of a correlation between serum CEA levels and tumour tissue CEA content in primary colorectal carcinoma patients. This was observed both in serum CEA-positive and -negative patients.

Quantitative analysis in tumour specimens obtained from serum CEA-negative patients showed a large variation in CEA content (up to 15,000 ng/ml), suggesting that serum CEA level is not an indicator of patients with CEA-positive tumours. Therefore, there is a high probability that the primary tumours of colorectal cancer patients will be targeted by an anti CEA radiolabeled MAb, independent of their pre-operative serum CEA levels. To verify this hypothesis, we investigated the potential diagnostic use of RIGS with the anti-CEA FO23C5 MAb fragment, in primary serum CEA-negative patients bearing colorectal adenocarcinomas. The results obtained demonstrated that, in all patients, the MAb localized to histologically confirmed tumour: this included 96% of primary tumour tissues, 29% of lymph-nodes and one occult liver metastasis. The impact of RIGS findings on surgical procedure was also considered. Major surgical changes were performed in 25% of patients, including re-definition of the limits of excision and liver resection in the patient in whom liver metastasis was not evident prior to operation. Therefore, serum CEA-positivity should not be used as a criterion for the use of anti-CEA MAbs for the diagnosis of colon cancer, since the serum CEA level is not indicative of CEA expression in tumours [22].
The quantitative expression of TAG-72 in primary colorectal cancer tissues has also been evaluated. The study was prompted by the need to identify those patients who may gain advantage from the RIGS procedure using anti TAG-72 MAbs, in particular the second generation CC49 MAb now in use in our Department. The study is still going on; at the end of accrual serum TAG-72, levels will be correlated with *in vivo* and *ex vivo* RIGS findings
Meanwhile, we used an autoradiography technique to identify the tissue distribution of the injected radiolabeled B72.3 first generation-Mab, in patients undergoing RIGS surgical resection of primary and metastatic colorectal cancer. The study was conducted in collaboration with the Department of Surgery and the Department of Pathology of the Ohio State University, and with The Laboratory of Tumour Immunology and Biology of the National Cancer Institute, NIH, Bethesda, MD, USA. The labeling pattern seen using autoradiography closely matched the pattern observed using immunohistochemical techniques. This was especially notable in the mucin-containing components of the different tumours. The 125I-B72.3 was also found associated with neoplastic cells, demonstrating good penetration and specificity of the radiopharmaceutic throughout the tumour masses. Regional nodes were the only tissue in which autoradiography and immunoperoxidase gave different results, i.e. TAG-72 antigen in parafollicular areas as shown by immunoperoxidase, contrasted with the silver deposition due to 125I-B72.3 in germinal centers. The presence of sinus histiocytosis and paracortical hyperplasia in regional nodes draining colon cancer has been correlated with improved survival, whereas increased germinal center activity has not. Recent studies indicate that the immune responses are directed towards tumour

associated sialomucins and that lymph-node processing of these antigens differs from that of CEA processing [7,23]. A significant increase in CD4 positive T cells in pericolic nodes lacking tumour, as compared with more distant mesenteric and extraregional nodes [24] with altered CD4:CD8 ratio in RIGS-positive nodes [25], has been found. Triozzi reported that the percentage of naive CD45RA positive T cells was highest in RIGS negative, pathology negative nodes, while antigen processing in RIGS-positive nodes was associated with a significant increase in CD45RO positive or "memory" T cells. This shift from "naive" to "memory" T cells is consistent with TAG-72 priming of cells. These findings suggest differences in the clearance pathways of TAG-72 antigen and B72.3 Mab.

Optimization of tumour targeting

Antigenic heterogeneity has been recognized as a problem in the development of clinical protocols using antibodies for diagnosis (immunoscintigraphy) as well as therapy (immunotherapy). Heterogeneity is a property of numerous phenotypes of tumour cell populations, especially solid tumours. These involve variation in morphology, hormone receptors, oncogene products, drug resistance, antigenic phenotype, etc. Obviously, tumour cells which do not express, or express a low level of, a given tumour antigen will most likely escape detection due to their failure to bind the MAb. One method currently under investigation for use in overcoming limitations imposed by antigenic heterogeneity or low antigenic expression, is the use of biological response modifiers, in particular, Interferons (IFNs), to upregulate expression of various surface antigens preferentially on tumour cells to produce more homogeneous tumour populations [26,30]. In vitro studies using both IFN–α and IFN–γ to treat human colorectal carcinoma, cells have demonstrated an increase in the percentage of cells expressing CEA or TAG-72 and in the amount of antigen expressed per cell, resulting in a more homogeneous expression of tumour antigen within the tumour population [31,33]. In vivo tumour localization studies using athymic mice bearing human tumour xenografts, pretreated with IFN–α or IFN–γ, showed increased localization [31,34]. Moreover, preclinical studies have provided evidence that adding IFN–γ to a protocol of radioimmunotherapy utilizing 131I-CC49, led to an improvement in the antitumour effect above that of administering the 131I-CC49 alone [34]. In some cases total eradication of the tumour xenografts was achieved. Additional evidence of the ability of IFN's to upregulate antigen expression was apparent from a Phase I trial [35] in which IFN–γ was administered intra-peritoneally to patients diagnosed with ovarian or gastrointestinal carcinoma and secondary ascites.

In the light of these considerations, it has been in our interest to study the possibility of overcoming antigen heterogeneity using interferon treatment, in the hope of optimizing the RIGS procedure. To this purpose, intramuscular IFN–α was utilized to determine whether systemic IFN–α administration could upregulate expression of TAG-72 and/or CEA at histologically confirmed sites of tumour [36]. Tumour and normal mucosa biopsies were obtained from each patient pre-IFN and post-IFN administration at surgery, and levels of TAG-72 and CEA were measured by immunohistochemistry (% of positive cells as well as relative staining intensity) and a quantitative radioimmunoassay. Only patients with gastric or colorectal adenocarcinomas entered into the study. At least 4 different areas from the tumour, including tumour center and periphery, and 4 from distant (i.e., > 10 cm from tumour) normal mucosa were biopsied before and after IFN–α. Following the first biopsy, each patient received i.m. injections of IFN–α, administered on one of 4 dose-schedules (cohort groups). In all cohorts, endoscopic biopsies were obtained on either Day -7 or Day -8, and surgery was performed on Day 0. In cohorts I and II, patients received two injections of 3 and 6 X 106 units of IFN–α, respectively. In cohort III, patients received three injections of 3 X 106. In cohort IV, patients received three injections of 6 X 106 units of IFN–α. Within a week following the first endoscopic biopsy, patients underwent surgery for resection of their carcinoma. Histologically-confirmed tumor tissue samples were obtained pre- and post-IFN–α and were analyzed for TAG-72 and CEA expression by the binding of the appropriate MAbs as determined by immunohistochemistry. An increase of 20% (i.e., 30 to 50%) of MAb-reactive tumour cells in the pre-IFN–α sample, together with an increase in the relative staining intensity, was required as an indicator for "increased" tumour antigen expression. The level of expression of both tumor antigens was increased in a higher percentage of tumour biopsies from patients of cohorts III and IV when compared with those in cohorts I and II. Following IFN–α administration, TAG-72 expression was elevated in the tumour biopsies of 8 out of 10 patients enrolled as part of cohorts III and IV. In contrast, tumour biopsies from just 1 of 8 patients of cohorts I and II had higher TAG-72 expression after IFN–α. Similar results were observed for CEA expression. Chi-square analysis revealed a highly significant difference ($p<0.001$) when cohorts I and II were combined, and compared with TAG-72 and CEA changes in cohorts III and IV. For the most part, the ability of IFN–α to enhance either TAG-72 or CEA in these tumour biopsies was accompanied by an increase in the other tumour antigen. However, in several cases, IFN–α selectively enhanced TAG-72 or CEA, indicating independent regulatory pathways for the two tumour antigens. An analysis of TAG-72 and CEA expression in adjacent histologically normal mucosa from those same patients revealed no significant changes in percentage of cells positive for either TAG-72 or CEA expression, or the relative amount of staining intensity after IFN–α administration. Quantitative RIA measurement of TAG-72 and CEA levels in those same samples confirmed those findings [36].

The fact that short-term, low dose IFN–α could upregulate TAG-72/CEA expression suggest that all patients selected for immunodiagnostic/ therapeutic intervention should be administered IFN–α. Our study also provided important insight into the dose and schedule of IFN–α which leads to tumour antigen upregulation. It appears, in fact, that the schedule of IFN–α treatment is more important than the dose, in order to induce a significant augmentation of TAG-72/CEA expression. The ability of IFN–α to augment tumour antigen expression, when systemically administered, may have immediate application to current and future clinical MAb-targeted diagnostic and therapeutic protocols. In particular, the use of IFNs might broaden the sensitivity of the detecting probe, and so reduce the number of RIGS-false negative sites.

Future Perspectives

It is evident that the future of the use of MAbs for radioimmunoguided surgery depends on biotechnological progress, which should lead to improvements in tumour targeting. For example, one major problem that has emerged with the use of radiolabeled MAbs is that the radiolabeled MAb not bound to a tumour remains in circulation with a half-life of several days, resulting in potential bone marrow toxicity. Another concern in the use of large molecules, such as immunoglobulins, is their inability to penetrate large tumour masses ; a smaller molecule would be expected to exhibit better penetration. The cloning of Ig genes, the generation of recombinant/chimeric immunoglobulin genes and their expression in a variety of systems, have led to the generation of several genetically engineered agents (single-chain antigen-binding proteins, VH-domain and hypervariable-region peptide molecules) capable of a more efficient binding. The availability of these new constructs is of particular interest, especially in making multiple dose administration regimens possible.

Antigen heterogeneity is still a major problem when dealing with solid tumours. Besides the above-discussed role of biological response modifiers, the use of MAbs cocktails has been proposed to increase tumour localization, as well. This possibility has been suggested through the finding of a complementary expression of tumour markers. In the case of colorectal cancer, for example, it has been reported that the simultaneous measurement of CEA and TAG-72 offers the possibility to increase significantly the percentage of patients in whom the course of disease can be monitored. This complementarity has been found not only in serum, but also in immunohistochemical studies, where the complementary properties of these two markers led to the detection of a greater number of tumour cells in the same tissue section, and demonstrated the different antigen location . These findings are of importance in selecting patients who may gain benefit from the RIGS procedure. However, as already discussed, serum marker determination is not sufficient, by itself, to provide information on the tissue antigen expression. Similar concerns also arise for immunohistochemical studies, that provide qualitative information only, but do not quantitate antigen content at the tumour level. For all these reasons, we propose the quantitative determination of tumour antigen content by radioimmunometric analysis of protein extracts of tumour tissue biopsies. This easy and reliable procedure may help in optimizing patients' recruitment, thus improving MAb-based diagnostic procedures, above all radioimmunoguided surgery.

References

1. Schottenfeld D. Epidemiology. In Cohen AM and Winawer SJ (ed): Cancer of the Colon, Rectum and Anus. New York: McGraw-Hill; 1995, pp 11-24.
2. Noguchi M, Miyazaki I. Extended lymph node dissection in gastrointestinal cancer. *J Surg Oncol* 1997;65:57-65.
3. Heald RJ,Ryall RD. Recurrence and survival after total mesorectal excision for rectal cancer. *Lancet* 1996; 2: 1479-82.
4. Roselli M, Guadagni F, Buonomo O, et al. Clinical value of radiolabeled monoclonal antibodies in the managent of carcinoma patients. *In Vivo* 1993,7: 615-22.
5. Thurston MO, Mojzisik CM. History and development of RIGS. *Semin Colon Rectal Surg* 1995; 6:185-91.
6. Kim JA. Obsetrvations on the immunologic basis of the radioimmunoguided surgery system. *Semin Colon rectal Surg* 1995; 6: 202-6.
7. Hitchcook CL. RIGS and staging of colorectal carcinoma. *Semin Colon Rectal Surg* 1995; 6:207-16.
8. Bertsch D, Burak W, Young D, et al. Radioimmunoguided surgery system improves survival for patients with recurrent colorectal cancer. *Surgery* 1995;118: 634-9.
9. Bertsch D, Burak W, Young D, et al. Radioimmunoguided surgery for colorectal cancer. *Ann Surg Oncol* 1996; 3:310-6.
10. Burek WE, Schneebaum S. RIGS recurrent clinical trials and application. *Semin Colon Rectal Surg* 1995; 6:226-33.
11. Nuti M, Teramoto YA, Mariani-Costantini R, et al. A monoclonal antibody (B72.3) defines patterns of distribution of a novel tumor-associated antigen in human mammary carcinoma cell populations. *Int J Cancer* 1982; 29:539-45 .
12. Stramignoni D, Bowen R, Atkinson B, et al. Differential relativity of monoclonal antibodies with human colon adenocarcinomas and adenomas. *Int J Cancer* 1983; 31: 543-52.
13. Thor A, Ohuchi N, Szpak CA, Johnston WW, et al. Distribution of oncofetal antyigen tumor-associated glycoprotein-72 defined by monoclonal antibody B72.3. *Cancer Res* 1986; 3118-24.
14. Martin Ewjr, Moijzisik CM, Hinkle GH, et al. Radioimmunoguided surgery using monoclonal antibody. *Am J Surg* 1988; 156. 380-92.
15. Choen AM, Martin EW jr, Lavery I, et al. Radioimmunoguided surgery using iodine 125 B72.3 in patients with colorectal cancer. *Arch Surg* 1991; 126: 349-51.

16. Arnold MW, Schneebaum S, Berens A, et al. Intraoperative detection of colorectal cancer with radioimmunoguided surgery and CC49, a second generation monoclonal antibody. *Ann Surg* 1992;216: 627-32.
17. Schneebaum S, Ritter DC, Burak WE Jr. RIGS primary clinical trials. *Semin Colon Rectal Surg* 1995;6: 217-25.
18. Arnold MW, Young D, Hitchcook CL, et al. Radioimmunoguided surgery in primary colorectal carcinoma: an intraoperative prognostic tool and adjuvant to traditional staging. *Am J Surgery* 1995;170:1-4.
19. Martinez D, Barbera-Guillem E, La Valle G, et al. Radioimmunoguided surgery for gastrointestinal malignancies: an analysis of 14 years of clinical experience. *Cancer Control* 1997;4 : 505-16.
20. Guadagni F, Roselli M, Amato T. Tumor-associated glycoprotein-72 (TAG-72) serum levels complement carcinoembryonic antigen (CEA) levels in monitoring patients with gastrointestinal carcinoma:A longitudinal study. *Cancer* 1991; 68: 2443-50.
21. Guadagni F, Roselli M, Cosimelli M, et al. TAG-72 (CA 72-4 Assay) as a complemenatry serum tumor antigen to carcinoenbryonic antigen in monitoring patients with colorectal cancer. *Cancer* 1993; 72: 2098-106.
22. Roselli M, Guadagni F, Buonomo O, et al. Intraoperative Radioimmunolocalization of an Anti-CEA Mab F(Ab')2 (FO23C5) in CEA serum-negative colorectal cancer patients. *Antic Res* 1996; 16: 883-90.
23. Mariani-Costantini R, Muraro R, Ficari R et al. Immunohistochemical evidence of immune responses to tumor-associated antigens in lymph nodes of colon carcinoma patients. *Cancer* 1991;67:2880-6.
24. Adduce W, Sugenoya A, Lida F. Immune competent cells of regional lymph nodes in colorectal cancer patients. I: Flow Cytometric analysis of lymphocyte subpopulation. *J Surg Oncol* 1991;46:110-6.
25. Triozzi PL, Kim JA, Aldrich W, et al. Localization of tumor-reactive lymph node lymphocytes in vivo using radiolabeled monoclonal antibody. *Cancer* 1994;73:580-9.
26. Attallah MM, Needy CF, Noguchi PD, et al. Enhancement of carcinoembryonic antigen expression by interferon. *Int J Cancer* 1979;24: 49-52.
27. Greiner JW, Hand PH, Noguchi P, et al. Enhanced expression of surface tumor-associated antigens on human breast and colon tumor cells after recombinant human leucocyte α-interferon treatment. *Cancer Res* 1984;44:3208-14.
28. Borden EC. Augmented tumor-associated antigen expression by interferons. *J Natl Cancer Inst* 1988;80:148-9.
29. Kantor J, Tran R, Greiner JW, et al. Modulation of carcinoembryonic antigen messanger RNA levels in human colon carcinoma cells by recombinant human γ-interferon. *Cancer Res* 1989;49: 2651-5.
30. Guadagni F, Witt P, Robbins P, et al. Regulation of carcinoembryonic antigen expression in differential human colorectal tumor cells by interferon–γ. *Cancer Res* 1990;50: 6248-55.
31. Nieroda CA, Milenic DE, Carrasquillo JA, et al. Improved tumor radioimmunodetection using a single chain Fv and γ-interferon: potential clinical applications for radioimmunoguided surgery and γ scanning. *Cancer Res* 1995;55: 2858-65.
32. Guadagni F, Schlom J, Johnston WW, et al. Selective interferon-induced enhancement of tumor-associated antigens on a spectrum of freshly isolated human adenocarcinoma cells. *J Natl Cancer Inst* 1989;81:502-12.
33. Greiner JW, Fischer PB, Pestka S, et al. Differential effects of recombinant human leukocyte interferons on cells surface antigen expression. *Cancer Res* 1986;46: 4984-90.
34. Greiner JW, Dansky Ullmann C, Nieroda C, et al. Improved immunotherapeutic efficacy of an anti-carcinoma monoclonal antibody (CC49) when given in combination with IFN–γ. *Cancer Res* 1993;53:600-8.
35. Greiner JW, Guadagni F, Goldstein D, et al. IP administration of Interferon-gamma to carcinoma patients enhances expression of tumor-associated glycoprotein -72 (TAG-72) and carcinoembryonic antigen (CEA) on malignant ascites cells. *J Clin Oncol* 1991;10:735-46.
36. Roselli M, Guadagni F, Buonomo O, et al. Systemic Administration of Recombinant Interferon in Carcinoma Patients Upregulates the Expression of the Carcinoma Associated Antigens TAG-72 and CEA. *J Clin Oncol* 1996;14: 2031-42.

CHAPTER 15

IMMUNOBIOLOGICAL APPROACH TO COLORECTAL CANCER STAGING: BIOLOGICAL MARKERS, CELLULAR "IN SITU" IMMUNOLOGICAL RESPONSE AND INTRANUCLEAR DNA IMAGING ANALYSIS. OLD AND NEW PARAMETERS. RETROSPECTIVE EVALUATION AND PROSPECTIVE TRIALS AFTER A FIFTEEN YEAR EXPERIENCE.

GIUSEPPE MIDIRI, *MARIA R.GIOVAGNOLI , ANTONINO TESORIERE *ENRICO GIARNIERI , AUGUSTO LOMBARDI, ANDREA BERTOLOTTI, *ALDO VECCHIONE , and MANUELE DI PAOLA

*4th Chair of Surgical Methodology, and *Department of Experimental Medicine, University of Rome "La Sapienza" , Rome, Italy*

Summary

The Authors consider whether it is possibile to classify and stage colo-rectal cancer not only on the grounds of its diffusion, histotype and grading, but also on the grounds of its biological expression.
In spite of the evaluation of new biomarkers, serum pre-operative and post-operative CEA evaluation is to date considered the most reliable test for improving staging, prognosis and treatment of colo-rectal cancer patients.
Pre and post-operative K – Ras serum evaluation is till now under discussion.
Retrospective and prospective studies of cellular "in situ" immunological response did not show any correlation with colon cancer staging.
High proliferative cell activity and aneuploidy, evaluated by intranuclear DNA imaging, appear to be connected with the extension of the primary tumor (T parameter) and with a severe prognosis, but through multiple full thickness sampling the Authors notice that different cell clones appear in different parts of the tumour, and multiclonality appears in samples taken from the infiltrating part of the tumour, close to the serosa of the colon.
After fifteen years experience on this topic, the Authors conclude that until it is possible to develop colon cancer heterogeneity, treatment planning, prognostic evaluation and follow-up protocols might be inadequate.
The question does not appear easy to solve, but it may be the keystone for improving biological knowledge of colo-rectal cancer.

Key Words: Biological Markers; cellular "in situ" immunological response; intranuclear DNA imaging.

E. Zanella (ed.), Advances in Abdominal Surgery, 163–173.

Introduction

The incidence of colo-rectal cancer is in constant increase in North America, North and West Europe, and Australia. Colo-rectal cancer represents about 15% of all malignant tumours, and in the United States approximately 150.000 new cases occur per year [4 ,21].

In spite of recent progress achieved in early diagnosis through endoscopy, in surgical treatment with the help of new technologies, and in adjuvant radio-chemo-therapy protocols,as a consequence of new developments,the cancer death-rate has not been reduced.

As a possible explanation of this failure, we consider the inadequacy of present colon cancer staging criteria, that do not allow characterization of the effective biological activity of the disease, which appears not to coincide with the neoplasm's natural history [13, 25].

In the last 20 years thanks to many clinical trials and immunobiological experiences, our knowledge of colon cancer development has increased.Still now there are many unsolved questions related to the complex antigenic architecture of colon cancer cells, their kinetic and intranuclear DNA content,the host's immunological response, adenoma-carcinoma sequence, and colon cancer family syndrome, from the point of view of genetics, invasive growth, recurrence or biological mechanisms of metastatic diffusion.

Nevertheless we stage colo-rectal cancer patients only by some unilateral parameters.

Duke's and TNM classifications are the staging system most applied all over the world. These staging methods express in alphabetical and numerical symbols, parameters which have been considered so far essential in order to refer to the stages of the disease in international language, but they are based exclusively on measurements of the tumour's anatomical extension. Clinical observation often leads us to conclude that for solid tumours, as in some mielolymphoproliferative diseases, different clinical evolutions correspond to different biological behavior, regardless of the neoplastic extension.

Consequently, we assert that a staging systems better able to define the evolution of a solid tumour, has to be based on parameters concerning the neoplasia's biological activity, and the host's immunological response, correlated with parameters concerning the neoplasia's anatomical extension [11,12 ,15].

Untill it is possible to develop such a system, over or understaging in colon cancer patients is possible, so that treatment-planning, prognostic evaluation and follow-up protocols might frequently be inadequate.

Even though such considerations have not yet altered the approach to colon cancer management, it is certainly changing the approach concerning staging, prognosis and treatment of some other neoplasms.

We can consider the study of monoclonal antibodies, which has made important headway in the identification and classification of the lymphocytes subpopulations,

and in the setting up of the lymphomas arising from them (ontogenetical stage of the disease). It is useful to examine the antigenic expression of tumours in the male and female genital spheres,the study of which has led to new trials of follow-up and adjuvant therapy.Above all we must bear in mind the disturbance caused in therapeutical and prognostic planning, by the introduction of the receptorial tissue evaluation, in patients affected with breast cancer [13,27].
Therefore when we started our experiments on this topic, the basic question was the following: is it possible to classify and stage colo-rectal cancer not only on the grounds of its diffusion, histotype and grading, but also on the grounds of its biological expression?

Biological markers

Colo-rectal cancer represented and still now represents a prototype for the building up of patterns, in the clinical application of oncological bio-markers.
For about ten years several reseachers have been trying to discover many cellular markers, by means of monoclonal or policlonal antibodies, and to typify the antigenic structure of the neoplastic cells.
Extreme sensitivity in discovering a minimum number of tumoral cells, specificity for a particular neoplasia, resolution strictly pertaining to the exsisting tumoral cells and simple, cheap and easily comparable study techniques are characteristics of an ideal marker. Even though Carcinoembrionic Antigen (CEA) cannot be considered an ideal marker, it was chosen as a colon cancer biological marker for our experiment.
At the outset, we tried to design experimental models by integrating serum and tissue CEA levels and standard staging parameters (TNM-UICC, Duke's classification, grading) in patients operated for colo-rectal cancer.
In 124 patients the pre-operative serum CEA level, determined through radioimmunological investigation, represented a laboratory parameter that, together with other instrumental clinical investigations, can provide information about the diffusion of the disease before surgical treatment [22,23].
In fact we can observe a directly proportional correlation between this evaluation and the disease's extension. From this point of view, the pre-operative serum CEA evaluation can reinforce the traditional clinical staging.
Some interesting considerations emerged from the post-operative serum C E A evaluation, in 69 patients surgically treated for colo-rectal cancer, obtained on the 14th day, fixed as clearance limit for this marker [12,24].
Only 18,5% of the patients with elevated post-operative serum C E A levels survived, versus 65,5% of the patients with a post-operative serum C E A within the normal range after a seven year follow-up. Such an observation leaves out personal evaluations concerning surgical radicality, kind of operation and stage of the disease. As a matter of fact, we concluded that the patients with post-operative

C E A levels within the normal range were those who underwent biologically radical surgery (tab. 1).

Table 1. Some interesting considerations emerged from the post-operative serum CEA evaluation in 69 patients surgically treated for colo-rectal cancer. Of the patients with elevated post-operative serum CEA levels survived only 18,5%versus 65,5% of the patients with a post operative serum CEA within the normal range, after seven year follow-up.

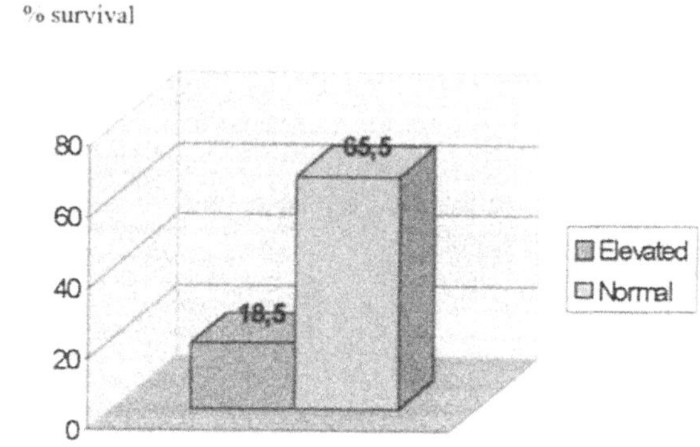

On the other hand elevated post-operative CEA levels lead to a severe prognosis [12,24].

From this point of view evaluation of post-operative serum CEA levels can be considered as a marker of the biological radicality in surgical treatment, and therefore a prognostic indication.

In order to improve the specificity of the test we evaluated the CEA level on tumoral tissue, by means of policlonal antibodies on 57 patients, and a monoclonal antibody prepared by our team on 138 patients, who had undergone surgical treatment for colo-rectal cancer.

This test was performed by Sterneberger's immunoperoxidase indirect method (PAP), but we did not achieve appreciable results from the point of view of staging and prognostic evaluation. The same test, performed on 39 colo-rectal polyps, showed a higher intensity of the staining reaction in severely displastic polyps [12,26].

The utility in monitoring patients affected and operated for colo-rectal neoplasia by means of CEA serum dosage, has been widely accepted.

The specificity of such a test in the future diagnosis of recurrences varies from 80 to 100% of cases, with a predictability of 6 months before the clinical instrumental appearance of metastases [13,17,25].

It is common knowledge that many Authors carry out second-look operations, or start chemotherapic protocols, only on the grounds of the increase in value of CEA, even though clinically neither recurrences nor metastases have been checked [12,15].

In the opinion of some Authors C E A scan affords high quality, same-day imaging, uses an inexpensive and readily-available radionuclide, adds clinically significant information in assessing extension and location of disease in colo-rectal cancer patients, and sometimes may represent a guide to surgical treatment [14,34]. In spite of the evaluation of several new serum biomarkers for the staging and monitoring of colon cancer patients, serum pre-operative and post-operative C E A evaluation is to date considered the most reliable test for clinical application in colo-rectal cancer.

In our opinion TPA and CA 19.9, though frequently evaluated in colon cancer patients' serum and tissue, have not shown more sensitivity and specificity than the CEA test.

Other biological markers are to day under evaluation in several studies.When we are able to solve the problems concerning the ways of synthesis and expression of the antigens(metabolism and serum clearance, the influence of repeating mitosis,cellular necrosis and circulating immunocomplex in vivo on the inhibition of such antigen expression) then probably the study of biological markers will open up new horizons in the staging and characterization of colo-rectal neoplasia [13,25,27,40].

Serum and tissue K-Ras evaluation as expression of an oncogene activation could in future be a parameter probably utilizable in the early diagnosis of colo-rectal cancer [7,38].

Cellular "in situ" immunological response

For several years many Authors have been interested in the possibility of understanding the etiopathogenesis of tumours in the immunological field, and so to control tumour growth and therapy immunologically.

Indeed in the last twenty years many clinical studies have proved the correlation between tumours and the host's immunitary defense [6,17,27,39].

The immune response to a certain antigen is the end-product of several biochemical messages active among different cellular populations, with the final effect of potentiating (cooperation) and/or inhibiting (suppression) immunity. In the oncological immunitary response both cellular and humoral immunity are involved .

But in recent studies some English Authors highlighted the importance for oncologists of "in situ" immunological response in cancer patients,with a retrospective analysis of 400 patients operated for colo-rectal cancer.

In particular a complex statistical analysis showed three parameters as being related to prognostic assessment: cellular "in situ" immunological response, metastatic rate in lymphatic space and regional spreading of colon cancer [19,20]

In some retrospective trials we tried to evaluate "in situ" cellular response by using paraffin preparates, traditional staining and microscopy, not only in colo-rectal cancer patients but also for breast and lung neoplasms. It was not a qualitative evaluation but a semi-quantitative assessment, which resulted in frequent mistakes by human error [9].

Then we isolated lymphocytic cell lines with no time for ischemic development from surgical specimens which taken from healthy intestinal mucosa and peritumoral mucosa of colo-rectal cancer patients; we cultivated and tested them for specific monoclonal antibodies.

This method was expensive and very difficult to follow because of the small number of vital cells and their frequent bacterial contamination. We stopped using this method [29].

From that point we evaluated a qualitative and quantitative method to be used in a prospective trial. The evaluation of cellular "in situ" immunological response was performed with traditional hysto-staining techniques, immunohystochemical analysis, and by incubating the specimens taken from healthy intestinal mucosa and peritumoral and intratumoral mucosa of colo-rectal cancer patients, with Mo Ab (Pan-Leu; Dak-Mac; CD 19; CD 3; CD 4; CD 8; CD 25; CD 45).

The data were related to N value, loco-regional spreading and intranuclear D N A imaging. The high cellular "in situ" immunological response, especially in neoplastic and perineoplastic tissue, was surprising, and we were able to observe a notable presence of macrophagic cells in intra and peritumoral tissue, and of T lymphocytic cells in peritumoral mucosa, while the percentage of B lymphocitic subpopulations was low.

No correlation was found with other parameters.

Therefore we concluded that, from the point of view of staging, only a higher number of cases and a longer follow-up could demonstrate the validity of such prospective studies [28,30].

However, it is possible that an inflammatory bowel disease related to colon cancer increases lymphocytic infiltration; therefore it is necessary to standardise a more reliable qualitative way of testing lymphocytic subpopulations.

Intranuclear DNA imaging

Cell kinetic evaluation and DNA content determination may be considered today as markers of the biological behavior of many neoplasias.

In particular in colon cancer patients there are many outstanding studies of pre-cancerous lesions, in primary tumours and in liver metastases.

But there are some unsolved questions, fundamentally related to: intranuclear DNA imaging analysis versus flow cytometric analysis;interpretation of the results; correlation with other hystomorphological and immunobiological parameters; effective significance of data; ploidy heterogeneity and tissue sampling, from the point of view of biological characterization, staging and prognostic evaluation of colon cancer [1,2,3,5,8,10,18,35,37].

We studied 20 patients surgically treated for colo-rectal cancer; 12 males and 8 females with a mean age of 60.
For each patient T N M - U I C C staging, grading and Intranuclear D N A imaging analyses were evaluated.The information potentially available from the correlation between present staging criteria, and ploidy determination by flow cytometric analysis, is up to now of very limited practical application for improving prognostic evaluation and treatment of colo-rectal cancer patients [2,5].
Intranuclear DNA imaging analysis was chosen for this study, because in our opinion this method is able to: allow visualization and determination of D N A ploidy directly in morphologically selected cells; permit selection of only viable neoplastic cells for analysis, and allow for the rejection of debris, degenerated cells and aggregates of tumour cells; better identify subpopulations of highly aneuploid cells and tumour multiclonality. In our opinion, with flow cytometry it is impossible to distinguish different cell clones in the same tumour, because they may be diluted by non neoplastic epithelial and inflammatory cells [1,16,33].
For each patient five glass slides were evaluated after touch imprinting on tumoral mass and staining by a modified Feulgen method, using a kit (DNA staining kit 102300-01 Becton-Dickinson Elmhurst, Illinois).
A CAS 200 was used for imaging analysis.
Highly proliferative cell activity and aneuploidy appear to be correlated with the extention of the primary tumour (T - parameter) (p = 0,022 Fisher test) and with a severe prognosis (tab. 2).

Table 2. High proliferative cell activity and aneuplody appear to be correlated with the extention of the primary tumour (T – parameter)

	T1	T2	T3	T4
Diploid	1	4	2	0
Tetraploid	0	1	2	0
Aneuploid	0	1	7	2

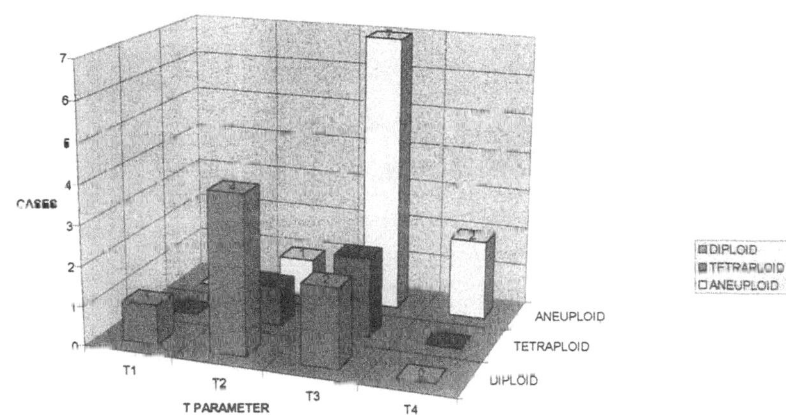

	T1	T2	T3	T4
DIPLOID	1	4	2	0
TETRAPLOID	0	1	2	0
ANEUPLOID	0	1	7	2

(p= 0,022 Fisher test)

No correlation was found with stage, N value,or grading and cellular "in situ" immunological response.
T3 and T4 tumours were mostly tetraploid or aneuploid (11/13) [31,32].
After a short follow-up (24 months on average) 100% of diploid versus 73% of tetraploid or aneuploid patients are still alive, not including three patients who underwent palliative resection [33].
Some Authors reported that aggressive colo-rectal tumours with a tendency to local recurrence more frequently revealed different cell populations.
These studies show that a policlonal condition influences lymphatic infiltration and haematic distant metastases, and it represents an additional significant prognostic indicator to aneuploidy [2,5,8,36].
We consider as a possible explanation of this conflict, the heterogeneity of colon cancer, in which invasive growth is characterised by an irregular distribution of the cellular multiplication. We suppose that ploidy might be an indipendent parameter with a further prognostic value. Cell multiplication is determined by different kinetic cellular activity and by local physico-chemical biological properties of the host, and it implies that tumours of the same histotype cannot be simply considered as a homogenous population of malignant cells [1,6].
A way to solve this problem may be to perform multiple full thickness sampling of the tumour. Therefore the eleven T3 colo-rectal cancer patients of this study were also evaluated by means of multiple full thickness sampling, performed by inserting a 14 gauge trucut from the outside of the sierosa through the tumour as far as the lumen [32,33] (Fig. 1).

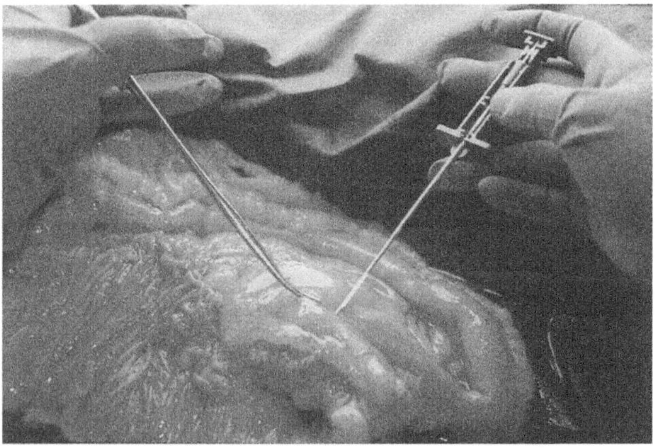

Figure 1. Therefore the eleven T3 colo-rectal cancer patients of this study were also evaluated by means of multiple full thickness sampling performed by inserting a 14 gauge trucut from the outside of the sierosa through the tumour as far as the lumen.
(see Color Plates, p. xix)

For each patient an average of 6 glass slides were prepared for the evaluation of the whole trucut biopsies at different levels.
Specimens were evaluated by the aforesaid method for intranuclear DNA imaging determination. Thanks to this preliminary experience we noticed that different cell clones appeared in different parts of the tumour, and multiclonality appeared in samples taken from the infiltrating part of the tumour, close to the sierosa of the colon. (Fig - 2)

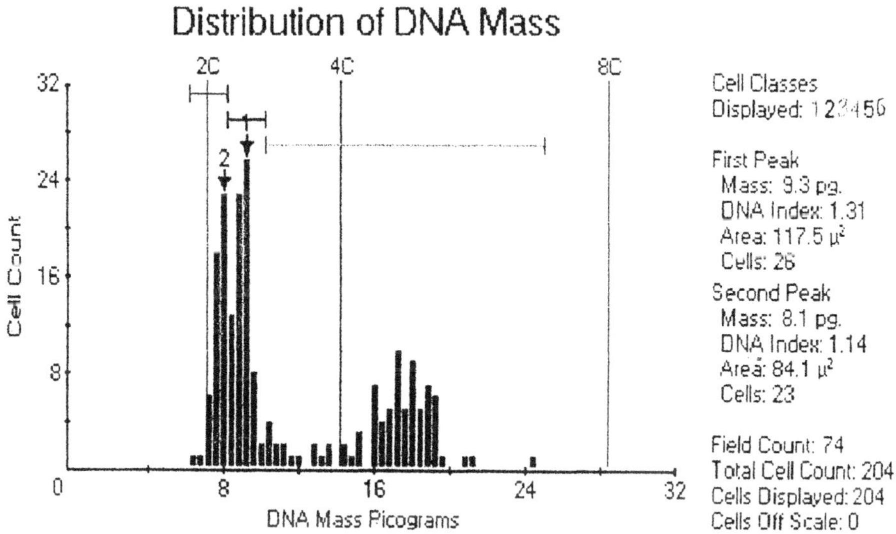

Figure2. Colon cancer tru-cut biopsy : sample taken close to the serosa –multiclonal pattern

Consequently ploidy heterogeneity and multiclonality appear to characterise invasive growth of colo-rectal cancer.
From this point of view, multiple full thickness sampling seems to be a promising methodology to be investigated.
However, we think that any final conclusions about the question related to the biological heterogeneity of colo-rectal cancer must be postponed.
This question is not easy to solve, but we think that it may be the keystone for a correct evaluation of colo rectal cancer staging and prognosis.

References

1. Alderisio M, Ribotta G, Giarnieri E, et al. Aneuploid polyclonality in image analysis: Clinical prognostic value in colorectal cancer. *Oncol Rep* 1996; 3: 567.
2. Allison DC, Piantadosi S, Hruban RH, et al. The National Cancer Data Base Report on colon cancer. *Cancer* 1996; 78: 918.
3. Aziz D, Peter SB. DNA ploidy and cell cycle analysis: tools for assessment of cancer prognosis. *J Clin Lab Anal* 1991; 5: 422.
4. Boring CC, Squireas TS, Tong T, et al. Cancer statistics 1994. *Cancer J Clin* 1994; 44: 7.
5. Bose KK, Allison DC, Hruban RH, et al. A comparison of flow cyrometry and absorption cytometric D N A value as prognostic indicators for pancreatic carcinoma. *Cancer* 1993; 71: 691.
6. Braun S, Pantel K. Immunodiagnosis and immunotherapy of isolated tumour cell disseminated to bone marrow of patients with colorectal cancer. *Tumori* 1995; 81:78.
7. Breivik J, Meling GI, Spurkland A, et al. K-Ras mutation in colorectal cancer: relations to patient, age, sex and tomor location. *Br J Cancer* 1994; 69: 367.
8. Chang KJ, Enker WE, Melamed M. Influence of tumor cell DNA ploidy on the natural history of rectal cancer. *Am J Surg* 1987; 153: 184.
9. Colizza S, Bertolotti A, Di Paola M, et al. The hosth defensive factor grade. *Dis Colon Rectum* 1978; 22: 93.
10. Danova M, De Renzis MR, Girino M, et al. DNA content and cell kinetics in colorectal carcinoma. *Tumori* 1995; 81: 12.
11. Di Paola M, Midiri G, Amanti C, et al. Concetti di stadiazione dinamica delle neoplasie del colon retto. *Min Chir* 1989; 44: 75.
12. Di Paola M, Midiri G, Bertolotti A, et al. Prognostic role of tissue and serum markers. *Exp Cl Cancer Res* 1989; 8: 102.
13. Di Paola M, Midiri G, Ramacciato G. Role of monoclonal antibodies in the management of colorectal carcinoma. in Current topics in Surgical Oncology ed. Masson Milano, 1991.
14. Doerr RI, Abdel - NABI H, Krag DN, et al. Radiolabeled antibody imaging in the management of colorectal cancer. *Ann Surg* 1991; 214: 118.
15. Galassi G, Midiri G, Pastore P, et al. Nuovi orientamenti nella stadiazione delle neoplasie solide. *Min Chir* 1989; 44: 79.
16. Giovagnoli MR, Lukic A, Muraro R, et al. Image cytometry for DNA analysis in endometrial carcinoma correlated with other prognostic parameters. *Int J Oncol* 1996 ;7 - 809.
17. Haferkamp O. Inflammatory stromal reaction in well differentiated adenocarcinoma of the large intestine in Metastatic tumor growth. ed. Verlag New York, 1980.
18. Harlow SP, Eriksen BL, Poggensee L, et al. Prognostic implication of proliferativa activity and DNA aneuploidy in Astler-Coller-Duke's stage C colonic adenocarcinoma. *Cancer Res* 1991; 51: 2403.
19. Jass SR, Loves S, Nothoner SMA. A new prognostic classification for rectal cancer. *Lancet* 1987; 1: 1303.
20. Jass SR, Morson BC. Reporting colo-rectal cancer. *Clin Pathol* 1987; 40: 1016.
21. Jessup JM, Mc Ginnis LS, Steele GD, et al. The National Cancer Data Base Report on colon cancer. *Cancer* 1996; 78: 918.
22. Midiri G, Amanti C, Benedetti M, et al. CEA tissue staining in colorectal cancer patients. *Cancer* 1985; 55: 2624.
23. Midiri G, Amanti C, Consorti F, et al. Usefulness of preoperative CEA levels in the assessment of colorectal cancer patient stage. *J Surg Onc* 1983; 22: 57.
24. Midiri G, Amanti C, Consorti F, et al. L'antigene carcinoembrionario CEA come indicatore di radicalità biologica di un intervento chirurgico. *Giorn Chir* 1988; 9 910.
25. Midiri G, Bertolotti A, Di Paola M, et al. La Stadiazione dinamica in funzione della prognosi delle neoplasie del colon retto. in "Il ruolo della terapia chirurgica in oncologia" ed. Monduzi Bologna, 1988.
26. Midiri G, Benedetti M, Campisi C, et al. Tissue CEA detection by immunoperoxidase PAP test in colorectal polyps: correlations with the degree of dysplasia. *J Surg Onc* 1988; 37: 13.

27. Midiri G, Bezzi M, Campisi C. La Reazione Immunitaria. in Manuale di Fisiopatologia Chirurgica ed. Masson Milano, 1993.
28. Midiri G, Di Massimo A, Verrico G, et al. Modelli clinico sperimentali per la definizione di parametri immunologici da integrare ai sistemi di stadiazione tradizionali delle neoplasie colo-rettali. *Giorn Chir* 1994; 15: 341.
29. Midiri G, Tesoriere A, Giarnieri E, et al. Immunità cellulare in situ e valutazione prognostica. Atti xviii Congr. SICO 1: 3 Varese 1994.
30. Midiri G, Tesoriere A, Lombardi A, et al. Cellular in situ immunological response and intranuclear DNA imaging evaluation in colorectal cancer patients. *It Rev Med Surg Res* 1995; 3: 29.
31. Midiri G, Giovagnoli MR, Tesoriere A, et al. E' possibile considerare l'analisi per immagine del DNA intranucleare come un nuovo parametro per la stadiazione del cancro colo-rettale ? *Giorn Chir* 1998; 19: 9.
32. Midiri G, Giarnieri E, Tesoriere A, et al. Is it possible to consider intranuclear DNA imaging as a new parameter for colo-rectal cancer prognostic evaluation ? 1 th World Congr Surg Onc San Diego USA March 1998.
33. Midiri G, Tesoriere A, Giarnieri E, et al. D N A ploidy and prognosis in colo-rectal cancer patients: preliminary report. *It J Coloproct* 1998 in press.
34. Moffat FL, Pinsky CM, Hammershaimb L, et al. Clinical utility of external immunoscintigraphy with the IMMU - 4 Technetium - 99m Fab antibody fragment in patients undergoing surgery for carcinoma of the colon and rectum: results of a pivotal, phase III trial. *J Cl Onc* 1996; 14: 2295.
35. Orfão A, Ruiz Arguelles A, Lacombe F. Flow citometry in application in haematology. *Haematologica* 1995; 80: 69.
36. Pietra N, Sarli L, Sansebastiano G, et al. Prognostic value of ploidy, cell proliferation kinatics and conventional clinicopathologic criteria in patients with colorectal carcinoma. *Dis colon cancer* 1996; 39: 494.
37. Scott N, Cross D, Plumb MI, et al. an investigation of different methods of cell cycle analysis by flow cytometry in rectal cancer. *Br J Cancer* 1995; 8: 10.
38. Spandidos DA, Kiaris H, Liondaki E, et al. Activating mutations in the K-Ras gene in ulcerative colitis and Crohn's disease. *Onc Rep* 1994; 1: 547.
39. Strauli P, Heammerli G. Interaction of locomotive and lytic activities of tumor cells in invasion. in Metastatic tumor growth ed. Verlag New York, 1980.
40. Vitelli CE, Ramacciato G, Midiri G, et al. Surgical management of recurrent colorectal carcinoma. in "Current topics in surgical oncology". Ed. Masson Milano, 1991.

CHAPTER 16

MINIMALLY INVASIVE SURGERY FOR ESOPHAGEAL DISEASES

ALBERTO PERACCHIA and *RICCARDO ROSATI

*Department of General Surgery and Surgical Oncology , University of Milan, Milan, and *Department of General and Minimally Invasive Surgery , Hospital "Humanitas" , Rozzano(Milan) , Italy*

Summary

In recent years laparoscopy and thoracoscopy have gained increasing popularity, becoming in some instances the first choice in the treatment of many benign esophageal diseases (gastroesophageal reflux, achalasia, epiphrenic diverticula, esophageal leiomyoma) in referral centers. Infact, in experienced hands, post-operative morbility is reduced when compared to open surgery. The operated patients benefit from better comfort, and the results are comparable to the traditional approach. Keys to a successful outcome of this procedure are: thorough pre-operative evaluation of patients, experience in open surgery of the esophagus, and remarkable skill in laparoscopy. Based on literature and on our personal experience, we can conclude that minimally invasive treatment of benign diseases of the esophagus is safe and effective. In some instances further follow-up is necessary to confirm the favourable initial results.

Key words: Esophagus; gastroesophageal reflux; achalasia; epiphrenic diverticula; leiomyoma.

Introduction

Minimal access surgery to treat benign and functional esophageal disease, has become very popular in recent years. Through laparoscopy, several authors reported the safety and effectiveness of antireflux surgery for gastroesophageal reflux disease GERD [1,6], of esophagomyotomy for treatment of achalasia [7,9], and of transhiatal diverticulectomy-myotomy-fundoplication for epiphrenic diverticulum of the esophagus [10]. In thoracoscopy, myotomy for motor disorders [11,13] and enucleation of leyomyomas [14,15] have become more and more popular, while the approach to thoracic diverticula [16,17] is controversial, and the indications of esophagectomy for benign diseases are very limited. Although the same technique well-established in open surgery should be reproduced through laparoscopy and thoracoscopy, some technical aspects are peculiar to the minimally invasive approach, where the lack of tactile perception may present more difficulties to the surgeon; intra-operative endoscopy is often

E. Zanella (ed.), Advances in Abdominal Surgery, 175–182.

helpful to facilitate the procedure.

Gastroesophageal reflux disease (GERD)

Gastroesophageal reflux disease is one of the most common gastrointestinal conditions in Western countries. Notwithstanding the frequency of this disease, surgical therapy of GERD has been neglected over the last decade. The reasons for a decrease in surgical indications might have been both fear of the consequences of aggressive operation, and good results obtained by new classes of drugs such as omeprazole and cisapride. The appearance of a controlled randomised trial which showed the superiority of surgery over medical therapy of severe GERD [17], and good results of laparoscopic fundoplication [1,6] have caused gastroenterologists to reconsider surgery in selected cases as an effective treatment, compared to lifelong patient commitment to medical therapy.

Careful selection of patients through complete pre-operative evaluation is mandatory to attain satisfactory post-operative results. Infact, only a thorough functional study can establish the correct indication for surgery and, even more important, the type of operation to be performed. This is the tailored approach to different surgical techniques, codified by the group of Tom DeMeester [19,20] on the basis of a pre-operative workup which includes: barium swallow, upper gastrointestinal endoscopy, stationary and, in some cases, 24-hour esophageal manometry, 24-hour pH monitoring and, in selected cases, radionuclide transit and evaluation of alkalyne reflux. Pre-operative study selects the patients that may benefit from a total fundoplication (those with good motility of the body of the esophagus), those that will have better results with partial fundoplication (in case of ineffective esophageal peristalsis), and those that need a more complex procedure for an acquired short esophagus.

Surgical technique in laparoscopy has been standardized after having first been described by Dallemagne in 1991 [1]. It consists in dissection of the diaphragmatic crura and of the lower esophagus, crural repair, and transposition of the gastric fundus to do either a short floppy total fundoplication (Nissen) or a partial posterior fundoplication (Toupet), according to the pre-operative workup.

Results of surgery are good in more than 90% of cases, both in clinical terms (control of symptoms), and in objectively solving reflux (healing of esophagitis - normalization of pH monitoring values) [3-6,21]. Cost effectiveness of the minimally invasive operation as compared to medical therapy and to open surgery has been demonstrated [18]. Side effects of surgery (dysphagia, gas and bloating, diarrhoea) account for less than 10% of patients and are cured in the vast majority of cases with a conservative therapy [6]. Complications of laparoscopic surgery have been reported, with an incidence of less than 5% of cases [3,6,21,22], a lower rate than after open surgery [23]. Moreover, it should be noticed that complications occur mainly at the surgeons "learning curve": they are generally due to errors of technique and indication, making it even more important that this surgery should be performed only by physicians with perfect knowledge of the pathophysiology of the esophagus and surgical techniques.

Esophageal achalasia

Esophageal achalasia is the major motor disorder of the esophagus, induced by an impaired swallowing-induced relaxation of the lower esophageal sphincter. Among non-surgical treatments, balloon dilatation of the cardia achieves only temporary relief, and involves risk of perforation [24] (and is thus reserved only to high-risk or elderly patients); botulinun toxin injection is still to be considered as experimental [25]. Extramucosal myotomy of the lower esophagus and cardia, combined with an anterior antireflux fundoplication, is in our opinion the ideal treatment for I to III degree achalasia. This technique has proved safe and effective through laparotomy and we have been using it satisfactorily for more than fifteen years [26]. In laparoscopy we have standardized the technique to respect the same surgical principles that we think are important during open surgery [7,27]: minimal dissection of the anterior aspect of the esophagus with no esophageal encircling, complete division of the longitudinal and circular muscle fibers for at least 6 cm above the esophagus and 1.5/2 cm above the stomach, under endoscopic control and guidance, anterior partial fundoplication to prevent gastroesophageal reflux, and sealing of the edges of the myotomy.

Morbility of this operation is negligible in our and other groups' experience. Long-term results have shown relief of dysphagia in over 90% of the patients, and an incidence of post-operative gastroesophageal reflux in less than 10% of patients [7,8]. Thus we believe that, in referral centers, laparoscopic myotomy and fundoplication is the first option in treating achalasia.

Epiphrenic esophageal diverticula

Diverticula are usually regarded as a consequence of some underlying functional disorder, and may cause dysphagia, regurgitation, chest pain and aspiration. Beyond radiological and endoscopic study, thorough functional evaluation with manometry and pH monitoring is essential in order to assess the motility disorder and choose the most suitable therapeutic option. Surgical treatment is indicated to relieve symptoms and to prevent aspiration (particularly in elderly or compromised patients with large diverticula), whereas close observation is recommended in asymptomatic cases, although some authors advocate systematic resection of esophageal diverticula [28,31]. The standard approach consists of resection of the diverticular pouch, combined with an extended myotomy and an antireflux procedure performed through left thoracotomy [29]. Low-situated epiphrenic

esophageal diverticula may be resected transhiatally with the use of an endoscopic stapler, then by combining a long esophageal myotomy and an antireflux procedure to treat the underlying motor disorder and avoid post-operative iatrogenic reflux. Due to the rarity of the disease, no extensive series have been reported. Our initial personal experience with this operation performed through laparoscopy accounts for five patients with good results [10].
In thoracoscopy, because of technical difficulty in performing the myotomy and fundoplication after resection of diverticulum, we replaced myotomy with pre-operative pneumatic dilation of the cardia, in patients with hypertensive or incordinated LES, reserving thoracoscopic diverticulectomy alone, for patients without any detectable abnormality at standard manometry [32]. This protocol, however, has been abandoned because of the high incidence of complications.

Esophageal motor disorders

Esophageal motor disorders causing dysphagia include hypertensive lower esophageal sphincter (LES), diffuse spasm, nutcracker esophagus and other nonspecific motor disorders. Differential diagnosis is made on standard esophageal manometry findings. A long myotomy of the thoracic esophagus is indicated in diffuse and segmental spasm: in such cases, surgical trauma related to the open approach is out of proportion to the relative simplicity of the operation, which may be easily achieved thoracoscopically with minimal discomfort for the patient. Through a left thoracoscopic approach the myotomy may be extended from above the gastroesophageal junction upwards, according to the level of the motor abnormality detected at manometry. Intra-operative esophagoscopy is of the utmost importance, since mild distension and transillumination of the mucosa help in identifying the muscular fibers, and check mucosal integrity. Fundoplication in thoracoscopic myotomy is not required because of the minimal hiatal dissection [8,11,13].

Benign esophageal tumors

Leiomyomas and other benign submucosal lesions such as congenital cysts are rare and often silent. Dysphagia is the most common complaint in symptomatic patients and its occurrence depends on the size and location of the mass [14]. Endoscopic ultrasonography (EUS) is usually diagnostic [33,34], whereas biopsy is contraindicated, since subsequent submucosal fibrosis may increase the risk of mucosal tear during tumor removal. Indication to surgical treatment relies on the presence of symptoms, and of associated disorders requiring surgery, rather than on the risk of complications or degeneration. Sometimes, malignancy may not be definitely ruled out with pre-operative imaging. Standard surgical treatment consists in simple enucleation of the mass through thoracotomy or laparotomy, depending on the location of the lesion. Esophageal resection may be required in patients with diffuse leiomyomatosis. Minimally invasive surgery appears to provide a valuable alternative to the open approach, since it allows the same operation to be performed with reduced post-operative discomfort [14].

Benign esophageal diseases requiring esophagectomy

Video-assisted techniques have been applied for esophagectomy both for cancer and for benign diseases. Oncological indications to esophagectomy leave just a small space to minimally invasive surgery [35]: through thoracoscopy both the removal of the esophagus and lymphonodal clearence are feasible [36,41] but with uncertain benefits [42]; through the transmediastinal access, video-assistance increases safety of the esophagectomy without thoracotomy [43], thus giving preference to this procedure rather than to blunt dissection. As for benign diseases, indication to esophagectomy is limited, in our opinion, to stage IV achalasia with dolicomegaesophagus, and to long-standing caustic stenosis after reconstruction with a retrosternal coloplasty. Evaluation of the results achieved with thoracoscopic esophagectomy should be made in terms of peri-operative morbidity. Operative mortality after thoracoscopic esophagectomy is comparable to open surgery, and does not seem to be directly related to the minimally invasive approach. The post-operative complication rate is comparable to traditional surgery, but it is not lessened by the minimal access afforded by thoracoscopy. Pulmonary infection, the most frequent complication after resective surgery of the esophagus [44], has infact a multifactorial etiology and its occurrence does not primarily depend on the extent of thoracotomy. On the other hand, thoracoscopic dissection of the esophagus might be longer than the open operation, thus requiring a prolonged lung exclusion. The benefits of the avoidance of thoracotomy on respiratory mechanics, and on reduced post-operative pain [45], may be overcome by longer one-lung ventilation, thus a final judgement on the real place of the procedure is not possible.

Comment

Minimally invasive surgery has gained increasing popularity over the last few years. Following the excellent results achieved with cholecystectomy, the laparoscopic approach was attempted, to perform other non-resective procedures for benign abdominal disease. Technical feasibility of laparoscopic fundoplication was first reported in 1991. Since then, several surgeons have applied laparoscopy for treatment of GERD and other benign diseases of the esophagus.
Two issues soon arose in the surgical community. The first was an apparent

broadening of indications, leading to a greater number of patients being subjected to surgical treatment. Apart from local situations and changing referral patterns, one basic principle is to keep to the indications that were stated before the laparoscopic era. Surgical treatment of GERD is indicated in patients with persistent symptoms or complications despite medical treatment. Esophagomyotomy should be regarded as the treatment of choice in patients with achalasia, since long-term results seem to be superior to endoscopic dilation of the cardia. As to epiphrenic diverticula, indication of surgical treatment and the choice of the procedure remain controversial. Diverticulectomy combined with selective myotomy for treatment of the underlying motor disorder seems to represent the correct approach in symptomatic patients. Improved patient comfort and minimal invasiveness of the laparoscopic approach may in future render surgery an even more attractive opportunity than lifetime medical treatment or repeated endoscopic dilation. All patients must undergo thorough functional evaluation in order to define the characteristics of the disease and select those who may benefit from surgery.

The second issue is the increase in iatrogenic complications and of functional failure following minimally invasive surgery of the foregut. Although this may be partly ascribed to the "learning curve" phenomenon, the incidence of malpractice, officially or unofficially reported, concerns a number of surgeons who are not familiar with gastroesophageal surgery.

These considerations, although of the utmost importance, do not compromise the role of minimally invasive surgery in the treatment of functional esophageal disease. Early post-operative results, in our experience as well as in other series, have clearly shown a reduction of morbidity and a shortening of hospital stay, thus resulting in improved patient comfort and, ultimately, in cost saving. Also, short-term functional outcome proved to be similar to the standard results of open surgical procedures, although longer follow-ups for a larger number of patients are required to confirm these observations. The clue for reproducing the functional results achieved in open surgery is to perform exactly the same operation through laparoscopy or thoracoscopy.

In conclusion, laparoscopic and thoracoscopic treatment of benign diseases of the esophagus are safe and effective. To ensure reliable results, including both accredited and investigational techniques, operations should be performed only by surgeons with solid experience in conventional treatment of esophageal disease, and adequate training in minimally invasive procedures.

References

1. Dallemagne B, Weerts J, Jehaes C, Markiewicz S, Lombard R. Laparoscopic Nissen fundoplication: preliminary report . *Surg Laparosc Endosc* 1991; 1: 138-43.

2. Nathanson LK, Shimi S, Cuschieri A. Laparoscopic ligamentun teres (round ligament) cardiopexy. *Br J Surg* 1991; 78: 947-51.

3. Dallemagne B, Taziaux P, Weerts J, Jehaes C, Markiewicz S. Chirurgie laparoscopique du reflux gastro-esophagien. *Ann Chir* 1995; 49: 30-6.

4. Cadière GB, Himpens J, Bruyns J. Fundoplicature selon Nissen par coelio-vidéoscopie. *Ann Chir* 1995; 49: 24-9.
5. Hinder RA, Filipi CJ, Wetscher G, Neary P, DeMeester TR, Perdikis G. Laparoscopic Nissen fundoplication is an effective treatment for gastroesophageal reflux disease. *Ann Surg* 1994; 220: 472-83.
6. Hunter JG, Trus TL, Branum GD et al . A physiologic approach to laparoscopic fundoplication for gastroesophageal reflux disease. *Ann Surg* 1996; 223: 673-87.
7. Rosati R, Fumagalli U, Bonavina L, Segalin A, Montorsi M, Bona S, Peracchia A. Laparoscopic approach to esophageal achalasia. *Am J Surg* 1995; 169: 424-7.
8. Anselmino M, Hinder RA, Filipi CJ, Wilson P. Laparoscopic Heller cardiomyotomy and thoracoscopic esophageal long myotomy for treatment of primary esophageal motor disorders. *Surg Laparosc Endosc* 1993; 3: 437-41.
9. Swanström LL, Pennings JL. Safe laparoscopic dissection of the gastroesophageal junction. *Am J Surg* 1995; 169: 507-11.
10. Rosati R, Fumagalli U, Bona S, Bonavina L, Peracchia A. Diverticulectomy, myotomy and fundoplication through laparoscopy: a new option to treat epiphrenic esophageal diverticula? *Ann Surg* 1997 (in press).
11. Cuschieri A. Endoscopic esophageal myotomy for specific motility disorders and non cardiac chest pain. *Endosc Surg Allied Technol* 1993; 1: 280-7.
12. Filipi CJ, Hinder RA. Thoracoscopic esophageal myotomy. A surgical technique for achalasia, diffuse esophageal spasm and "nutcracker esophagus". *Surg Endosc* 1994; 8: 921-6.
13. Peters JH, DeMeester TR. Thoracoscopic myotomy of the lower esophageal sphincter and esophageal body. In: Peters JH, DeMeester TR. Minimally Invasive Surgery of the Foregut. St. Louis, Quality Medical Publishing, 1994: 83-102.
14. Bonavina L, Segalin A, Rosati R, PavanelloM , Peracchia A. Surgical therapy of esophageal leiomyoma. *J An Coll Surg* 1995; 181: 257-62.
15. Gayet B. Vidéo-chirurgie et oesophage . *Chirurgie* 1994-1995; 120: 153-5.
16. Peracchia A, Bonavina L, Rosati R, Bona S. Thoracoscopic resection of epiphrenic esophageal diverticula. In: Peters JH, DeMeester TR. Minimally Invasive Surgery of the Foregut. St. Louis, Quality Medical Publishing, 1994: 110-6.
17. Eypasch E, Barlow A. Surgery for esophageal diverticula. In Modern approach to benign esophageal disease, Bremner CG, DeMeester TR and Peracchia A eds, QMP Inc. St. Louis (Missouri - USA) 1995; 143-55.
18. Spechler SJ. Gastroesophageal Reflux Study Group. Comparison of medical and surgical therapy for complicated gastroesophageal reflux disease in veterans. *N Engl J Med* 1992; 326: 786-92.
19. Stein HJ, DeMeester TR. Who benefits from antireflux surgery? *World J Surg* 1992; 16: 313-19.
20. Peters JH, Kauer WKH, DeMeester TR. Tailored antireflux surgery. In Modern approach to benign esophageal disease, Bremner CG, DeMeester TR and Peracchia A eds, QMP Inc. St. Louis (Missouri - USA) 1995; 57-68.
21. Champault G. Reflux gastroesophagien. Traitement par laparoscopie 940 cas- experience française. *Ann Chir* 1994; 48. 159-64
22. Weerts JM, Dallemagne B, Hamoir F. Laparoscopic Nissen Fundoplication: detailed analysis of 132 patients. *Surg Laparosc Endosc* 1993; 3: 359-64.
23. DeMeester TR, Bonavina L, Albertucci M. Nissen fundoplication for gastroesophageal reflux disease. Evaluation of primary repair in 100 consecutive patients. *Ann Surg* 1986; 204: 9-20.
24. Csendes A, Braghetto I, Henriquez A, Cortes C. Late results of a prospective randomized study comparing forceful dilation and esophagomyotomy in patients with achalasia. *Gut* 1989; 30: 299-304.
25. Parischa PJ, Ravich WJ, Hendrix TR, Sostre S, Jones B, Kalloo AN. Intrasphinteric botulinum toxin for the treatment of achalasia. *N Engl J Med* 1995; 333, 73.
26 Bonavina L, Nosadini A, Bardini R, Baessato M, Peracchia A. Primary treatment of esophageal achalasia. Long-term results of myotomy and Dor fundoplication. *Arch Surg* 1992; 127: 222-7.
27. Rosati R, Fumagalli U, Bona S, Chella B, Peracchia A. A special instrument for a safe and effective esophageal myotomy. *Surg Laparosc Endosc* 1996; 6: 385-7.

28. Benacci JC, Deschamps C, Trastek VF, Allen MS, Daly RC, Pairolero PC. Epiphrenic diverticulum: results of surgical treatment. *Ann Thorac Surg* 1993; 55: 1109-14.
29. Orringer MB. Epiphrenic diverticula: fact and fable. *Ann Thorac Surg* 1993; 55: 1067-8.
30. Altorki NK, Sunagawa M and Skinner DB. Thoracic esophageal diverticula. Why is operation necessary? *J Thorac Cardiovasc Surg* 1993; 105: 260-4.
31. Streitz JM, Glick ME, Ellis FH. Selective use of myotomy for treatment of epiphrenic diverticula. Manometric and clinical analysis. *Arch Surg* 1992; 127: 585-8.
32. A.Peracchia, L.Bonavina, R.Rosati, S.Bona. Thoracoscopic resection of epiphrenic esophageal diverticula. In "Minimally-invasive Surgery of the Foregut" J. Peters, T.R.DeMeester Eds., Quality Medical Publishing Inc. St Louis, 1994: 110-6.
33. Tio TL, Tytgat GNJ, Den Hartog J. Endoscopic ultrasonography for the evaluation of smooth muscle tumors in the upper gastrointestinal tract: an experience with 42 cases. *Gastrointest Endosc* 1990; 36: 342-50.
34. Boyce GA, Sivak MV Jr, Rosch T. Evaluation of submucosal upper gastroeintestinal lesions by endoscopic ultrasound. *Gastrointest Endosc* 1991; 37: 449-54.
35. Akiyama H, Tsurumaru M, Udagawa H, Kajiyama Y. Radical lymph node dissection for cancer of the thoracic esophagus. *Ann Surg* 1994, 220: 364-73.
36. Gossot D, Fourquier O, Celerier M. Thoracoscopic esophagectomy: technique and initial result. *Ann Thorac Surg* 1993; 56: 667-70.
37. Fumagalli U, Rosati R, Bonavina L, Bona S, Chella B, Cioffi U, Montorsi M, Peracchia A. Thoracoscopic dissection of the esophagus: an experimental study and preliminary clinical experience. *Endosurgery*, 1993; 1: 71-4.
38. Collard JM, Lengele B, Otte JB, Kestens PJ. En bloc and standard esofagectomies by thoracoscopy. *Ann Thorac Surg* 1993; 56: 675-9.
39. Descottes B, Valleix D, Sodji M, Thognon Ph, Breuille G. Oesophagectomie sous thoracoscopie. Proceedings XVI Journées Niçoises de Pathologie et Chirurgie Digestive et Video-laparoscopie. Nice, 11-12 février 1993: 4.
40. Azagra JS, Ceuterick M, Goergen M. Thoracoscopy in oesophagectomy for oesophageal cancer. *Br J Surg* 1993; 80: 320-1.
41. McAnena OJ, Rogers J, Williams NS. Right thoracoscopically assisted oesophagectomy for cancer. *Br J Surg* 1994; 81: 236-8.
42. Collard JM. Chirurgie vidéo-endoscopique et cancer de l'oesophage: réflexions. *Chirurgie* 1994-1995; 120: 426-9.
43. Bumm R, Holscher AH, Feussner H, Tachibana M, Bartels H, Siewert JR. Endodissection of the thoracic esophagus. Technique and clinical results in transhiatal esophagectomy. *Ann Surg* 1993; 218: 97-104.
44. Croizier TA, Sydow M, Siewert JR, Braun U. Postoperative pulmonary complication rate and long-term changes in respiratory function following esophagectomy with easophagogastrostomy. *Acta Anaesthesiol Scand* 1992; 36: 10-5.
45. Landrenau RJ, Hazelrigg SR, Mack MJ. Postoperative pain-related morbidity: videoassisted thoracic surgery versus thoracotomy. *Ann Thorac Surg* 1993; 56: 1285-9.

CHAPTER 17

COMPARISON BETWEEN RECTOPEXY BY LAPAROSCOPY AND LAPAROTOMY FOR COMPLETE RECTAL PROLAPSE : CLINICAL AND FUNCTIONAL RESULTS.

PAOLO BOCCASANTA and ALBERTO PERACCHIA

Department of General Surgery and Surgical Oncology ,University of Milan, Milan , Italy

Summary

Purpose The aim of this rectrospective study was to compare functional and clinical results of rectopexy by laparotomy and laparoscopy in 2 homogeneous groups of patients with complete rectal prolapse and fecal incontinence.

Methods Between November 1992 and June 1997, 21 patients underwent abdominal rectopexy. Thirteen patients (Group A) (12 females and 1 male, mean age 52.9 years, range 28-70), and 8 patients (Group B) (8 females, mean age 58.2, range 20-76) were submitted to Well's rectopexy by open technique and laparoscopy respectively, without dividing lateral rectal ligaments. The allocation to each group was done at random. Before the operation a detailed clinical history was collected and patients were studied with inspection and digital examination of the anorectum, proctosigmoidoscopy, pancolonic transit time, dynamic defecography, anorectal manometry and anal electromyography. After the operation all patients underwent perineal physiotherapy, external electric stimulation, and perineal biofeedback. Mean follow-up time was 29.5 months (range 6-54) in Group A and 25.7 months (range 8-45) in Group B patients. Values were compared by Chi square, Mann-Whitney U, and Wilcoxon tests,as appropriate; differences were considered significant at $p<0.05$.

Results In both groups dyschezia and faecal incontinence improved significantly ($p<0.05$) after the operation; basal pressure of anal sphincter, squeezing pressure and recto-anal reflex improved, without significance, and anal-perineal pain was not significantly reduced. In Group B post-operative hospital stay was lower than in Group A, with a sensible reduction of costs.

Conclusion Well's laparoscopic rectopexy produces the same clinical and functional results as laparotomy, with shorter post-operative hospital stay and fewer costs.

Key words: Rectal prolapse; faecal incontinence; laparoscopic colonic surgery; abdominal rectopexy.

Introduction

Complete rectal prolapse is an invalidating disease not only due to the prolapse itself, but also because of associated faecal incontinence [1].
Since 1939, when Pemberton and Stalker [2] described the first abdominal suspension and fixation of the rectum for the treatment of rectal prolapse, many

E. Zanella (ed.), Advances in Abdominal Surgery, 183–191.

techniques have been performed, and many variations of rectal fixation have been described, all involving a mobilization of the rectum and its fixation to the pre-sacral fascia, with different levels of pelvic dissection, with or without division of lateral ligaments. The fixation may be done with sutures, or a mesh of absorbable (Vicryl or Dexon) or non-absorbable (Mersilene, Prolene, Marlex) foreign material.

In a recent review of abdominal rectopexy the recurrence rate was 3.8%, continence improved significantly after operation, particularly in patients under 70 years of age and nulliparous women, and bowel function was generally unchanged after rectopexy. The mean follow-up period was 36.7 months [3].

In 1992 Berman [4], and Senagore [5] in 1993, published the first results of laparoscopic rectopexy.

In the present study we compared 2 groups of patients, similar in age-range, who were submitted to laparotomic and laparoscopic rectopexy respectively for complete rectal prolapse and faecal incontinence.

Patients and methods

Between November 1992 and June 1997, 20 females and 1 male with complete full-thickness rectal prolapse and variable degrees of faecal incontinence, underwent abdominal rectopexy by the same surgical equipe. They ranged in age between 22 and 76 years (average 57.3 years). The patients were allocated at random to be submitted either to open technique or laparoscopy. The size and weight of patients in both groups were similar. Thirteen patients (group A), (12 females and 1 male, mean age 52.9 years, range 28-70), were submitted to Well's [6] laparotomic (Pfannenstiel incision) rectopexy without dividing lateral rectal ligaments, using mersilene in 6 cases and marlex in 7. Eight patients (group B),(8 females, mean age 58.2, range 20-76) underwent Well's stapled laparoscopic rectopexy with marlex. In both groups evacuation habits were studied prior to operation with a questionnaire, as follows:

A = Incontinence degree:

1) anal soiling;
2) loss of liquid matter;
3) loss of solid matter.

B = Frequence of incontinence:

1) less than once a week;
2) more than once a week;
3) daily.

Adding A+B yielded a score of 0 to 6. The same score was used after the operation to evaluate the results [7].

In all patients a full clinical investigation, including inspection and digital examination of the ano-rectum, proctosigmoidoscopy, pancolonic transit time, dynamic defecography, anorectal manometry and anal electromyography, was then performed. No patients had neoplastic or inflammatory bowel disease at proctoscopy. Colonic transit study with radiopaque markers (Sapimed, Alessandria, Italy) was done, as suggested by Hinton and Lennard-Jones [8]. Defecography was performed according to Mahieu [9], with lateral spot films taken at rest, during straining without evacuation, and with forced evacuation. The pathological perineal descent was studied radiologically evaluating the Posterior Rectal Inclination (PRI) (described by the angle between the horizontal plane passing through the end point of the coccyx and the plane passing from the end point of the coccyx to the anorectal junction) at rest, and during maximum evacuation straining. The variation in the PRI (vPRI) was defined as the difference expressed in degrees between these two angles. As described by Costalat and Garrigues [10], the patients were classified in three stages in relation to the PRI and vPRI: stage 1 or solid perineum with PRI at rest < 20 degrees, vPRI < 20 degrees; stage 2 or descending perineum with PRI at rest < 20 degrees, vPRI > 20 degrees; stage 3 or descended perineum with PRI at rest > 20 degrees.

Anorectal manometry was perfomed prior to operation, then 6 and 12 months after rectopexy: resting and squeezing pressures, rectal capacity, rectoanal inhibitory reflex, threshold volume and painful reflex to rectal stretching, were measured with open-ended continuously perfused catheters (infusion rate 1ml/min) and air-filled balloon probes (Beckmann R601, Shiller Park, IL.U.S.A.).

A Medelec MG6 instrument with MCD50 electrode wires (Woking U.K.) (length 50 mm, caliber 0.45 mm) was used to obtain a complete electromyography evaluation of the external sphincter; fine electrode wires were placed percutaneously in the posterolateral commissure 1 cm and 3-4 cm in depth. After the operation all patients underwent perineal physiotherapy, external electrical stimulation, and perineal biofeedback. Values were compared by Chi square, Mann-Whitney U, and Wilcoxon tests, as appropriate; differences were considered significant at $p<0.05$.

Operative Tecnique

All patients underwent conventional pre-operative bowel preparation with a hypertonic saline solution for 24 h prior to surgery, and received routine antibiotic prophylaxis; in all patients nasogastric tubes and urinary catheters were placed after anesthesia induction. All procedures were performed with the patients in the Lloyd-Davis position with a 30° Trendelenburg.

Laparotomy

Laparotomy was performed through a Pfannenstiel incision, and an accurate dissection of the left peritoneum reflexion, the rectovaginal septum, and the posterior mesorectum. Mobilization was extended in the front to the elevator muscles in order to perform a Douglassectomy, at the back to the same level, and laterally to the rectal ligaments to avoid resecting them. A polyphropylene mesh

(10 cm x 6 cm) was fixed to the sacral promontory and to the right and left wall of the rectum, with 3 non-absorbable stitches.

Laparoscopy

Pneumoperitoneum was created by using a standard closed technique for insufflation through a Veress needle, and mantained at 10 to 12 mmHg. The angled scope was inserted through a 10 mm into the umbelical scar and initial inspection was performed. Two other 10 mm trocars were inserted into the left and right iliac fossa and a further 12 mm port was inserted suprapubically. To expose the operative field, the uterus was suspended from the abdominal wall, with a transfixed stitch, and the small bowel was dislocated, from the pelvis to the upper abdomen. By grasping and elevating the middle third of the rectum, the ureter was identified, and the left peritoneal reflexion of the mesorectum was sectioned with coagulation scissors. Dissection was continued at the front in the rectovaginal septum and then to the posterior mesorectum, in the avascular plane between the fascial capsule and the fascia, in order to create a wide retrorectal window. A rectangular polypropylene mesh (10 cm x 6 cm) was then inserted into the peritoneal space through the 12 mm port and fixed to the sacrococcigeal area with an Endo- Hernia stapler; the free lateral margins of the mesh were finally sutured to the rectal lateral wall with non-absorbable interrupted stitches, knotted with intra or extracorporeal techniques. The procedure was completed with peritoneal reapproximation and port sides closure. No drainage was left.

Results

Pre-operative

Five days after ingestion, four patients (50%) of Group A and 1 (12.5%) of Group B, had more than 30% of the radiopaque markers in the left colon.

Eight patients (61.5%) of Group A and 5 (62.5%) of Group B had pathological perineal descent at rest (descended perineum, 3rd degree), 4 (30.8%) of Group A and 2 (25.0%) of Group B during maximum evacuation straining (descending perineum, 2nd degree), and 1 patient of Group A (7.7%) and 1of Group B (13,5%) had a normal perineum (1th degree).

In 10 patients of Group A (77.0%) and in 6 patients of Group B (75.0%), anal sphincter pressure was lower than normal at rest and during contraction.

Fibrillation of recruitment units, due to neurogen suffering with peripheral denervation and reduced voluntary contraction, was found in 11 patients of Group A (84.6%) and in 6 of Group B (75.0%).

Operative

There were no operative deaths and no intra-operative complications in the two groups; in the laparoscopic series no conversion to open technique was necessary.

Post-operative

Mean follow-up was 29.5 months (range 6-54) in Group A and 25.7 months (range 8-45) in Group B patients. Long term results in Group A and B are reported in Tables 1-2.

Dyschezia and faecal incontinence improved significantly in both groups ($p<0.05$), while ano-perineal pain was not significantly reduced. In Group A severe post-operative constipation rose from 15.4% to 38.5% ($p<0.05$). In Group B only 1 patient (12.5%) had severe pre-operative and post-operative constipation.

Table 1. Laparotomic Vs laparoscopic rectopexy for complete rectal prolapse with faecal incontinence: operative results.

	Laparotomic rectopexy (n = 13)	Laparoscopic rectopexy (n = 8)	p*
Operation time (minutes)	190(190-270)	273(190-300)	ns
Hospital stay (days)	9(7-12)	7(5-12)	ns
Return of bowel function (days)	5(4-7)	3(2-5)	ns

Values are expressed as means (Range)
*Mann Whitney U test

Table 2. Comparative clinical long-term results of laparotomic Vs laparoscopic rectopexy for complete rectal prolapse with faecal incontinence.

	Laparotomic rectopexy (n =13)		Laparoscopic rectopexy (n = 8)	
	Pre-operative	Post-operative	Pre-operative	Post-operative
Dyschezia	9(69.2)[a]	3(23.1)[b]	8(100)[c]	1(12.5)[d]
Anal-perineal major pain	4(30.1)	2(15.4)	1(12.5)	1(12.5)
Serious constipation	2(15.4)[e]	5(38.5)[f]	1(12.5)	1(12.5)
Faecal incontinence (score)	34[g]	10[h]	24[i]	9[l]

Values are expressed as number of cases (%).
a vs b, c vs d, e vs f, g vs h, i vs l $p<0.05$ by Chi square test[1]

One year after the laparotomic operation, 1 patient was submitted to subtotal colectomy with cecorectostomy due to subocclusive symptoms; 1 patient had a mucosal recurrence and was submitted to perineal mucosectomy.

In Group B compared to Group A , there was a reduction of post-operative hospital stay, with a non-significant prolongation of the operative time. The return of bowel function was not significantly modified In 1 patient of Group B with persistent dyschezia, a perineal reparation of rectocele was performed 1 year after the first operation,with good results.

Table 3 compares pre-operative and post-operative results of anorectal manometry in both groups.

After operation, basal pressure of anal sphincter, squeezing pressure and recto-anal reflex improved insignificantly in both groups.

The analysis of economic costs [11] of the two procedures is reported in Table 4. Costs of surgical materials were obviously higher in laparoscopy, due to the use of disposable trocars and staplers; nevertheless, the shorter post-operative hospital stay determined a considerable reduction of the total amount of laparoscopic rectopexy (1873$ vs 3369$ in laparotomy). In our department hospitalization costs about 400$ a day.

Table 3. Pre and post-operative results of anorectal manometry in 21 patients submitted to laparotomic rectopexy (Group A-13 patients) and laparoscopic rectopexy, with complete rectal prolapse and faecal incontinence (Group B- 8 patients).

Laparotomic rectopexy - Manometric values	pre-operative	6 months	12 months
Basal Pressure (mmHg)	34.3 (2.4)	42.6(2.1)	47.2 (6.2)
Squeezing pressure (mmHg)	88.7 (4.8)	100.3 (5.2)	97.4 (2.7)
Rectal capacity (ml)	180.3 (3.4)	175.2 (3.1)	170.4 (2.8)
Recto-anal inhibitory reflex (ml)	15.4 (0.9)	16.1 (1.0)	17.3 (0.9)
Threshold volume (ml)	16.2 (0.4)	15.2 (0.9)	14.9 (0.7)
Painful reflex to rectal stretching (ml)	30.6 (1.6)	34.1 (1.4)	30.9 (1.0)
Laparoscopic rectopexy - Manometric values	pre-operative	6 months	12 months
Basal Pressure (mmHg)	32.3 (13.8)	43.6 (11.1)	47.2 (16.3)
Squeezing pressure (mmHg)	87.9 (27.1)	101.3 (30.5)	98.4 (14.9)
Rectal capacity (ml)	180.5 (20.1)	176.2 (18.1)	171.4 (15.2)
Recto-anal inhibitory reflex (ml)	16.4 (4.4)	17.1 (4.6)	15.3 (7.5)
Threshold volume (ml)	16.7 (2.1)	16.2 (4.3)	15.1 (3.4)
Painful reflex to rectal stretching (ml)	31.6 (8.2)	33.1 (7.2)	31.9 (4.9)

Values are expressed as means (SEM) and compared by the Wilcoxon test

Table 4. Analysis of economic costs of laparotomic Vs laparoscopic rectopexy in U.S. dollars (mean/range).

	Laparotomic rectopexy (n = 13)	Laparoscopic rectopexy (n = 8)
Surgical materials	231$	927$
Hospital stay	3600$ (2800-4800)	2800$ (2000-4800)
Total	3369$ (2569-4569)	1873$ (1073-3873)

Discussion

Among possible operations for external rectal prolapse, rectopexy performed with different techniques represents a safe and effective procedure, with very satisfactory results regarding faecal incontinence and dyschezia. In the series of Farouk [12], 91.7 % of the patients became continent of solid and liquid stool within six months after surgery. Actually 78.5% of our patients are still continent.

Apart from the Ripstein operation, the different surgical techniques of rectal fixation to the sacrum demonstrated the same results on bowel transit time. We preferred the Well's technique that is easy and safe, eliminates the problems of stenosis and can be performed by laparoscopy.Unlike Speakman et al. [13], we preserved the lateral rectal ligaments, in order to avoid further nerve injury to the pelvic floor, that is already partially denerved due to the prolapse itself. In our experience ligament preservation did not increase the incidence of prolapse recurrency.

Rectopexy is not advisable for patients with obstinate constipation, due to prolonged colonic transit time with dolicocolon (colonic inertia), or distal constipation due to rectal inertia: the operation could in fact result in a worsening of the colo-recto-anal transit time, and in causing serious chronic constipation. In these patients we prefer a laparoscopic left colon resection [14], or subtotal colectomy. Blatchford et al. [15], reported an increase in constipation from 48% to 71% after suture rectopexy, Mann and Hoffmann from 29% to 47% after extended Ivalon rectopexy [16], and Yoshioka , Heyen and Keighley from 24% to 44% after Marlex mesh rectopexy [17]. In our series (Group A) the increase was from 15.4 % to 38.5%. In Group B only 1 patient had constipation, both prior to and after operation; it was therefore not possible to assess whether laparoscopy may worsen or not pre-operative constipation.

The mechanism of recovery of continence after prolapse surgery has been considerably debated. The exact mechanism of incontinence in such patients appears to be related to inhibition of the internal sphincter and neurogenic damage to the external sphincter. 82.3% of our patients had neurogen suffering revealed by EMG of the external sphincter.

Voluntary contraction of the external sphincter must be carefully evaluated by EMGraphy: if it is reduced, surgical repair of the anatomic defect will improve continence; otherwise, if major neurological impairment is detected, rectopexy will obtain no effect on faecal incontinence, and post-anal repair should be carried out. Farouk studied 49 patients with rectal prolapse and faecal incontinence [18]. They had reduced resting and squeeze pressures, shortened sphincters, prolonged pudendal latencies, and a relatively non-compliant rectum. The recto-anal inhibitory reflex was found in only 5 patients. This would suggest that the internal sphincter is already fully inhibited in patients with rectal prolapse.

As suggested by other Authors [19], the unsatisfactory results regarding anal perineal pain were probably due to pudendal nerve distress in the Alcock channel [20].

The laparoscopic approach to rectopexy provides the recognized advantages of laparoscopic surgery. The surgical technique of laparoscopic rectopexy is the same as in the open procedure, and can be combined with colonic resection, cystopexy [21] and Douglassectomy. Darzy [22] (in 29 cases of laparoscopic stapled rectopexy with marlex without division of lateral ligaments) and Milson [23] (in 20 cases with laparoscopic direct sutured rectopexy) had an average hospital stay of 5 and 6 days respectively, with length of operation from 95' to 180'. Milson reported a 5% recurrence with an average follow-up of 27 months, and two major complications requiring relaparotomies.

Even if a longer follow-up and a larger patient population are required to assess our preliminary results, laparoscopy seems to afford a successfull approach to pelvic floor operations,with shorter hospital stays and lower cost than laparotomy. The good functional results are also due to physiotherapy and external electric and biofeedback stimulation, that we strongly recommend in order to improve functional results, for 6 months after surgery and every time we suspect an alteration of the automatic process of defecation, during the follow-up period.

Conclusion

Laparoscopic rectopexy gives the same clinical and functional results as laparotomy, a shorter hospital stay, and lower costs.

Well's laparoscopic stapled technique with the conservation of rectal lateral ligaments, provides the same results on prolapse and continence as the other rectopexy procedures, after an adequate pelvic floor rehabilitation.

Up till now preservation of lateral ligaments of the rectum have not increased the incidence of prolapse recurrency in our patients.

References

1. Keighley MRB, Fielding JWT, William JA. Results oh Marlex Mesh abdominal rectopexy for rectal prolapse in 100 consecutive patients. *Br J Surg* 1983;70:229-32.
2. Pemberton J, Stalker LK. Surgical treatment of complete rectal prolapse. *Ann Surg* 1939;109:799.
3. Mc Cue JL, Thomson JPS. Clinical and functional results of abdominal rectopexy for complete rectal prolapse. *Br J Surg* 1991;78:921-3.
4. Berman IR. Sutureless laparoscopic rectopexy for procidentia: technique and implications. *Dis Colon Rectum* 1992;35:689-93.
5. Senagore AJ, Luchtefeld MA, Mac Keigan JM. Rectopexy. *Surg Laparosc Endosc* 1993;3:339-43.
6. Wells C. New operation for rectal prolapse. *J R Soc Med* 1959; 52:805-13.
7. Pescatori M, Anastasio G, Bottini C, Mentasti A. New grading and scoring for anal incontinence.Evaluation of 335 patients. *Dis Colon Rectum* 1992; 35:482-7.
8. Hinton JM, Lennard-Jones JE, Young AC. A new method for studying gut transit time using radiopaque markers. *Gut* 1969; 10:842-7.
9. Mahieu P, Pringot J, Bodart P. Defecography. Contribution to the diagnosis of defecation disorders. *Gastrointest Radiol* 1978; 75:623-31.

10. Costalat G, Garrigues JM, Drawed F, Veyrac M, Vernhet J. Rectopexie antero-posterieure pour troubles de la statique rectale: resultats cliniques et radiologiques.Interet de la rectographie numerisée. A propos de trente cas. *Ann Chir* 1989; 43:733-43.
11. Greenhalgh T. Papers that tell you what things cost (economic analyses). *BMJ* 1997; 315:596-9.
12. Farouk R, Duthie GS, Bartolo DCC, Mac Gregor AB. Restoration of continence following rectopexy for rectal prolapse in associated with recovery of the internal anal sphincter electromyogram. *Br J Surg* 1992;79:107-13.
13. Speakman CT, Madden MV, Nicholls RJ, Kamm MA. Lateral ligament division during rectopexy causes constipation but prevents recurrences: results of a prospective, randomized study. *Br J Surg* 1991;78:1431-3.
14. Frykman HM, Goldberg SM. The surgical treatment of rectal procidentia. *Surg Gynecol Obstet* 1969; 129:1225-30.
15. Blatchford GJ, Perry RE,Christiansen MA, Thorson AG. Rectopexy without resection for rectal prolapse. *Am J Surg* 1989;158:574-6.
16. Mann CV, Hoffman C. Complete rectal prolapse:the anatomical and functional results of treatment by extended abdominal rectopexy. *Br J Surg* 1988;75:34-7.
17. Yoshioka K, Heyen F, Keighley MRB. Functional results after posterior abdominal rectopexy for rectal prolapse. *Dis Colon Rectum* 1989;32:835-8.
18. Farouk R, Duthie GS, Mac Gregor AB, Bartolo DCC. Rectoanal inhibition and incontinence in patients with rectal prolapse. *Br J Surg* 1994;81:107-13.
19. Shafik A. Pudendal canal syndrome decompression in the treatment of idiopatic faecal incontinence. *Dig Surg* 1992; 9:265-71.
20. Shafik A. Pudendal canal syndrome. Description of a new syndrome and its treatment.Report of seven cases. *Coloproctology* 1991; 13:102-9.
21. Liu CY. Laparoscopic treatment for genuine urinary stress incontinence. *Clin Obstet Gynecol* 1994; 8:789-98.
22. Darzy A, Henry MM, Guillou PJ, et al. Stapled laparoscopic rectopexy for rectal prolapse. *Surg Endosc* 1995;9:230-6.
23. Milson JW. Current role of laparoscopy in rectal prolapse. Proceedings of The Eighth Annual Colorectal Disease in 1997, Cleveland Clinic Florida - Fort Lauderdale1997;651-7.
24. Wexner SD, Cheope JD, Jose MN Jorge, Heyman S, Jagelman DC. Biofeedback for costipation. *Dis Colon Rectum* 1992; 35:145-50.

CHAPTER 18

RENAL FUNCTION IN PATIENTS WITH ORTHOTOPIC LIVER TRANSPLANTATION.

GIORGIO SPLENDIANI , CARMELA TOZZO, VALENTINA MAZZARELLA , *GIUSEPPE TISONE , FRANCO PISANI , ORESTE BUONOMO, and CARLO UMBERTO CASCIANI

*Department of Surgery, University of Rome "Tor Vergata", Rome, and *CNR, Rome, Italy*

Introduction

Since 1980 the introduction of Cyclosporine (CyA) into clinical practice has broadened the indications for orthotopic liver transplantation (OLT), because of improved patient and graft survival.

Unfortunately, this improvement in patient survival has been accompanied by the frequent occurrence of CyA associated nephrotoxicity [1].

Furthermore, renal dysfunction is a common occurence in patients undergoing OLT; in fact patients with chronic and acute liver disease can manifest the entire spectrum of renal abnormalities (from functional renal impairment to chronic renal failure)[2].

It is well-known that pre-transplant renal impairment contributes significantly to post-transplant morbidity[3]. The association of liver cirrhosis and renal failure (hepato-renal syndrome) is a severe clinical condition associated with a negative prognosis and a mortality rate close to 100%. In such cases liver transplantation or a double transplant, liver-kidney, represents an extreme solution [4].

In this retrospective study we reviewed the course of renal function in a selected group of liver transplant recipients, with normal renal function before and one week after OLT, in order to evaluate the impact of OLT on renal function.

Patients and methods

At our unit between June 1992 and December 1997, we performed 120 liver transplants, of which patients 75 are actually alive, and being followed up in our

E. Zanella (ed.), Advances in Abdominal Surgery, 193–196.

Outpatients' Day Hospital. We selected for study the 26 patients who had received LT at least 6 months previously, with normal renal function prior to operation, and up to a week after (creatinine in the normal range), and good graft function in the observation period. Immunosuppression was based on Cya, prednisolone and azathioprine. Up to March 1996 patients received Sandimmun Cya iv. and orally and subsequently Neoral, from the first post-operative day.
Cyclosporine whole blood levels were monitored by a polyclonal assay (Abbott TDX) and trough blood levels were to be maintained between 350 and 400 ng/ml for up to 4 months, and after from between 200 and 250 ng/ml. Renal function was assessed before and after liver transplantation (months 6,12,24 and 48) by measurements of serum creatinine (tab. 1). Renal failure after LT was defined as serum creatinine which was higher or equal to 1.8 mg/dl in at least three consecutive tests.
Statistical analysis was calculated by the paired t-test.

Results

Our results showed a significative increment of creatinine values 6 months after operation, in comparison with those recorded before and one week after OLT (tab. 1).

Table1.

Pre-LT(a)	7gg (b)	6m (c)	1 a (d)	2 a (e)	3 a (f)	4 a (g)
0.88±0.32	1.00±0.42	1.58±0.45	1.41±0.37	1.52±0.38	1.54±0.35	1.50±0.32

d vs b,c vs b : $P<0.05$
d vs c : NS

Creatinine values recorded in the subsequent observation period did not differ significantly from those recorded during the initial 6 months. None of the patients had creatinine values above 1.8 mg/dl during the observation period.

Discussion

Renal dysfunction often complicates the clinical course of liver transplant recipients [4].
The main topic of this paper was to study renal function in the post-transplant period, in OLT recipients with a normal function before and immediately after the surgical procedure. This selection allowed us to exclude the effects on renal function of concomitant nephropathy and / or surgical complications.

We observed in our patients a significative increase of serum creatinine levels during the first six post-operative months. This may be connected to the higher doses and serum levels of Cya in the first months after transplant. Subsequently, we noted that the significative increase of creatinine values observed at six months after OLT remained stable during the next period (12,24,36 and 48 months). This could be explained by the usual improvement of renal function after a successful liver transplant, because of the normalization of venous splancnic circulation, with the disappearance of porto-systemic shunts and vasodilator factors[5,6].
The use of CyA is associated with an increment of creatinine values and changes in renal histology, as is shown by many studies on human and animal models[5,7]. CyA causes a reduction of GFR and consequently creatinine clearance, induces tubular changes and arterial hypertension, increases body weight and causes hypercalcemia [8].
The true mechanism of CyA is not well-known. Actually the pathogenesis of CyA nephrotoxicity seems to be due to the vasoconstrictive effects on renal circulation, followed by interstitial fibrosis and vascular sclerosis [9]. In a study conducted on heart and liver transplant recipients, Falkenhaim demonstrated that the histological damage of the kidney increases in relation to the time of exposure to CyA and the total dose of CyA received [10].
During the use of CyA an increase of arachidonic acid metabolism, prostanoid urinary elimination and cytochines release has been observed [11]. A temporary increase of the novel vasoconstrictor peptide, endothelin, that can contribute to the hemodynamic alterations caused by CyA [12,13], has also been recently demonstrated.
Our results agree with those reported by Gonwa [14] et al., who showed that the trend of renal function after the third year in OLT recipients is to remain stable without further deterioration.
However, the histological changes due to CyA can evolve, inducing a chronic deterioration of renal function.
Actually at our unit there are ongoing trials to obtain the optimization of CyA dosage, and to test newer immunosuppressants in order to reduce the long-term side effects of chronic use of CyA.

References

1. Iwatsuki S, Esquivel CO, Klintmain GB, Gordon RD, Shaw BW, Starzl TE. Nephrotoxicity of Cyclosporine in liver transplantation. *Transplant Proc* 1985; 17:S 191-5.
2. Vaamonde CA. Selected renal and electrolyte abnormalities in liver disease. *AKF* Nephrol Lett 1992;9:13 -28.
3. Rimola A, Gavaler JS, Schade RR, El-Lankany S, Starzl TE, Van Thiel DH. Effect of renal impairment on liver transplantation. *Gastroenterology* 1987; 93:148-56.
4. Hauters P, De Hemptine B, Carlier M, Ottobrelli A, Delaby J, Balducci G, Kestens PJ. Long-term analysis of glomerular filtration rate and hypertension in adult liver transplant recipients treated with cyclosporine A. *Transplant Proc* 1991; 23: 1458-9.

5. Tegress AM, Doorenbos BM, Minderhound JM, Donker AJ. Prospective serial renal function studies in patients with non-renal disease treated with cyclosporine A. *Transplant Proc* 1988; 20(suppl 2): 390-3.
6. Ayres R, Ismail T, Angrisani L, Buckels J, Elias E, McMaster P, Neuberger J. Long-term renal function in renal transplantation. *Transplant Proc* 1991; 23: 1469 -70.
7. English J, Evan A, Houghton DC, Bennett WM. Cyclosporine-induced acute renal dysfunction in the rat : evidence of arteriolar vasoconstriction with preservation of tubular function. *Transplantation* 1987; 44: 135-41.
8. Mihantsch MJ, Thiel G, Ryffel B. Cyclosporine nephrotoxicity. *Adv Nephrol* 1988; 17 : 303 - 20.
9. Wheatley HC, Datzman M, Williams JW, Miles DE, Hatch FE. Long-term effects of cyclosporine on renal function in liver transplant recipients. *Transplantation* 1987 ; 43 : 641 - 7.
10. Falkenhain ME, Cosio FG, Sedmak DD. Progressive histologic injury in kidneys from heart and liver transplant recipients receiving cyclosporine. *Transplantation* 1996; 62: 364-70.
11. Mason J, Muller-Schweinitzer E, Dupont M. Cyclosporine and the renin-angiotensin system. *Kidney Int* 1991; 32 : S28.
12. Bennett WM, Elzinga L, Kelley V. Pathophysiology of cyclosporine neprhrotoxicity: role of eicosanoids. *Transplant Proc* 1988; 20: 628-33.
13. Coffman TM, Carr DR, Yarger WE, Klotman PE. Evidence that renal prostaglandin and thromboxane production is stimulated in chronic cyclosporine.
14. Gonwa TA, Morris CA,Goldstein RM, Husberg BS, Klintmalm GB. Long term survival and renal function following liver transplantation in patients with and without hepatorenal syndrome. Experience in 300 patients. *Transplantation* 1991; 51:428-30.

CHAPTER 19

NATIONAL SURVEY OF PRIMARY SCLEROSING CHOLANGITIS : AN EMERGENT INDICATION FOR NEW THERAPEUTIC STRATEGIES.

MARCO BACOSI, MARCO DELLE MONACHE, FRANCESCA RUSSO and GIOVANNI L. RICCI

Department of Gastroenterology, University of Rome "La Sapienza", Rome, Italy

Summary

Primary sclerosing cholangitis is a scattered, fibrosis causing stenosis of the whole biliary tree, which follows the progressive atrophy of the biliary epithelium for reasons yet unknown. A variable type of immunological reaction is present as well as a genetical component as is confirmed by both histotype and the report of this disease occurring at a very young age. The disease is nearly always associated to an IBD (Inflammatory Bowel Disease), usually ulcerative colitis, and both represent a risk for the development of cancer.

The progression of the disease may be slowed down, and there is no relationship between the clinical outcome of ulcerative colitis, and primary sclerosing cholangitis; orthotopic liver transplantation is the definite cure, and immunosuppressive treatment may be beneficial for the IBD.

Introduction

Primary sclerosing cholangitis (PSC) is the fibrosing inflammation around the bile ducts which follows the alteration and atrophy of bile duct cells. The reasons for the begining of this process in the biliocytes is totally unknown.

The pathology of inflammation is somehow typical of this disease and allows its identification [1]; a comparison with chronic non-suppurative, destructive cholangitis [2,3] and chronic active hepatitis [4,6] has focused the attention that the mechanism is not a lympho-plasmacellular aggression toward target cells, but rather a lymphocyte reaction elicited by damaged biliocytes [7,8].

The apparent rarity of primary sclerosing cholangitis is worsened by: a) the lack of a specific serological marker [9], b) the clinical predominance of the often associated inflammatory bowel disease, c) the cholestatic pattern overlapping with that of other affections [10].

E. Zanella (ed.), Advances in Abdominal Surgery, 197–221.

The term was used for the first time by Delbet in 1924 [11] to depict a cholestatic syndrome with narrowing and obliteration of bile ducts; indeed the term is appropriate for a certain range of diseases in which the fibrosing inflammation of bile ducts of different sizes, causes a definite similarity to the clinical course of cancer, infections, morphological abnormalities forming either from drug injury or congenital, and stones in the biliary tree. In this syndromic situation clinical variants are due to the localization, not to the etiology [2,12].
The term primary is reserved for the syndrome often associated to an inflammatory bowel disease, in which some of the above etiologies have been ruled out, although stones, strictures and cholangiocarcinoma may be rather common consequences. Primary sclerosing cholangitis is not a consequence of an intestinal disease, but may share with some common mechanisms, e.g. ischemia [13,14], activation of Th1 lymphocytes [15,17]; in this sense idiopathic would probably be a better term.

Clinical epidemology

About one-hundred-ten cases of primary sclerosing cholangitis were reported in medical literature up till the middle of the seventies: a very rapid increase in the number of cases has been reported by many Authors, who described the radiological features of the disease and recognized the intrahepatic localization.
The perspective search for the disease has changed its geographical and racial distribution: it is now well acknowledged that primary sclerosing cholangitis exists in African [18,19] and Asiatic [20,21] countries. We do not yet know whether the clinical pattern, associated to IBD, stones, infections and cholangiocarcinoma is similar in Western countries [22,29]. It is feasible that environmental factors play a role as well as genetic factors [30,31].

Source of data
Data on the prevalence of the disease come from different sources, and are not comparable: 1) Gastroenterology Units (G.U) and institutions devoted to the management of inflammatory bowel diseases (IBD) where the diagnostic algorithm is prompted by the finding of an increased serum alkaline phosphatase (sALP); 2) referral Centers for liver disease. None of these is capable of assessing the prevalence of the disease and all have a strong selection bias.
In the first type of institution, although about 1% of patients with IBD have a biochemical abnormality, all portal and/or peribiliary lesions found either in liver biopsy, or surgical, wedge specimens, are regarded as primary sclerosing cholangitis, or early lesions of the disease [32,33]. The term pericholangitis has been misleadingly used to indicate any edema and inflammation around the bile

ducts, thus causing erroneous reports on the association of these diseases [25,27,34,37].

In the Liver Centers the need for staging the disease has caused some confusion between intrahepatic lesions, and hepatic consequences of cholestasis due to stenosing fibrosis of the large ducts [38]. The improvement of hepatic histology after endoscopic or surgical treatment of large duct stenosis [39,42], can only be explained as a relief of the bile stasis, not remission of PSC [43]. In the same Centers the association PSC-IBD is also lower than in G.U. departments.

Occurence of disease

In Western countries PSC is thought to show a prevalence of 0.2-1/100.000; the inconsistence of this datum in different series is due either to the type of Center, or the population sampled. In the North-European series the ages of patients go from 8 to 80 years [23], so suggesting the presence of subgroups, with a preponderance of different determinants for the evolution of the disease: the younger group has strong genetic connections, and a more rapid evolution towards liver insufficiency and orthotopic liver transplantation [44,45].

The Italian National survey [22] allows a statistical projection of 0.5 cases/100.000 equally spread all over the Country, with a slowly progressive course.

The other series do not permit a true evaluation of prevalence, either because they are not perspective studies, or they come from referral Centers for Liver disease, and are the result of statistical overcalculation. The prevalence in United States has been approached by the frequent association of PSC to ulcerative colitis (in the Mayo Clinic series of about 70%) [35] and a reported prevalence of PSC in ulcerative colitis of 2.4 to 7.5% [26,27]: using this proportion and the prevalence of ulcerative colitis ranging from 40 to 225 case /100.000 in different countries [25,27,29,46] the same Authors came up with a figure of 2-7 PSC cases/100.000. The estimate almost correlates with an epidemiological study from Sweden, which reported a prevalence of ulcerative colitis and PSC of respectively 171 and 6.3 cases /100.000. American and North European Authors claim that these data may be underestimateed since PSC can occur in patients with normal sALP. The issue is due to remain unresolved for a long time as the diagnosis is always initiated by an increased sALP, since other laboratory tests produce a large proportion of false positives, and confirmation is rather invasive, i.e. liver biopsy and ERCP. It is possible that a wider use of NMR cholangiography could increase the number of investigated patients, and so change these figures.

PSC is a disease in young men (about 70%) with a mean age of 39 at the time of diagnosis; the reason for age and sex distribution is unknown [19], while the proportion of complications, cirrhosis, portal ipertension and IBD is the same for both sexes.

Association with other disease

While the association with IBD has been known for a long time, an increasing number of diseseas have been found to be associated with PSC, and the continuous search is greatly linked to the fact that the pathogenesis of PSC is largely undefined. Some of the associated diseases are autoimmune or have a disfunction of a specific line of immunocytes, thus supporting the hypothesis that PSC is an autoimmune disease [69] (Tab.1).

Table 1. Diseases associated and related with PSC. Associated diseases may be a consequence of cholestasis and/or impaired biliary secretion, either flow or composition; related to disorders in which the undelying mechanisms (inflammatory, interleukine production, Th differentiation, etc.) might share a common path with PSC.

Associated Diseases
- Chronic pancreatitis
- Gallbladder disease
- Intra-abdominal adenopathy

Related Diseases
- Inflammatory Bowel Disease
- Celiac disease
- Rheumatoid arthritis
- Retroperitoneal fibrosis
- Peyronie's disease
- Thyroiditis
- Bronchiectasis
- Sjögren's syndrome
- Systemic sclerosis
- Autoimmune chronic active hepatitis
- Membranous nephropathy
- Lupus erytematosus
- Pseudotumor of the orbit
- Vasculitis
- Autoimmune hemolytic anemia
- Immune thrombocytopenic purpura
- Angioblastic Lymphadenopathy
- Histiocystosis X
- Cystic fibrosis
- Eosinophilia

Chronic pancreatitis [47,48], intra-abdominal adenopathy [49], and diseases of the gallbladder including cholecystitis and gallstones [50,51], have also been reported as common occurences during PSC: they might be regarded as consequences of the altered transit through the biliary tree and of adifferent localization of the disease.

The association of PSC with IBD is by far the strongest and the one known about for a longer time: it was reported in the sixties by Mistilis [52], Warren [53] and Thorpe [54]. Relatively recent studies reported an association of IBD between 54% and 100% in most patients having ulcerative colitis.

The situation in our Country has been investigated by the Italian PSC Group which reported an association of 54% [22], and this will be dealt with in section 2. The association with Crohn's disease has been reported in up to 13% of patients [55,58], and in 10.3% in the Italian series: in all these patients there was a colonic localization, and an association with terminal ileitis alone has never been reported [9,22,58,60].

Among the disease which might share a common path in the dysfunction of T-lymphocytes some interest has been raised by the association with celiac sprue [61,63] and sarcoidosis [64]. The relation to Hodgking lynphomas [65] and eosinophilia [66] might have something in common with the association to vasculitis [67,68]: the inflammation of the arteriolar peribiliary plexus may produce an ischemic disease of bile ducts followed by inflammation and fibrosis.

Screening for PSC

The opportunity of screening for PSC in the general population arises from the consideration that this is a discase wich is easily controlled at its beginning, with a rather innocuous therapy, in terms of known side effects. The cost of screening could thus be weighed against the costly expenditure of therapies in advanced stages.

Serum alkaline phosphatase appears to be the only adequate test for screening, and the specificity and sensitivity changes at the risk of the investigated population: the diagnostic algorithm always starts with an altered sALP. In a group of IBD [9] the accuracy of sALP is high; in other selected populations - e.g. relatives of patients, young males - the test retains its specificity and sensitivity, although the risk of disease is slightly higher than in the general population.

Unfortunately other tests which really describe the disease [81,83,85], and are prognostic for the onset of complications or worsening in follow-up [80], do not appear as good for screening. The use of antineutrophil cytoplasmic antibodies, with a typical perinuclear staining pattern (pANCA), is expensive, describes the disease [70,71,73,75], and is not able to reveal a population group at risk [74,76]. Any type of screening test would be able to identify an individual at risk,but the diagnosis needs however to be confirmed by more invasive tests, such as retrograde cholangio-pancreatography (ERCP) and/or liver biopsy [77,78]. The relative importance of these two tests is minor when a diagnosis should be issued, and even less than during follow up of any patient with well-established diagnosis. An additional problem is in the ability to reveal the disease at its very beginning, i.e. before the destruction of bile ducts has produced cholestasis.

With all these drawbacks, a promising screening test, at least for selected populations, is cholescintigraphy: recent achievements can show focal areas of radioactivity within the hepatic area, likely to be due to stenosis and dilatation of the biliary tree [79].

Performances of different diagnostic tests

The diagnosis of PSC is multidisciplinary and the performance of a given test strongly depends on a proper diagnostic algorithm. The sensitivity and specificity of sALP are respectively 57% and 64% in the general population and 88% and 91% in patients with IBD [9,22]. On the other hand in a group of random patients with raised sALP the chances of finding patients with PSC can be calculated as less than 1%. Once the disease has been morphologically demonstrated, the role of sALP becomes less important: at the beginning of the natural history of PSC, with a well-functioning parenchima, sALP is actively synthetised; at a later stage this does not happen any more, and the impairment of bile secretion is better described by the serum concentration of bilirubin.

Gamma-glutamil-transpeptidase is too sensitive and of less specificity: it must be confined to define the source of sALP in questionable situations. Serum transaminases describe the damage of hepatocytes as a consequence of cholestasis, and their role is important in the later stages of the disease.

Cholangiography, in particular ERCP, reveals the presence of an extraparenchimal PSC: the prevalence of altered morphology, and/or specific changes in the presence of other risk factors (male, young age, IBD, high sALP), is not known. The disease could be better observed in the wall of bile ducts, even before the development of a stenosis and narrowing of lumen: it is possible that further refinements in the resolution of NMR-cholangiography will identify the disease , by overcaming several problems due to: a) scattering of lesions, b) presence of micro and macro-lesions detected at the same time; c) detection of risk factors predicting the evolution of the disease, besides the non-invasivity and good reproducibility of the test.

Natural history of primary sclerosing cholangitis

The great difficulty encountered in tracking the natural history of PSC lies in its rarity. Indeed several Authors have identified the disease at different stages, ranging from the very odd "pericholangitis" to a cholangiocarcinoma in the esplanted liver, but links between the different stages were missing. The task was partially achieved through different steps: the first was to identify the variables determining the course of disease. The so-called prognostic variables taken into account were: age, presence or absence of IBD, hepatomegaly, splenomegaly, serum bilirubin, serum alkaline phosphatase, haemoglobin, hepatic histological stage, and the extension of biliary system involvement at cholangiography [90,94,100]. The next step consisted in using a statistical approach according to Kaplan-Meyer analysis, to assess the natural history of the disease [95,99].

The national survey of PSC

Sixteen Italian Centers have recently reported retrospective data regarding 117 unselected patients with PSC,controlled between January 1973 and December 1993, using a mixed type of record, of fixed and free format. The time of onset was either from the presence of symptoms, signs, or abnormality of laboratory data, and the definition of asymptomatic and symptomatic was based on the association of laboratory and physical signs. Among those regarded as specific were: fatigue, pruritus, jaundice, abdominal pain, weight loss, anorexia, nausea, vomiting, fever, hepatomegaly, skin hyperpigmentation, xanothomas, arthralgia, gastrointestinal bleeding, ascites and/or acute cholangitis.

Liver biopsy was also performed within one year from presentation in 64 patients, and repeated in 45 during follow-up. The following features were assessed: periductal inflammation and fibrosis, bile ductular proliferation, portal inflammation with lymphocytic aggregation and fibrosis, fibrous-obliterative cholangitis, piecemeal necrosis, paucity of bile ducts and their disappearance, cirrhotic nodules.

At presentation there was a wide range of ages (from 12 to 74 years, average 35 years); most were males (73 patients, 62,4% of total), younger than females (33.6 $\pm$ 12.6 vs.38.3 $\pm$ 13.9 years). Thirty five patients (29.9%) were asymptomatic at presentation; of those who were symptomatic, the most common feature was fatigue (40,2%), while both pruritus and jaundice were recorded in 30.8% of the cases. Hepatomegaly was detected in 34.2% of patients. Less common symptoms were anorexia (17.9%), abdominal pain (16.2%) fever (12.8%) and weight loss (10.3%). Disease complications, such as acute cholangitis, ascites and gastrointestinal bleeding, were rarely the first manifestation (1.7 – 5.1%).

Abnormal levels of sALP were observed in all but two cases at presentation, with an average of four times the upper normal value for the whole group. Serum transaminases showed abnormal levels in the great majority of patients, with an average of three to four times the upper normal value. The serum level of total bilirubin was increased (>19 mmol/l) in 52.4% of the cases, and the mean was 50 mmol/l for 103 patients in whom it was reported. Total serum cholesterol was abnormal (>6.22 mmol/l)in 47.9% of patients (mean 6.99 mmol/l). Impairment of albumin synthesis of prothrombin activity was not common at first observation (31..1% and 10.8% of the patients, respectively), and neither was anaemia (17,2%) or thrombocytopenia (15.5%).

Cholangiograms were recorded in 98 patients, mainly as ERCP (n=93): 46% showed both intrahepatric and extrahepatic disease, 28% had extrahepatic disease only, and 26% had PSC confined to the intrahepatic biliary system.

Multifocal short annular narrowings were the most common feature, found in 44.9% of both intrahepatic and extrahepatic bile ducts. Band-like strictures were present both in the extrahepatic (33.7%) and in the intrahepatic (25.5%) biliary

tree; localized dilated segments were found in the intrahepatic (27.6%) and in the extrahepatic (15.3%) biliary system. In four patients (4.1%) diverticular-like outpouchings were detected in the extrahepatic bile ducts.
Pathology showed the following distribution in terms of severity: 15.6% of cases were stage I, 20.3 stage II, 46.9% stage III, and 17.2% stage IV. Portal inflammation (67,2%), portal fibrosis (51.6%) and bile ductular inflammation (46.9%) were the most frequent hystological features, while the diagnostic gold standard – fibrous obliterative cholangitis – and characteristic bile ductular proliferation occurred in 35.9% of patients. Other features related to progression of histological damage, such as paucity of bile ductules (34.4%) piecemeal necrosis (17.2%) and cirrhotic nodules (17.2%), were less commonly reported. Symptomatic patients were more frequently classified as stage III-IV(74.3%) compared with asymptomatic patients (57.9%); this difference was not statistically significant, but resulted in an odds ratio of 2:1.

Association with IBD and other diseases
The close association between PSC and IBD has been recognized for several years, and studies over the last decade have reported a 54-100% prevalence of IBD in PSC [1,90,92,112,113]. In the Italian survey the prevalence of IBD was about 54% and ulcerative colitis was seen in only 36% of total patients (Tab.2).

Table 2. Prevalence of IBD in several reported series.
IBD = inflammatory bowel disease; **CUC** = chronic ulcerative colitis; **CD** = Crohn's disease.

Study	N	IBD	CUC	CD
		%	%	%
Wiesner and La Russo, 1980	50	54	48	6
Chapman et al., 1980	29	72	72	0
Sivak et al., 1981	13	85	77	8
Lebovics et al., 1987	38	61	47	13
Helzberg et al., 1987	53	62	58	4
Aadland et al., 1987	45	100	82	13
Stockbrugger et al., 1989	44	98	82	5
Wiesner et al.,1989	174	71	--	--
Rabinowitz et al., 1990	66	71	59	12
Fausa et al., 1989	66	98	78	13
Delle Monache et al., 1992	37	91	81	10
Okolicsanyi et al., 1996	117	53	36	10
Totals / mean	732	76	65	9

It seems there is a rather obvious bias:the rate of IBD was understimated since endoscopy or barium enema were not performed in patients asymptomatic for the presence of an intestinal disease. In another series from the Mediterranean area ulcerative colitis was detected in 44.2% of cases [25].

Ulcerative colitis (35.9%) was more common than Crohn's disease (10.3%). In nine patients (7.7%) a non-specific non-ulcerative form of chronic colitis was reported. IBD activity was mainly moderate (52.2%), and was severe in only 13% of cases.

Among other associated diseases (Tab.3) chronic pancreatitis and chronic thyroiditis were seen in five and three PSC patients respectively, whereas sarcoidosis, breast cancer and scleroderma were all seen in one individual. In the remaining 48 patients entering the survey (41%) no associated pathologies were reported.

Table 3. Prevalence of associated and related diseases in the Italian Survey for PSC. One hundreed and seventeen patients have been repored by 16 Centers.

	n	%
Chronic ulcerative colitis	42	35.9
Crohn's disease	12	10.3
Chronic non-ulcerative colitis	9	7.7
Chronic pancreatitis	5	4.3
Chronic thyroiditis	3	2.6
Sarcoidosis	1	0.8
Breast cancer	1	0.8
Scleroderma	1	0.8
No associated disease	48	41.0

Factors influencing the course of IBD

For many years it has been believed that there was no relationship between the clinical course of PSC and IBD, or even an inverse correlation: once the colitis retreads towards remission the liver disease flares up.

In the Italian series no significant difference was found in survival, among patients with or without manifest IBD, or according to distribution of biliary tract disease in agreement with data from other groups [90,114].

According to one European study patients with ulcerative colitis and PSC underwent milder course than those with IBD alone, under the same maintenance tratment for the colonic disease: patients with ulcerative colitis were hospitalized because of significantly more frequent colonic activity ($p<0.02$) [115]. No difference was recorded in the number of patients undergoing colectomy in the two groups.

A retrospective review of 24 records of patients with IBD and PSC who underwent colectomy at the Cleveland Clinic, showed that the cirrhotic stage of the disease was a significant risk factor for post-operative death [143].

The treatment for PSC was evaluated for effects on IBD in a group of 35 patients randomly allocated to cyclosporin or placebo: a remission or a mild course of colitis was present in 94% of patients under cyclosporin vs. 60% in the placebo group [150]. The number of episodes of recurrence of both diseases was also significantly decreased.

An analysis of factors influencing the course of IBD was also performed in 55 patients who underwent orthotopic liver transplantation for PSC [149]: patients who had severe acute rejection and 5 patients who had recurrent PSC were younger at the time of diagnosis of IBD. Regarding the intestinal problem the younger age was a risk factor for a worse outcome of IBD after transplantation.

Analysis of survival and risk factors

The conflicting results concerning the assessment of prognostic variables in PSC are largely due to their heterogeneity: data describing cholestasis may be different from those relative to hepatic failure, and the presence of the latter may affect the former. The presence of IBD and malabsorption/malnutrition may change the clinical pattern by increasing the importance of certain variable.

In several studies the following independent risk factor of death/transplantation were considered in PSC: age [93,94,99,100], hepatomegaly [90,91], splenomegaly [94,99], presence of IBD [93], serum level of bilirubin and ALP [94], haemoglobin, histological stage, anti-neutrophil cytoplasmic antobodies [86,101,102], and association with HLA DR4 [103].

In the Italian survey 91 patients had an average follow-up, from time of presentation to the last updates of 4 years (range 6 months-20 years). Fifteen (16.3%) of the 91 patients underwent liver transplantation or died of liver disease. Liver transplantation was performed in 10 patients (11%) at an average,of 4 years after presentation (range 3-12 years). There were 5 deaths in the series, which occurred after an average of 5.5 years (range 2-13 years): 3 by cholangiocarcinoma, 1 by variceal bleeding and another by toxic megacolon.

The survival curve obtained from Kaplan-Meyer analysis gives extimated survivals at 5 years and 10 years as 88.4% and 74,4%, respectively: average survival time could not be extimated because the proportion of patients surviving remained more than 50% when all liver deaths and liver transplantation had occurred.

The univariate analysis, the log-rank test and the multivariate analysis on the Cox proportional hazards model, points to six features as risk for the poorest prognosis: low haemoglobin, raised AST, high cholesterol, total bilirubin, albumin and age.

The 74.4% estimated survival at 10 years is a result with several possibilities of bias. One is the time of onset of PSC defined as the time of first symptom or first biochemical abnormality, while the actual cholangiographic definition could have been made years later (lead time bias). A second problem is linked to the fact that in some patients (16.2%) PSC had been diagnosed as small duct disease on the basis of liver biopsy, without the classical cholangiographic findings (lead investigational bias). A third one is the difference in patient selection and disease characteristics of any multicenter study.

Treatment

The first decision is related to whether any therapeutic intervention should be made. The goals of therapy should be clearly identified: treatment should be directed ether towards symptoms, complications, or the underlying hepatobiliary disease.

It is totally unknown whether any treatment should be established for the asymptomatic patient with mild liver test abnormalities and early disease on liver biopsy; prognosis is reasonably good, no established specific therapy is available, and the decision to use ursodiol, (although one which does not rceibly involves the physician), should be weighed against the increased prevalence of colonic carcinoma in these patients.

Therapy for symptoms and complications

Complications which are relatively specific for PSC include: recurrent cholangitis and bacteraemia, dominant strictures and cholangiocarcinoma.

Patients with recurrent episodes of cholangitis without dominant strictures should be treated with broad-spectrum antibiotics as needed. Prophylactic antibiotics are favoured in some patients with frequent episodes of cholangitis, but the efficacy of this approach has not been firmly established.

Patients may develop dominant strictures in the biliary tract, which can lead to rapid increases in serum bilirubin levels,wich account for recurrent episodes of cholangitis, and precipitate or aggravate pruritus. Dilatation of these strictures in the symptomatic patient is reasonable, particularly in patients with non-cirrhotic disease; depending upon their location, a transhepatic or endoscopic approach with or without stent placement may be useful. Indeed, recent data of the transhepatic approach in symptomatic patients with PSC and dominant strictures suggest that balloon dilatation is very effective in alleviating pruritus and diminishing the frequency of secondary cholangitis.

Cholangiocarcinoma develops perhaps in 10 to 15 per cent of patients with PSC. The treatment of a suspected or established cholangiocarcinoma superimposed on PSC is complicated, and is currently being evolved. If the cholangiocarcinoma is surgically resectable, and the patient is not candidate for liver transplantation, an attempt at surgical resection would seem reasonable. Alternatively, if the cholangiocarcinoma is not surgically resectable, or if it is but the patient has advanced liver disease, consideration should be given to orthotopic liver transplantation, although results have been poor. The reason for this might be the

relatively early onset of cancer in PSC: the discovery of a cholangiocarcinoma in explanted livers without any sign of a complicating cancer is constant.
Pruritus and fat-soluble vitamin deficiencies are common problems in patients with PSC; conventional approaches to management of these problems, which will not be reviewed here, are reasonable. Also, when complications such as variceal bleeding develop, appropriate intervention such as sclerotherapy should be considered.

Surgical approach
An aggressive surgical approach in the treatment of PSC itself, using a variety of procedures for internal or external biliary drainage has been proposed; no controlled trials have, however, been performed. Such procedures might provide transient and symptomatic benefit in the occasional patient with jaundice and pruritus secondary to a dominant stricture of the common bile or common hepatic duct. There is absolutely no evidence that any of these procedures will alter the natural history of PSC which seems to be a disease of the whole biliary tract, and when letal because of parenchimal failure. Many patients already have cirrhosis at the time of operation and this will not be affected by improving biliary drainage. It seems more reasonable to consider biliary tract reconstructive procedures in the same category as balloon dilatation, i.e. as palliative procedures to alleviate symptoms, but which are unlikely to affect the natural history of the disease. Unfortunately, only limited and uncontrolled published data are currently available to allow confident evaluation of the role of biliary tract reconstructive procedures in the treatment of the underlying liver disease in PSC.
Some workers have suggested that proctocolectomy in a patient with PSC and chronic ulcerative colitis may favourably affect the hepatobiliary disease. This is an important issue, not only because beneficial treatment for PSC is needed, but because a proctocolectomy in a patient with PSC and chronic ulcerative colitis may be associated with considerable morbidity. Moreover, proctocolectomy for the latter disease with a conventional or continent ileostomy results in the development of varices around the ostomy stoma in at least 25% of patients with PSC. In nearly 50% of these patients, major and often life-threatening bleeding occurs from these varices. A recently published study in patients with PSC and chronic ulcerative colitis, which evaluated the effects of proctocolectomy on progression of clinical, biochemical, cholangiographic and hepatic histological features demonstrated that a new onset of complications, serial changes in biochemical tests, histological progression of liver biopsy, and survival, were not affected by proctocolectomy. It was concluded from the study that proctocolectomy for chronic ulcerative colitis is not beneficial for PSC in patient with both diseases. Clearly, however, if a patient with PSC and chronic ulcerative colitis demonstrates colitic indications for proctocolectomy, such as rectal bleeding,

stricture formation, or intractability, a proctocolectomy should be considered.
In contrast, it seems reasonable to treat symptomatic cholelithiasis or choledocholithiasis surgically in some patients with PSC, even though the presence of underlying parenchymal disease may result in increased operative morbidity and mortality.
In some patients with PSC and choledocholithiasis, particularly if they have had a cholecystectomy, endoscopic sphincterotomy may be preferable to surgical choledocholithotomy. Other forms of non-surgical treatment for cholelithiasis, such as direct solvent or oral dissolution agents and extracorporeal shock wave lithotripsy, remain to be evaluated in patients with PSC and cholelithiasis.

Medical approach
Medical approaches for the treatment of parenchimal disease in PSC have included the use of cupriuretic, immunosuppressive, antifibrogenic, and choleretic agents. Unfortunately, no medical therapy has been shown to induce complete clinical, biochemical, radiological, and histological remission [118,119].
The finding of elevated hepatic copper levels in PSC, and early reports showing apparent biochemical improvement induced by D-penicillamine in primary biliary cirrhosis, another chronic cholestatic liver disease with many similarities to PSC, suggested a similar therapeutic trial.
In a randomized prospective double-blind trial, 39 patients received penicillamine (250 mg, three times a day), and 31 received a placebo [117]. Although a predictable decrease in levels of hepatic copper was achieved, there was no beneficial effect on disease progression or on overall survival. Progressive symptoms and pathology progression were similar in both groups. Moreover the development of major side-effects led to permanent discontinuation of penicillamine in 21 per cent of the patients taking the drug.
A variety of uncontrolled studies on small numbers of patients have assessed the effect of immunosuppressive agents including prednisone, azathioprine, and, most recently, cyclosporin A. Corticosteroids have been used both topically [124] and systematically [125,128] in several small studies in PSC. A small controlled trial of nasobiliary lavage with corticosteroids versus placebo was recently reported; the results were negative [124]. Uncontrolled observation in a small number of patients with marked inflammatory activity in liver biopsy, has shown good responses to orally-administered corticosteroids. In one study, 7/10 patients with PSC showed objective biochemical improvement and some beneficial effect on liver histology while receiving long-term corticosteroid therapy [125].
Azathioprine was used in at least two instances without apparent benefit [131,153].
Recently, use of low dose methotrexate has been reported in two patients with PSC; in this small study, methotrexate therapy was associated with an

improvement in biochemical studies, apparent stabilization of bile duct scarring and improvement in liver histology [126]. More data are now available on this therapy, alone or in combination with ursodiol [134,142]: the drug should however only be used in controlled trials till more data is available.

Cyclosporin, which inhibits the production of interleukin-2 by T lymphocytes resulting in decreased T-lymphocyte activation and proliferation, is currently under investigation in several centres in double-blind, controlled trials [140]. Results are quite good, both alone or in combination with ursodiol and several papers and abstracts are in print.

The use of colchicine is based on encouraging data concernig in its primary biliary cirrhosis [139]. Whether the apparent biochemical benefit will be sustained and whether this drug will prevent histological progression and improve survival in PSC or other chronic liver diseases must await results of controlled trials.

The potential benefit of ursodeoxycholic acid in the treatment of chronic liver diseases [130,133,137] is based on its aspecific effects on membrane fluidity, involving ribosomes turnover and alkaline phosphatase production, expression of antigens and epitopes from different sources on plasmamembranes, etc.

Ursodiol has a proven, good effect on primary biliary cirrhosis and some reports suggest its rolein treating PSC.

Currently, a number of controlled trials assessing the efficacy of ursodeoxycholic acid in curing PSC are under way: the goal is to measure the effect of the progression of the disease.

Orthtopic liver transplantation and outcome

Orthotopic liver transplantation is probably the definite therapeutic option for a patient with PSC. Indeed, at many major transplantation centres, PSC is one of the three most frequent indications for liver transplantation in adults. The outcome is quite similar in different Centers with a 5-year survival rate of approximately 80 per cent. However, special problems may be encountered in patients with PSC who undergo liver transplantation. For example, primary duct-to-duct anastomosis is always difficult, and often impossible, because of disease in the common bile duct. Therefore, the donor's bile duct is usually anastomosed to the limb of the recipient's jejunum. Such an anastomosis may create a greater number of postoperative problems than a direct duct-to-duct anastomosis. In addition, up to 60 per cent or more of patients with PSC have undergone previous abdominal surgical procedures such as proctocolectomy or a choledochoenterostomy. Such surgical procedures are likely to increase difficulty with the technical aspects of liver transplantation. Finally, it is important to emphasize that only limited published data are available on several aspects of liver transplantation in patients with PSC, including the recurrence of PSC after successful liver transplantation, or the effect of active inflammatory bowel disease on the transplanted liver in patients with both diseases. A recent preliminary publication has raised the possibility that PSC may actually recur in the transplanted liver; this observation requires confirmation.

Peculiar pattern of PSC

Asymptomatic PSC at diagnosis is now being identified with increasing frequency. In the early 1980s such patients ranged from 7 to 10% of study cohorts [1,35,112,113] but most recent data report frequencies between 20 and 30% [37,114]. However most patients (nearly 60%) seem to have a II-III hystological stage pointing to the fact that PSC could already have progressed to significative histological damage, even in the absence of symptoms. Survival rate does not seem related to symptoms.

Indeed there are some differences in reported series: Wiesner et al. [93] reported that asymptomatic patients have better survival than symptomatic patients at diagnosis; furthermore, in the series of Martin et al. [101] only two of the 28 asymptomatic patients died of liver disease, with an average follow-up of 10.3 years. In contrast, Porayko et al. [37] studied 45 patients without symptoms at presentation and found that the progressive nature of their disease became evident with close follow-up over a 6 to 7 year period. No major difference in the prognosis of symptomatic and asymptomatic patients was demonstrated by Schrumpf [100].

From the Italian survey a peculiar pattern emerged of high serum cholesterol at presentation. Both by univariate and multivariate analysis this seems a risk factor for a poor outcome in PSC: 48% of patients had elevated serum levels of total cholesterol, with a mean value of approximately 7 mmol/l. Indeed one could link the high serum cholesterol to the pathogenetic mechanisms of the disease: it is known from morphological studies that the biliary tree is particularly vulnerable to ischaemic injury [104]. In analogy to hepatic allografts where biliary strictures often results from arterial occlusion [105], one could speculate that the presence of a damage to the arterial wall of the peribiliary plexus.

Quite a curiosity is the association of habitual smoking with a relatively lower risk of PSC [154,156]: the figures are there but the meaning is uncertain.

Risk factors for developing cholangiocarcinoma

Adenocarcinoma arising in the biliary system of patients with pre-existing PSC is well-acknowledged complication [100,107,108]. As a matter of fact, PSC must be considered as a premalignant lesion much the same as ulcerative colitis is considered a premalignant condition of the colon [157,159,160]. The frequency of cholangiocarcinoma is known to be increasing in relation to the general population; however, absolute numbers are erratic. Autopsy studies suggest a frequency of somewhere between 33 and 42 per cent, whereas clinical reviews, including experience with PSC patients undergoing orthotopic liver transplantation, suggest an even wider frequency even ranging from 10 to 100%. Although risk factors for the development of adenocarcinoma of the bile duct in patients with PSC are currently being evaluated, patients with both PSC and adenocarcinoma of the bile duct usually, but not always, have cirrhosis, portal hypertension, and long-standing IBD; they will generally be older at the time of diagnosis of PSC and may show progressive changes on cholangiography. Nevertheless, young patients have also been identified with early PSC and this devastating complication [158,161]. Cholangiocarcinoma should be a primary consideration in any PSC patient who experiences a sudden, rapid decline in clinical or biochemical status. The outcome of cholangiocarcinoma in patients with PSC is virtually always death, with an overall average survival of approximately 5 months. In recent studies [109,111], the diagnostic use of a tumor marker Ca19-9 was evaluated in PSC patients. Using a lower cut-off value of 100 U/ml the sensitivity and specificity of Ca19-9 in detecting cholangiocarcinoma was 89 and 86 per cent, respectively. Significant elevations in Ca19-9 were seen in several patients prior to the clinical diagnosis of cholangiocarcinoma [163,165]. This observation implies that the tumor may be identified while it is at an occult and potentially treatable stage. However, a normal Ca19-9 level in a patient with PSC may not exclude the diagnosis of cholangiocarcinoma. Other altered pathophysiological states might be associated to the development of cancer [166,167], and represent quite good insight into the inner mechanisns for the development of neoplasia [163], although they are not of real value, from the point of view of clinical epidemiology.

In the Italian survey only three cases of cholangiocarcinoma among 91 PSC patients with a known follow-up (3.3%)were identified. Since cholangiocarcinoma is detected in the later stage of PSC, its apparently low rate in the National series could be ascribed to a shorter period of follow-up (median 4 years) as compared with other studies, with follow-up periods of approximately 10 years.

PSC as an increased risk for developing colonic cancer

Proctocolectomy was initially regarded as a possible treatment for PSC associated to IBD: it is now clear that there is no beneficial effect, and that the course of the two diseases have different determinants [114,120].

More recently, another reason for colectomy in PSC patients has been proposed, e.g. the increased prevalence of colonic neoplasias. A population-based cohort consisting of 125 patients with PSC, perspectively studied for the occurrence of colorectal cancer [168], both had a prevalence of 6 cases before the diagnosis of PSC was established, and a 25% risk at 10 years. A cross sectional study [170], and one based on post-operative examination [169], found an occurrence of displasia and cancer ranging from 29 to 66%, when the patients had both ulcerative colitis and PSC, against a 9-12% in patients with colitis alone.

Another comprehensive study [160,173] demonstrated an increased prevalence of both colonic and biliary cancer in patients having the associated disease. Similar data are available from other series, all very sound from the statistical point of view [171,174,175].

Prophylactic surgery could thus be proposed as well,in the presence of intractable IBD, toxic megacolon and dysplasia, and there is no evidence of worse clinical outcome of IBD patients due to the concomitant PSC [120] The procedure of choice seems to be a proctocolectomy followed by reconstruction of anal contention with an ileal-pouch: permanent ileostomy was reported to be followed by the development of peristomal varices in patients with PSC. More recent data are consistent with a similar prevalence of varices in other types of surgery [114,172], as a likely consequence of the cirrhotic stage.

References

1. Chapman RW, Arborg BA, Rhodes JM et al. Primary sclerosing cholangitis: a review of its clinical features, cholangiography, and hepatic histology. *Gut* 1980; 21:870-7.

2. Wiesner RH, LaRusso NF, Ludwig J, and Dickson ER. Comparison of the clinicopathologic features of primary sclerosing cholangitis and primary biliary cirrhosis. *Gastroenterology* 1985; 88:108-14.

3. Ludwig J, Barham SS, LaRusso NF, Elvebacë LR, Wiesner RH and McCall JT. Morphologic features of chronic hepatitis associated with primary sclerosing cholangitis or chronic ulcerative colitis. *Hepatology* 1981; 1:623-40.

4. Lindor KD, Wiesner RH, LaRusso NF, Dickson ER. Chronic active hepatitis overlap with primary biliary cirrhosid and primary sclerosing cholangitis. In Czajá AÊ and Dickson ER, Eds.Chronic Active Hepatitis: The Mayo Clin Experience, New York, Marcel Dekker Inc. 1986, pp:171-87.

5. Gohlke F, Lohse AW, Dienes Hp, Lohr H, Mrker-Hermann F, Gerken G, Meyer zum Buschenfelde KH. Evidence for an overlap syndrome of autoimmune hepatitis and primary sclerosing cholangitis. *J Hepatol* 1996, 24: 699 705.

6. Boberg KM, Fausa O, Haalnd T, Holter E, Mellbye OJ, Spurkland A, Schrumpf E. Features of autoimmune hepatitis in primary sclerosing cholangitis: an evaluation of 114 primary sclerosing cholangitis patients according to a scoring system for the diagnosis of autoimmune hepatitis. *Hepatology* 1996; 6:1369-76.

7. Dienes HP, Lohse AW, Gerken G, Schirmacher P, Gallati H, Lohr HF, Meyer zum, Buschenfelde KH. Bile duct epithelia as target cells in primary biliary cirrhosis and primary sclerosing cholangitis. *Virchows Arch* 1997; 431: 119-24.

8. Broome I, Scheynius A, Hultcrantz R. Induced expression of heat-shock protein on biliary epithelium in patients with primary sclerosing cholangitis and priamry biliary cirrhosis. *Hepatology* 1993; 18: 298-303.

9. Delle Monache M, Salvio A, Fiocca F, Basoli A, Ricci GL. Primary sclerosing cholangitis: an

analysis of 37 retrospective cases. *Ital J Gastroenterol* 1992; 24:484-7.
10. Okolicsanyi L, Fabris L. Diagnostic approach to primary sclerosing cholangitis: open questions. *Ital J Gastroenterol* 1991; 23:436-41.
11. Delbet P. Retrecissement du choledoque cholecystoduodenostomie. *Bull Mem Soc Chir Paris* 1924; 50:1144-6.
12. Wiesner RH, LaRusso NF. Clinicopathologic features of the syndrome of primary sclerosing cholangitis. *Gastroenterology* 1980; 79:200-6.
13. Terasaki S, Nakanuma Y, Unoura M, Kaneko S, Kobayashi K. Involvement of peribiliary glands in primary sclerosing cholangitis: a histopatologic study. *Ann Intern Med* 1997; 36:766-70.
14. Castellano G, Moreno-Sanchez D, Gultierrez J, Moreno-Gonzalez E, Colina F, Solis-Herruzo JA. Caustic sclerosing cholangitis. Report of four cases and a cumulative review of the literature. *Hepatogastroenterology* 1994; 41:458-70.
15. Broome U, Grunewald J, Scheynius A, Olerup O, Hultcrantz R. Preferential V beta3 usage by hepatic T lymphocytes in patients with primary sclerosing cholangitis. *J Hepatol* 1997; 26:527-34.
16. Martins EB, Graham AK, Chapman RW, Fleming KA. Elevation of gamma delta T lymphocytes in peripheral blood and livers of patients with primary sclerosing cholangitis and other autoimmune liver diseases. *Hepatology* 1996; 23:988-93.
17. Hashimoto E, Lindor KD, Homburger HA, Dickson ER, Czaja AJ, Wiesner RH, Ludwing J. Immunohistochemical characterization of hepatic lymphocytes in primary biliary cirrhosis in comparison with primary sclerosing cholangitis and autoimmune chronic active hepatitis [see comments]. *Mayo Clinic Proc* 1993; 68:1049-55.
18. Kalgalwalla AF, Altraif I, Shamsan L, Omojola M, Khan H, Kagalwalla YA. Primary sclerosing cholangitis in Arab children: report of four cases and literature review. *J Pediatr Gastroenterol Nutr* 1997; 24:146-52.
19. Kelly P, Patchett S, McCloskey D, Alstead E, Farthing M, Fairclough P. Sclerosing cholangitis, race and sex. *Gut* 1997; 41:688-9.
20. Takikawa H, Manabe T. Primary sclerosing cholangitis in Japan-analysis of 192 cases. *J Gastroenterol* 1997; 32: 134-7.
21. Kochhar R, Goenka MK, Das K, Nagi B, Bhasin DK, Chawla YK, Vaiphei K, Singh K, Dilawari JB. Primary sclerosing cholangitis: an experience from India. *J Gastroenterol Hepatol* 1996; 11: 429-33.
22. Okolicsanyi L, Fabris L, Viaggi S, Carulli N, Podda M, Ricci GL. Primary sclerosing cholangitis: clinical presentation, natural history and prognostic variables: an Italian multicentre study. The Italian PSC Study Group. *Eur J Gastroenterol Hepatol* 1996; 8: 685-91.
23. Broome U, Olsson R, Loof L, Bodemar G, Hultcrantz R, Danielsson A, Prytz H, Sandberg-Gertzen H, Wallerstedt S, Lindberg G. Natural history and prognostic factors in 305 Swedish patients with primary sclerosing cholangitis. *Gut* 1996; 38:610-5.
24. Bansi DS, Fleming KA, Chapman RW. Importance of antineutrophil cytoplasmic antibodies in primary sclerosing cholangitis and ulcerative colitis: prevalence, titre, and Ig G subclass. *Gut* 1996; 38:384-9.
25. Escorsell A, Pares A, Rodes J, Solis-Herruzo JA, Miras M, de la Morena E. Epidemiology of primary sclerosing cholangitis in Spain. Spanish Association for the Study of the Liver. *J Hepatol* 1994; 21:787-91.
26. Schrumpf E, Fausa O, Elgjo K, Kolmannskog F. Hepatobiliary complications of inflamatory bowel disease. *Sem Liver Dis* 1988; 8:201-9.
27. Shepherd HA, Selby WS, Chapman RWG, Nolan D, Barbatis C, McGee J O'D, Jewell DP. Ulcerative colitis and persistent liver dysfunction. *Q J Med* 1983; 52:503-13.
28. Stonnington CM, Phillips SF, Melton LJ III, Zinmaister AL. Chronic ulcerative cholitis:incidence and prevalence in a community. *Gut* 1987; 28:402-9.
29. Bonnevie O, Riis P, Anthonisen P. An epidemiologic study of ulcerative cholitis in Copenhagen. *Scand J Gastroent* 1968, 3:432-8.
30. Chapman RW, Varghesr Z, Gaul R. Association of primary sclerosing cholangitis with HLA-B8. *Gut* 1983; 24:38-41.
31. Prochazká EJ, Terasaké PI, Parë MD. Association of primary sclerosing cholangitis with HLA-Drw52a. *N Engl J Med* 1990; ii:1842-4.

32. Ludwig J. Small-duct Primary Sclerosing Cholangitis. *Seminars in Liver Disease* 1991; 11:11-7.
33. Wee A, Ludwig J. Pericholangitis in Ulcerative cholitis: small duct primary sclerosing cholangitis? *Ann Internal Med* 1985; 102:581-7.
34. Ludwig J, LaRusso NF, Wiesner RH. Primary sclerosing cholangitis, in: Peters RL and Craig JR Eds, Liver Pathology -Contemporary Issues in Surgical Pathology, NewYork, Churchill Livingstone, 1986, pp:193-214.
35. LaRusso NF, Wiesner RH, Ludwig J, MacCarty RL. Primary sclerosing cholangitis. *New England Journal of Medicine* 1984; 310:899-903.
36. Lindor KD, Wiesner RH, MacCarty R et al. Advances in primary sclerosing cholangitis. *Am J Med* 1990; 89:73-80.
37. Poraykï MK, Wiesner RH, LaRusso NF. Patients with asymptomatic primary sclerosing cholangitis frequently have a progressive disease. *Gastroenterology* 1990; 98:1594-602.
38. Wiesner RH, Grambsh PM, Dickson ER, Ludwig J, McCarty RL, Hunter EB, Fleming TR, Fisher LD, Beaver SJ, Larusso NF. Primary sclerosing cholangitis: natural history, prognostic factors and survival analysis. *Hepatology* 1989, 10:430-6.
39. van Milligen de Wit AW, van Bracht J, Rauws EA, Jones EA, Tytgat GN, Huibregste K. Endoscopic setnt therapy for dominant extrahepatic bile duct strictures in primary sclerosing cholangitis. *Gastrointest Endscop* 1996; 44 : 293-9.
40. van Milligen de Wit AW, Rauws Ea, van Bracht J, Mulder CJ, Jones EA, Tytgat GN, Huibregtse K. Lack of complications following short-term stent therapy for extrahepatic bile duct strictures in primary sclerosing cholangitis. *Gastrointest Endosc* 1997; 46: 344-7.
41. Wanger S, Gebel M, Meier P, Trautwein C, Bleck J, Nashan B, Manns MP. Endoscopic management of biliary tract strictures in primary sclerosing cholangitis [see comments]. *Endoscopy* 1996; 28: 546-51.
42. van Laethem JL, Deviere J, Bourgeois N, Love J, Gelin M, Cremer M, Adler M. Cholangiographic findings in deteriorating primary sclerosing cholangitis. *Endoscopy* 1995; 27: 223-8.
43. van Milligen de Wit AW, Rauws Ea, van Bracht J, Mulder CJ, Jones EA, Tytgat GN, Huibregtse K. Lack of complications following short-term stent therapy for extrahepatic bile duct strictures in primary sclerosing cholangitis. *Gastrointest Endosc* 1997; 46 : 344-7.
44. Amedee-Mannesme O, Brunelle F, Hadchouel M, Bernard O, Alagille D. Sclerosing cholangitis in infancy. *Hepatology* 1984, 4:786.
45. El-Shabrawi M, Wilkinson ML, Portmann B, Mieli Vergani G, Chong SKF, Williams R, Mowat AP. Primary sclerosing cholangitis in childhood. *Gastroenterology* 1987, 92:1226-35.
46. Mendeloff AI. The epidemiology of inflamatory bowel disease. In: Kirshner JB, Shorter RG, Eds .Inflamatory bowel disease, 2nd ed, Lea & Febirger, Philadelphia 1980, pp 5-19.
47. Borkje B, Vetvik K, Odegaard S, Schrumpf E, Larssen TB. Chronic pancreatitis in patients with sclerosing cholangitis and ulcerative cholitis. *Scand J Gastroenterol* 1985; 20:539-42.
48. Epstein O, Chapman RWG, Lake Bakaar G, Foo AY, RosalkJ SB, Sherlock S. The pancreas in primary biliary cirrhosis and primary sclerosing cholangitis. *Gastroentrology* 1982; 83:1177-82.
49. Alberti-Flor JJ, Kalemeris G, Dunn CD, Avant GR. Primary sclerosing cholangitis associated with massive intra-abdominal lymphadenopathy. *Am J Gastroenterol* 1986; 81:55 60.
50. Brandt DJ, McCarty RL, Charbonau JW, Larusso NF, Wiesner RH, Ludwig J. Gallbladder discase in primary sclerosing cholangitis. *Am J Radiol* 1988; 150:571 4.
51. Jeffrey GP, Reed WD, Carrello S, Shilkin KB. Histological and immunohistochemical study of the gallbladderlesion in primary sclerosing cholangitis. *Gut* 1991; 32:424-9.
52. Mistilis SP, Skyring AP, Goulston SJM. Effect of long term tetracyoline terapy, steroid therapy and cholectomy in pericholamgytis associated with ulcerative cholitis. *Aust Ann Med* 1965; 14:286-94.
53. Warren KW, Athanassiades S, Monge JL. Primary sclerosing cholangitis. a study of fourty-two cases. *Am J Surg* 1966; 111:23-38.
54. Thorpe MEC, Scheuer PJ, Scherlock S. Primary sclerosing cholangitis, the biliary tree and ulceratice cholitis. *Gut* 1967; 8:435-48.
55. Aadland E, Schrumpf E, Fausa O, Eljo K, Heiko A, Aakus T, Gjone E. Primary sclerosing cholangitis: a long-term follow-up. *Scand J Gastroenterol* 1987; 22:655-64.
56. Fausa O, Schrumpf E, Elgjo K. Relationship of Inflammatory Bowel Disease and Primary Sclerosing Cholangitis. *Seminars in Liver Disease* 1991;11:31-9.

57. Dew MG, Thompson H, Allan RN. The spectrum of hepatic disfunction in inflamatory bowel disease. *Quart J Med* 1979; 48:113-35.

58. Thobias R, Wright JP, Kottler RE, Bornman PC, Price SK, Hathfield A, Marks IN. Primary sclerosing cholangitis associated to inflamatory bowel disease in cape-Town: 1975-1981. *S Afr Med J* 1983; 63:229-35.

59. Rabinovitz M, Gavaler JS, Schade RR, Dindzans VJ, Chien M-C, Van Tjhiel DH. Does primary sclerosing cholangitis occurring in association with inflamatory bowel disease differ from that occurring in absence of inflamatory bowel disease? A study of sixty-six subjects. *Hepatology* 1990; 11:7-11.

60. Rasmussen HH, Fallingborg JF, Mortensen PB, Vyberg M, Tage-Jensen U, Rasmussen SN. Hepatobiliary dysfunction and primary sclerosing cholangitis in patients with Crohn's disease. *Scand J Gastroenterol* 1997; 32 : 604-10.

61. Tysk C. Concurrent ulcerative colitis, celiac sprue, and primary sclerosing cholangitis. *J Clin Gastroenterol* 1994; 18 : 241-2.

62. Haj JE, Wiesner RH, Shorter RG, LaRusso NF, Baldus WP. Primary sclerosing cholangitis and celic disease: a novel association. *Ann Intern Med* 1988; 109:713-7.

63. Lewis HM, Goldin R, Leonard JN. Dermatitis herpetiformis and primary sclerosing cholangitis. *Clin Exp Dermatol* 1993; 18 : 363-5.

64. Ilan Y, Rappaport I, Feigin R, Ben-Chetrit E. Primary sclerosing cholangitis in sarcoidosis. *J Clin Gastroenterol* 1993; 16 : 326-8.

65. Man KM, Drejet A, Keeffe EB, Garcia-Kennedy R, Imperial JC, Esquivel CO. Primary sclersosing cholangitis and Hodgkin's disease. *Hepatology* 1993; 18 : 1127-31.

66. Shimomura I, Takase Y, Matsumoto S, Kuyama J, Nakajima T, Maeda H, Sugase T, Hata M, Okuno M. Primary sclerosing cholangitis associated with increased peripheral eosinophils and serum IgE. *J Gastroenterol* 1996; 31:737-41.

67. Barquist ES, Goldstein N, Zinnere MJ. Polyarteritis nodosa presenting as a biliary stricture. *Surgery* 1991; 109:16-9.

68. Wenger J, Gingrich GW, Mendeloff J. Sclerosing cholangitis: a manifestarion of systemic disease. *Arch Intern Med* 1965; 116:509-14.

69. Chapman R.W. Role of immune factors in the pathogenesis of Primary Sclerosing Cholangitis. *Seminars in liver disease* 1991, 11:1-4

70. Zauli D, Baffoni L, Cassani F, Fusconi M, Lenzi M, Ballardini G, Luigi M, Bianchi FB, Schrumpf E. Antineutrophil cytoplasmic antibodies in primary sclerosing cholangitis, ulcerative colitis, and autoimmune diseases. *Gastroenterology*. 1992, 99:1088-90.

71. Bansi DS, Bauducci M, Bergqvisit A, Boberg K, Broome U, Chapman R, Fleming K, Jorgensen R, Lindor K, Rosina F, Schrmpf E. Detection of antineutrophil cytoplasmic antibodies in primary sclerosing cholangitis: a comparison of the alkaline phosphatase and immunofluorescent techniques. *Eur J Gastroenterol Hepatol* 1997; 9:575-80

72. Peen E, Almer S, Bodemar G, Ryden BO, Sjolin C, Tejle K, Skogh T. Anti-lactoferrin antibodies and other types of ANCA in ulcerative colitis, primary sclerosing cholangitis, and Crohm's disease. *Gut* 1993; 34:56-62.

73. Lo SK, Fleming KA, Chapman RW. A 2-year follow-up study of anti-neutrophil antibody in primary sclerosing cholangitis: relationship to clinical activity, liver biochemistry and ursodeoxycholic acid treatment. *J Hepatol* 1994; 21:974-8.

74. Olerup O, Olsson R, Hultcrantz R, Broome U. HLA-DR and HLA-DQ are not markers for rapid disease progression in primary sclerosing cholangitis. *Gastroenterology* 1995; 108:870-8.

75. Vidrich A, Lee J, James E, Cobb L, Targan S. Segregation of pANCA antigenic recognition by Dnase treatment of neutrophils: ulcerative colitis, type 1 autoimmune hepatitis, and primary sclerosing cholangitis. *J Clin Immunol* 1995; 15:293-9.

76. Bansi DS, Lo S, Chapman RW, Fleming KA. Absence of antineutrophil cytoplasmic antibodies in relatives of UK patients with primary sclerosing cholangitis and ulcerative colitis. *Eur J Gastroenterol Hepatol* 1996; 8:111-6.

77. Olsson R, Hagerstrand I, Broome U, Danielsson A, Jarnerot G, Loof L, Prytz H, Ryden BO, Wallerstedt S. Sampling variability of percutaneous liver biopsy in primary sclerosing cholangitis. *J Clin Pathol* 1995; 48:933-5.

78. MacCarty RL, LaRusso NF, Wiesner RH, Ludwig J. Primary sclerosing cholangitis findings on cholangiography and pancreatography. *Radiology* 1983, 149:39-44.
79. Ziessman HA. Atlas of cholescintigraphy: selected update. In: Ziessman HA and Van Nostrand D Editors, Selected Atlas of gastrointestinal scintigraphy. Springer Verlag New York 1992, pp 1-34.
80. van Laethem JL, Deviere J, Bourgeois N, Love J, Gelin M, Cremer M, Adler M. Cholangiographic findings in deteriorating primary sclerosing cholangitis. *Endoscopy* 1995; 27:223-8.
81. Aaseth J, Thomassen Y, Aadland E, Fausa O, Schrumpf E. Hepatic retention of copper and selenium in primary sclerosing cholangitis. *Scand J Gastroenterol* 1995; 30:1200-3.
82. Gross JB, Ludwig J, Wiesner RH, McCall JT, LaRusso NF. Abnormalities in tests of copper metabolism in primary sclerosing cholangitis. *Gastroenterology* 1985, 89:272-8.
83. Jorgensen RA, Lindor KD, Sartin JS, LaRusso NF, Wiesner RH. Serum lipid and fat-soluble vitamin levels in primary sclerosing cholangitis. *J Clin Gastroenterol* 1995; 20: 215-9.
84. Bloom S, Fleming K, Chapman R. Adhesion molecule expression in primary sclerosing cholangitis and primary biliary cirrhosis. *Gut* 1995; 36:604-9.
85. Kowdley KV, Knox TA, Kaplan MM. Hepatic copper is normal in early primary biliary cirrhosis and primary sclerosing cholangitis. *Dig Dis Sci* 1994; 39: 2416-20.
86. Pokorny CS, Norton ID, McCaughan GW, Selby WS. Anti-neutrophil cytoplasmic antibody: a prognostic indicator in primary sclerosing cholangitis. *J Gastroenterol Hepatol* 1994; 9:40-4.
87. Garred P, Lyon H, Christoffersen P, Mollnes TE, Tranum-Jensen J. Deposition of C3, the terminal complement complex and vitronectin in primary biliary cirrhosis and primary sclerosing cholangitis. *Liver* 1993; 13:305-10.
88. Lo SK, Chapman RW, Fleming KA. Tissue distribution of autoantigen specific for primary sclerosing cholangitis. *J Clin Pathol* 1993; 46:246-9.
89. Broome U, Hultecrantz R, Scheynius A. Lack of concomitant expression of ICAM-1 and HLA-DR on bile duct cells from patients with primary sclerosing cholangitis and primary biliary cirrhosis. *Scand J Gastroenterol* 1993; 28:126-30.
90. Helzeberg JK, Petersen JM Boyer JL. Improved survival with primary sclerosing cholangitis: a review of clinicopathologic features and comparison of symptomatic and asymptomatic patients. *Gastroenterology* 1987, 92:1869-75.
91. Aadl E, Schrumps E, Fausa O, Elgjo K, Heilo A, Aakhus T, et al. Primary sclerosing cholangitis:a long term follow up study. *Scand I Gastroenterol* 1987, 22: 655-64.
92. Lebovics E, Palmer M, Woo J, Shaffner F. Outcome of primary sclerosing cholangitis. Analysis of long-term of 38 patients. *Arch Intern Med* 1987, 147: 729-31.
93. Wiesner RH, Grambsh PB, Dickson ER, Ludwig J, MacCarthy RL, Hunter EB, et al. Primary sclerosing cholangitis: natural hystory prognostic factors, and survival analysis. *Hepatology* 1989, 10: 430-6.
94. Farrant JM, Hayllar KM, Wilkinson ML, Karani J, Portmann BC, Westaby D. Natural history and prognostic variables in primary sclerosing cholangitis. *Gastroenterology* 1991, 100:1710-7.
95. Kaplan EL, Meyer P. Non-parametric estimation from incomplete observation. *J Am Stat Assoc* 1958, 53: 457 – 81.
96. Cox DR. Regression models and life-tables. *J R Stat Soc B* 1972, 34: 187-202.
97 Harrington DP, Fleming TR. A class of rank test procedures for censored survival data. *Biometrika* 1982, 69: 553-66.
98. Christensen E. Multivariate survival analysis using COX's regression model. *Hepatology* 1987, 1346 58.
99. Dickson ER, Murtaugh PA, Wiesner RH, Grambsh PM, Fleming TR, Ludwig J et al. Primary sclerosing cholangytis. Refinement and validation of survival models. *Gastroenterology* 1992, 103: 1893-1901.
100. Schrumpf E, Abdelnoor M, Fausa O, Elgjo K, Jenssen E. Kolmannskog F. Risk Factors in primary sclerosing cholangitis. *J of Hepatology* 1994 21: 1061-6.
101. Duerr RH, Targan SR, Landers CI, Larusso NF, Lindsav KL, Wiesner RH et al. Neutrophil cytoplasmic antobodies: a link between primary sclerosing cholangitis and ulcerative colitis. *Gastroenterology* 1991, 100: 1385-91.
102. Mehal WZ, Lo SK, Chapman RW, Fleming KA. The immunogenetic basis for antineutrophil

cytoplasmic antibody production in primary sclerosing cholangitis and ulcerative colitis. *J of Hepatology* 1994, 21:910-1.
103. Mehal WZ, Dennis Lo Y-M, Wordsworth BP, Neuberger JM, Hubscher SC, Fleminf KA et al. HLA DR4 is a marker for rapid disease progression in primary sclerosis cholangitis. *Gastroenterology* 1994, 106:160-7.
104. Terblanche J, Allison HF, Northerover JMA. An ischemic basis for biliary strictures. *Surgery* 1983, 94:52-8.
105. Greif f Bronsther OL, Van Thiel DH, Casavilla A, Iwatsuki S, Tzakis A, et al. The incidence, timing and management of biliary tract complication after orthopic liver transplantation. *Ann Surg*. 1994, 219:40-5.
106. Fausa O, Schrumpf E, Elgjo K. Inflammatory bowel disease occurs in almost al patients with primary sclerosing cholangitis. *Scand J Gastroenterol* 1989; 24(suppl. 159):53.
107. Wee A, Ludwig j, Coffey RJ, Larusso NF, Wiesner RH. Hepatobiliary carcinoma associated with primary sclerosing cholangitis and chronic ulcerative colitis. *Hum Pathol* 1985; 16:719-26.
108. Martinis EBG, Fleming KA, Garrido MC, Hine Kr, Chapman RW. Superficial thrombophlebitis, dyspleasia, and cholangiocarcinoma in primary sclerosing cholangitis. *Gastroenterology* 1994; 107:537-42.
109. Rosen CB, Nagorney DM, Wiener RH, Coffey RJ, Larusso NF. Cholangiocarcinoma complicating primary sclerosing cholangitis. *Ann Surg* 1991, 213:21-5.
110. Miros M, Kerlin P, Walker N, Harper J, Lvnch S, Strong R. Predicting cholangiocarcinoma in patient with primary sclerosing cholangitis before transplantation. *Gut* 1991; 32:1369-73.
111. Fausa O, Schrumpf E. Cholangiocarcinoma occurs with high frequency in primary sclerosing cholangitis. *Scand J Gastroenterol* 1989; 24 (supp.159): 54.
112. Ludwig J, Larusso NF, Wiesner RH. The syndrome of primary sclerosing cholangitis. *Prog liver Dis* 1990; 9: 555-6.
113. Thopson HH, Pitt, HA, Tomkins RK, Longmire WP. Primary sclerosing cholangitis. A heterogenous disease. *Ann Surg* 1982; 196: 127-36.
114. Martin FM, Rossi RL, Nugent FW, Scholz FJ, Jenkins RL, Lewis WD, Gagner M, Foley E, Braasch JW. Surgical aspects of sclerosing cholangitis: results in 178 patients. *Ann Surgery* 1990; 212:551-6.
115. Lundquist K, Broome U. Differences in colonic disease activity in patients with ulcerative colitis with and without primary sclerosing cholangitis: a case control study. *Dis Colon Rectum* 1997; 40:451-6.
116. Springer DJ, Gaing AA, Siegel JH. Radiologic regression of primary sclerosing cholangitis following combination therapy with an endoprosthesis and ursodeoxycholic acid. *Am J Gastroenterol* 1993; 88: 1957-9.
117. LaRusso NF, Wiesner RH, Ludwig J, MacCarty RL, Beaver SJ, Zinsmeister AR. Prospective trial of penicillamine in primary sclerosing cholangitis. *Gastroenterology* 1988; 95:1036-42.
118. Lindor KD, Wiesner RH, LaRusso NF. Recent advanced in the management of primary sclerosing cholangitis. *Seminars in Liver Disease* 1987; 7:322-7.
119. Kaplan MM. Medical approaches to Primary Sclerosing Cholangitis. *Seminars in Liver Disease* 1991; 11:56-63.
120. Cangemi JR, Wiesner RH, Beaver SJ, Ludwig J, McCarty RL, Dozois RR, Zinmeister AR, LaRusso NF. Effect of proctocolectomy for chronic ulcerative colitis on the natural history of primary sclerosing cholangitis. *Gastroenterology* 1989; 96:790-4.
121. Wiesner RH, Porayko MK, Dickson ER, Ludwig J, LaRusso NF. Selection and timing of liver transplantation in primary biliary cirrhosis and primary sclerosing cholangitis. *Hepatology* 1992; 16:1290-9.
122. Esquivel CD, March JW, VanThiel DH. Liver transplantation for chronic cholestatic liver disease in adults and children. *Gastroenterol Clin North Am*. 1988; 17:145-55.
123. Marsh JW, Iwatsuky S, Makowka L et al. Orthoptic liver transplantation for primary sclerosing cholangitis. *Annals of Surgery* 1988; 207:21-5.
124. Allison M, Burroughs AK, Noone D, Summerfield JA. Biliary lavage with corticosteroids in primary sclerosing cholangitis. A clinical cholangiographic and bacteriological study. *J Hepatol* 1986; 3:118-22.
125. Burgert SL, Brown BP, Kirkpatrick RB, LaBrecque. Positive corticosteroid response in early

primary sclerosing cholangitis. *Gastroenterology* 1984; 86:1037.
126. Kaplan MM, Arora S, Pincus SH. Primary sclerosing cholangitis and low dose oral pulse methotrexate: clinical and histological response. *Ann Intern Med* 1987; 106:231-5.
127. LaRusso NF, Wiesner RH, Beaver SJ. Combined antifibrogenic and immunosuppressive therapy in primary sclerosing cholangitis. *Gastroenterology* 1987; 92:1493.
128. Lindor KD, LaRusso NF, Wiesner RH. Prednisone and colchicine are not of benefit after two years in patients with primary sclerosing cholangitis. *Hepatology* 1989; 10:638.
129. Lindor KD, Wiesner RH, Colwell LJ, Steiner B, Beaver S, LaRusso NF. The combination od prednisone and colchicine in patients with primary sclerosing cholangitis. *Am J Gastroenterol* 1991; 85:57-61.
130. Stiehl A, Rudolph G, Sauer P, Benz C, Stremmel W, Walker S, Theilmann L. Efficacy of ursodeoxycholic acid treatment and endoscopic dilatation of major duct stenoses in primary sclerosing cholangitis. An 8-year prospective study. *J Hepatol* 1997; 26: 560-6.
131. Javett SL. Azathioprine in primary sclerosing cholangitis. *Lancet* 1971; 1:810
132. Chazouilleres O, Poupon R, Capron JP. Ursodeoxycholic acid for primary sclerosing cholangitis. *Journal of Hepatology* 1990; 11:120-3.
133. Lirussi F, Okolicsanyi L. Cytoprotection with ursodeoxycholic acid: effect in chronic non-cholestatic and chronic cholestatic liver disease. *Ital J Gastroenterol.* 1992; 24:31-5.
134. Lindor Kd, Jorgensen RA, Anderson ML, Gores GJ, Hofmann AF, LaRusso NF. Ursodeoxycholic acid and methotrexate for primary sclerosing cholangitis: a pilot study. *Am J Gastroenterol* 1996; 91:511-5.
135. Goss JA, Shackleton CR, Farmer DG, Arnaout WS, Seu P, Markowitz JS, Martin P, Stribling RJ, Goldstein LI, Busuttil RW. Orthotopic liver transplantation for primary sclerosing cholangitis. A 12-year single center experience. *Ann Surg* 1997; 59:472-81.
136. Lindor KD. Ursodiol for primary sclerosing cholangitis. Mayo Primary Sclerosing Cholangitis-Ursodeoxycholic Acid Study Group. *N Engl J Med* 1997; 336:691-5.
137. De Maria N, Colantoni A, Rosenbloom E, Van Thiel DH. Ursodeoxycholic acid does not improve the clinical course of primary sclerosing cholangitis over a 2-year period. *Hepatogastroenterol* 1996; 43:1472-9.
138. Jorgensen RA, Lindor KD, Sartin JS, LaRusso NF, Wiesner RH. Serum lipid and fat-soluble vitamin levels in primary sclerosing cholangitis. *J Clin Gastroenterol* 1995; Apr 20: 215-9.
139. Olsson R, Broome U, Danielsson A, Hagerstrand I, Jarnerot G, Loof L, Prytz H, Ryden BO, Wallerstedt S. Colchicine treatment of primary sclerosing cholangitis. *Gastroenterology* 1995; 108:1199-203.
140. Kyokane K, Ichihara T, Horisawa M, Suzuki N, Ichihara S, Suga S, Nakao A, Morise K. Successful treatment of primary sclerosing cholangitis with cyclosporine and corticosteroid. *Hepatogastroenterol* 1994; 41:449-52.
141. Van Thiel DH, Carroll P, Abu-Elmagd K, Rodriguez-Rilo H, Irish W, McMichael J, Starzl TE. Tacrolimus (FK 506), a treatment for primary sclerosing cholangiotis: results of an open-label preliminary trial. *Am J Gastroenterol* 1995; 90:455-9.
142. Knox TA, Kaplan MM. A double-blind controlled trial of oral-pulse methotrexate therapy in the treatment of primary sclerosing cholangitis. *Gastroenterology* 1994; 106: 494-9.
143. Post AB, Bozdech JM, Lavery I, Barnes DS. Colectomy in patients with inflammatory bowel disease and primary sclerosing cholangitis. *Dis Colon Rectum* 1994; 37: 175-8.
144. Dodd GD 3rd, Niedzwiecki GA, Campbell WL, Baron RL. Bile duct calculi in patients with primary sclerosing cholangitis. *Radiology* 1997; 203:443-7.
145. Shetty K, Rybicki L, Carey WD. The Child-Pugh classification as a prognostic indicator for survival in primary sclerosing cholangitis. *Hepatology* 1997; 25:1049-53.
146. Janczewska I, Olsson R, Hultcrantz R, Broome U. Pregnancy in patients with primary sclerosing cholangitis. *Liver* 1996, 16:326-30.
147. van de Meeberg PC, Portincasa P, Wolfhagen FH, van Erpecum KJ, VanBerge-Henegouwen GP. Increased gall bladder volume in primary sclerosing cholangitis. *Gut* 1996; 39:594-9.
148. Ludwig J, Colina F, Poterucha JJ. Granulomas in primary sclerosing cholangitis. *Liver* 1995; 15:307-12.

149. Miki C, Harrison JD, Gunson BK, Buckels JA, McMaster P, Mayer AD. Inflammatory bowel disease in primary sclerosing cholangitis: an analysis of patients undergoing liver transplantation. *Br J Surg* 1995; 82:1114-7.
150. Sandborn WJ, Wiesner RH, Tremaine WJ, LaRusso NF. Ulcerative colitis disease activity following treatment of associated primary sclerosing cholangitis with cyclosporin. *Gut* 1993; 34: 242-6.
151. Strasser S, Sheil AG, Gallagher ND, Waugh R, McCaughan GW. Liver transplantation for primary sclerosing cholangitis versus priamry biliary cirrhosis: a comparison of complications and outcome. *J Gastroenterol Hepatol* 1993; 8:238-43.
152. Sheng R, Campbell WL, Zajko AB, Baron RL. Cholangiographic features of biliary strictures after liver transplantation for primary sclerosing cholangitis: evidence of recurrent disease. *Am J Roentgenol* 1996; 166: 1109-13.
153. Wagner A. Azathioprine treatment in primary sclerosing cholangitis. *Lancet* 1971, 2:663-4.
154. Cohen RD, Hanauer SB. Protection from primary sclerosing cholangitis: smoke trails of just coattails? *Gastroenterology* 1996; 110: 1658-62.
155. van Erpecum KJ, Smits SJ, van de Meeberg PC Linn FH, Wolfhagen FH, vanBerge-Henegouwen GP, Algra A. Risk of primary sclerosing cholangitis is associated with nonsmoking behavior. *Gastroenterology* 1996; 110: 1503-6.
156. Loftus EV Jr, Sandborn WJ, Tremaine WJ, Mahoney DW, Zinsmeister AR, Offord KP, Melton LJ 3d. Primary sclerosing cholangitis is associated with nonsmoking: a case-control study. *Gastroenterology* 1996; 110: 1496-502.
157. Wee A, Ludwig J, Coffey RJ, LaRusso NF, Wiesner RH. Hepatobiliary carcinoma associated with primary sclerosing cholangitis and chronic ulcerative colitis. *Human Pathology* 1985;16:729-6.
158. Kornfeld D., Ekbom A, Ihre T. Survival and risk of cholangiocarcinoma in patients with primary sclerosing cholangitis. A population-based study. *Scand J Gastroenterol* 1997; 32: 1042-5.
159. Harnois DM, Gores GJ, Ludwing J, Steers JL, LaRusso NF, Wiesner RH. Are patients with cirrhotic stage primary sclerosing cholangitis at risk for the development of hepatocellular cancer? *J Hepatol* 1997; 27: 512-6.
160. Broome U, Lofberg R, Veress B, Eriksson LS. Primary sclerosing cholangitis and ulcerative colitis: evidence for increased neoplastic potential. *Hepatology* 1995; 22:1404-8.
161. Nashan B, Schlitt HJ, Tusch G, Oldhafer KJ, Ringe B, Wagner S, Pichlmayr R. Biliary malignancies in primary sclerosing cholangitis: timing for liver transplantation. *Hepatology* 1996; 23:1105-11.
162. Rizzi PM, Ryder SD, Portmann B, Ramage JK, Naoumov NV, Williams R. p53 Protein overexpression in cholangiocarcinoma arising in primary sclerosing cholangitis. *Gut* 1996; 38:265-8.
163. Ramage JK, Donaghy A, Farrant JM, Iorns R, Williams R. Serum tumor markers for the diagnosis of cholagiocarcinoma in primary sclerosing cholangitis. *Gastroenterology* 1995; 108:865-9.
164. Rogers SA, Podolsky DK. Predicting cholangiocarcinoma in patients with primary sclerosing cholangitis: an analysis of the serological marker CA 19-9. *Hepatology* 1994;19: 543-5.
165. Nichols JC, Gores GJ, LaRusso NF, Wiesner RH, Nagorney DM, Ritts RE Jr. Diagnostic role of serum CA 19-9 for cholangiocarcinoma in patients with primary sclerosing cholangitis. *Mayo Clin Proc* 1993; 68: 874-9.
166. Martins EB, Fleming KA, Garrido MC, Hine KR, Chapman RW. Superficial thrombophlebitis, dysplasia, and cholangiocarcinoma in primary sclerosing cholangitis. *Gastroenterology* 1994; 107: 537-42.
167. D'Costa DF. Cholangiocarcinoma associated with hypercalcaemia and ascites presenting as sclerosing cholangitis. *Br J Clin Pract* 1994; 48: 217-8.
168. Kornfeld D, Ekbom A, Ihre T. Is there an excess risk for colorectal cancer in patients with ulcerative colitis and concomitant primary sclerosing cholangitis? A population based study. *Gut* 1997; 41: 522- 5.
169. Marchesa P, Lashner BA, Lavery IC, Milson J, Hull TL, Strong SA, Church JM, Navarro G, Fazio VW. The risk of cancer and dysplasia among ulcerative colitis patients with primary sclerosing cholangitis. *Am J Gastroenterol* 1997; 92:1285-8.
170. Leidenius MH, Farkkila MA, Karkkainen P, Taskinen EI, Kellokumpu IH, Kockerstedt KA. Colorectal dysplasia and carcinoma in patients with ulcerative colitis and primary sclerosing cholangitis.

Scand J Gastroenterol 1997; **32**:706-11.
171. Penna C, Dozois R, Tremaine W, Sandborn W, LaRusso N, Schleck C, Ilstrup D. Pouchitis after ileal pouch-anal anastomosis for ulcerative colitis occurs with increased frequency in patients with associated primary sclerosing cholangitis. *Gut* 1996; **38**:234-9.
172. Wiesner RH, Beaver SJ, Dozois RR, LaRusso NF. Peristomal varices after proctocolectomy in patients with primary sclerosing cholangitis. *Gastroenterology* 1986; 90:316-22.
173. Brentnall TA, Haggitt RC, Rabinovitch PS, Kimmey MB, Bronner MP, Levine DS, Kowdley KV, Stevens AC, Crispin DA, Emond M, Rubin CE. Risk and natural history of colonic neoplasia in patients with primary sclerosing cholangitis and ulcerative colitis. *Gastroenterology* 1996; 110: **331-8**.
174. Gurbuz AK, Giardiello FM, Bayless TM. Colorectal neoplasia in patients with ulcerative colitis and primary sclerosing cholangitis. *Dis Colon Rectum* 1995; 38:37-41.
175. D'Haens GR, Lashner BA, Hanauer SB. Pericholangitis and sclerosing cholangitis are risk factors for dysplasia and cancer in ulcerative colitis. *Am J Gastroenterol* 1993; 88: 1174-8.

CHAPTER 20

PANCREATIC ISLET CELL-TRANSPLANTATION.

DOMENICO MARRANO, VINCENZO MARIA GRECO, and ANDREA CONTI

Department of Surgery and Anesthesiology, 1st Surgical Clinics, University of Bologna, Bologna, Italy

Summary

Pancreatic islet cell-transplantation is currently used in major transplant centers as an alternative to total pancreas transplant, in the surgical treatment of insulin-dependent diabetes mellitus. Pancreatic islet cell-transplantation was first considered in the past century, but the first satisfactory results were obtained in 1990, after Ricordi had developed an automated procedure for islet isolation from the surrounding parenchyma. While developing an effective isolation technique, several islet purification procedures have been tested, the most effective of which has been found to be the one based on the use of Ficoll solutions with different density gradients. The transplanted cells must necessarily be introduced into a heterotopic site, the best one so far identified being the liver. Almost all clinically successful islet cell-transplantations have been obtained by means of intraportal islet embolization. Pancreatic islet cells can be transplanted in association with other organs, and the best results have been obtained with simultaneous kidney-islet cell-transplantation. We shall present an overview on this subject based on our experience as well as on the experience of the most important centers included in the International Registry.

Support therapy with exogenous insulin is the basis for medical treatment of Type I diabetes mellitus (IDDM); insulin administration has certainly increased diabetic patients' life expectancy, but it has been found to be incomplete and ineffective in preventing chronic and degenerative complications of the disease. In fact, exogenous insulin does not have physiological pharmacokinetics, and is not able to reproduce the sophisticated autoregulatory mechanisms which control pancreatic β–cell secretory activity [1]. This kind of insulin treatment, even if enhanced by implementing pre-determined infusion algorithms, and by using micropumps, is not able to guarantee an ideal glycemic control. In order to obtain a more physiological insulin secretion activity, and prevent long-term complications of diabetes, two different surgical strategies can be adopted: total pancreas transplantation or pancreatic islet cell-transplantation. It is currently possible to perform pancreatic islet cell- transplantation intrahepatically, by means of intraportal embolization. This method is used in major transplant centers [2,3,4,5,6,7,8] as a valid alternative to total pancreas transplantation, since the procedure is easier, there are fewer surgical risks and less immunogenetic activity, and the operation can easily be repeated, in case of functional deficit or functional failure.

Historical data on islet cell-transplantation

Pancreatic islet cell-transplantation was first attempted in Bristol in 1893 by Williams and Harsant [9], who unsuccessfully introduced sheep pancreatic tissue fragments subcutaneously into a 15-year old boy in ketoacidosic coma (the only

E. Zanella (ed.), Advances in Abdominal Surgery, 223–241.

xenograft ever performed). In 1922, after insulin had been introduced into clinical practice, research on transplants was abandoned, since diabetes treatment seemed to have become readily available. Later on, when the correlation was discovered between long-term complications of diabetes and non physiological control of exogenous insulin-induced glycemia, interest in transplantations recommenced. In 1965, Moskalewski [10] discovered that the collagenase enzyme was able to digest pancreatic connective matrix and that it was possible to separate the islet component from the acinar one. Later on, Lacy e Kostianowsky [11] discovered that the pancreas could be usefully distended by injecting collagenase into the Wirsung duct, to achieve better pancreatic islet cell retrieval. In 1972, Lacy [12] successfully performed the first pancreatic islet cell- transplantation on a small mammal. In 1988, Ricordi [13] developed an automated pancreatic islet cell-isolation technique, and laid the foundations for the currently-used procedure in all transplant centres dealing with the issue.
As a result of the joint efforts of Pittsburgh, Milan and Miami transplant centres the first unequivocally successful islet cell allograft was performed in 1990, which made simultaneous liver and pancreatic islet cell-transplantation possible in the same recipient [14].Since 1990, international results have been encouraging, and the procedure has been more extensively used both at clinical and experimental level, as shown in the International Islet Transplant Registry (ITR)[15].

Indications and advantages

Indications for pancreatic islet cell-transplantation that are unanimously accepted by different Authors [16], are similar to those developed for total pancreas transplant, and are currently often used in combination with renal transplant:

1) Type I diabetic patients with renal failure where simultaneous kidney-islet transplantation is indicated by harvesting organs from the same donor. This is the largest group and the one in which the best results are obtained in terms of transplanted islet functional survival.
2) Successful renal transplant Type I diabetic recipients, with progressively deteriorating endocrine pancreatic function, where islet transplantation could help protect the transplanted kidney against additional hyperglycemia-induced damage, by stabilizing glycemic control.
3) Rare cases of hyperlabile diabetes (even without complications) that are resistant to insulin treatment, and where islet transplantation can be performed with no simultaneous renal transplant.
4) A few, well-selected patients who have undergone total pancreatectomy for benign disorders,and can be subjected to pancreatic islet auto-transplantation.

Hopefully, in the future, pancreatic islet cell-transplantation can also be performed in uncomplicated juvenile diabetes, in order to prevent degenerative evolution of the disease. This solution is not currently feasible, since chronic immunosuppresion-induced complications outweigh the advantages offered by the procedure [17].

Compared with total pancreas transplant, islet cell-transplantation offers a number of advantages: an easier harvesting and transplanting technique, lower surgical risk, transplant can be repeated in case of islet functional failure and, last but not least, several donors can be used in order to obtain a sufficient number of cells (using cultured or cryopreserved islet cells).

Duodeno-pancreatic en bloc removal without intact vascular pedicles is possible, by means of a simple surgical procedure during which the pancreatic capsule must be carefully preserved; this is essential in order to obtain a good collagenase-induced glandular distension. Using this procedure, the pancreas can always be removed, even in those cases where vascular abnormalities are present in the hepatic graft [18] (Fig.1).

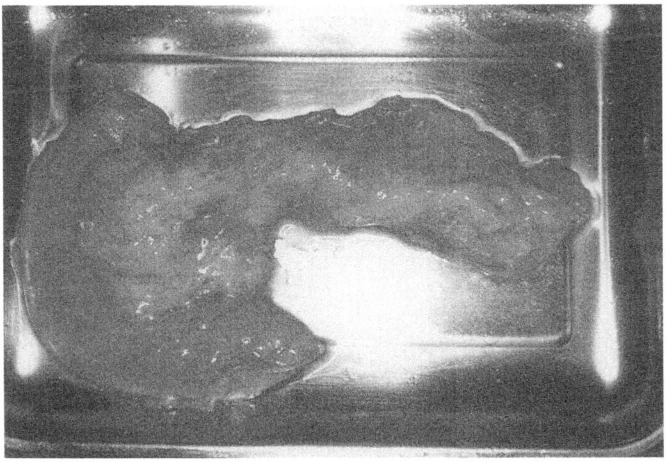

Figure 1. Duodeno-pancreatic bloc without vascular pedicles, at the end of the harvesting phase. (see Color Plates, p. xx)

Processing method

Pancreatic islet cells can be obtained from the harvested organ by means of several procedures to be performed in adequately equipped laboratories. Materials and instruments will be described, by making particular reference to our own experience.

Pancreas cleaning: the pancreas is initially separated from the duodenum and then cleaned by carefully removing peripancreatic fat tissue, lymph-nodes and vascular segments. This phase requires special attention so as not to damage the capsule,the integrity of which is essential in order to perform successfully the following distension and digestion of the gland.

Distension and digestion: before starting pancreas distension, electrolytic and enzymatic solutions needed for the procedure [i.e. HBSS (Hanks solution) and Collagenase (type P, Boheringer)] must be prepared in a sterile environment by working in a laminar flow room; the latter solution is necessary for pancreas fibroconnective tissue digestion [11]. After collagenase preparation, the pancreas digestion circuit is assembled according to Ricordi's automated method [13]. The circuit to be assembled inside a sterile laminar flow room is made up of the stainless steel digestion chamber developed by Ricordi, a mechanical shaker to be connected to the above chamber, a 37°C bath to heat the circuit and silicon tubing for fluid circulation by means of a peristaltic pump (Fig.2).

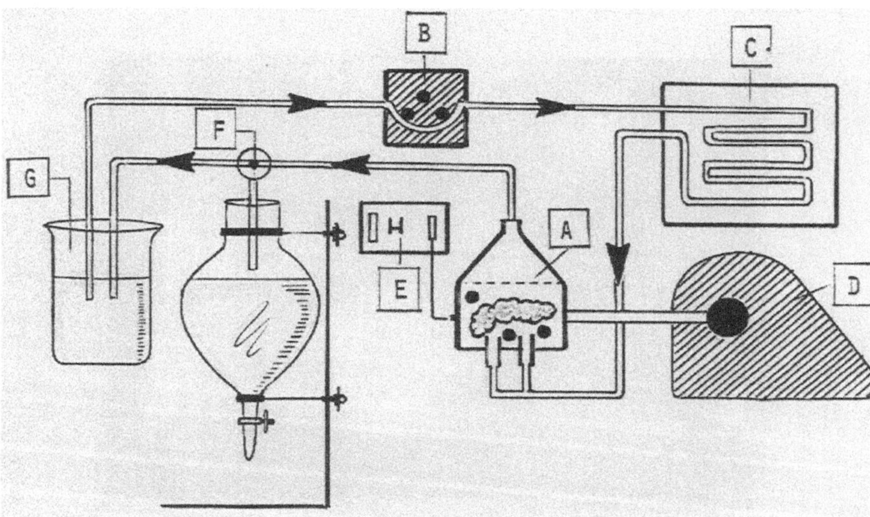

Fig. 2 ; Schematic representation of Ricordi's automated method for pancreatic islet isolation.
Flow diagram:
a) isolation chamber
b) peristaltic pump
c) heating circuit
d) mechanic shaker
e) thermometer
f) collection tank
g) recirculation cylinder

The next step is pancreas dissection at the level of the isthmus and cannulation of the Wirsung duct by means of a small venous catheter. Then, 250 ml of pre-heated collagenase are injected intraductally, which will induce considerable organ distension (Fig.3).

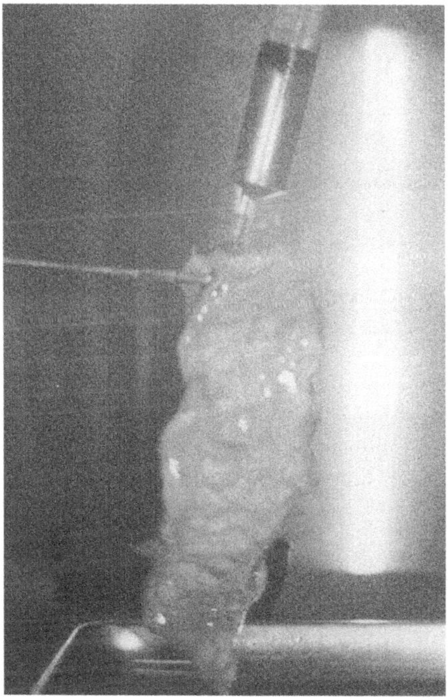

Figure 3. Marked gland distension induced by intraductal collagenase injection.
(see Color Plates, p. xx)

Isolation. after dissection, the pancreas is loaded into the digestion chamber, which is then perfectly closed (Fig.4 a/b). The peristaltic pump must be adjusted to provide a 100 ml/min flow, continuous shaking is started, and chamber temperature is maintained at a physiological level of 37°C by means of a thermostat, in order to keep collagenase active. Fluid is sampled every two minutes approximately, and observed under inverted microscopy after dithizone

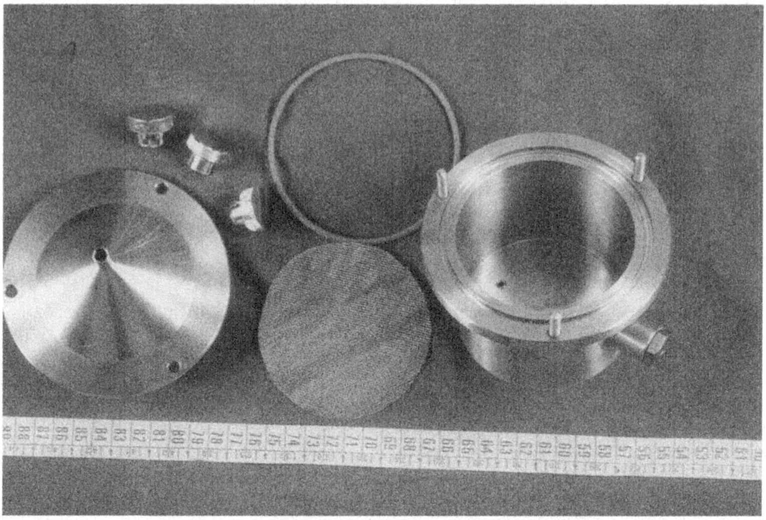

a

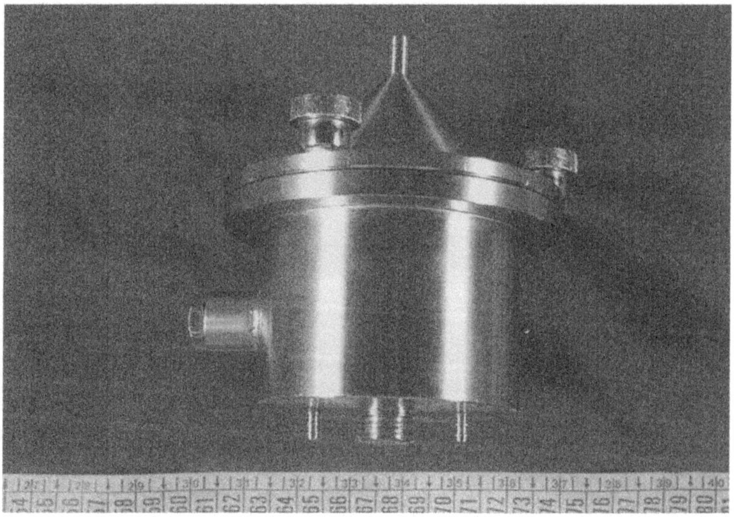

b

Figure 4. Upper and lower components of stainless steel isolation chamber, separated by a micropore screen allowing passage of particles below 400 micron in size (a). Assembled chamber (b).

(see Color Plates, p. xx)

Staining [19]: DTZ is a specific stain for detection of islet tissue which is a characteristic orange colour, while the remaining exocrine parenchyma is black (Fig.5).

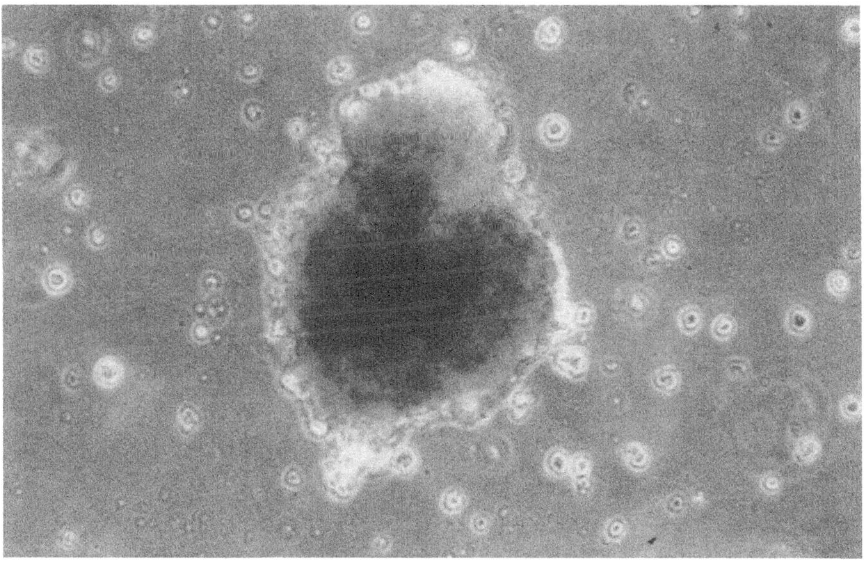

Figure 5. Dithizone stained pancreatic islet observed with inverted light microscopy at the end of digestion. (see Color Plates, p. xxii)

When free pancreatic islet cells with no exocrine acinar tissue can be observed through the microscope, the harvesting phase can be started. Temperature must therefore be reduced in the circuit, and the islet containing outflowing fluid is collected in Corning type 250 ml tubes which will then be stored in ice before centrifugation is started. Tubes containing digested pancreatic tissue are then pelleted by centrifugation at 4 °C, and the pancreatic tissue is washed 2 or 3 times in order to completely remove collagenase from the cells, and pellet the remaining tissue (Fig.6).

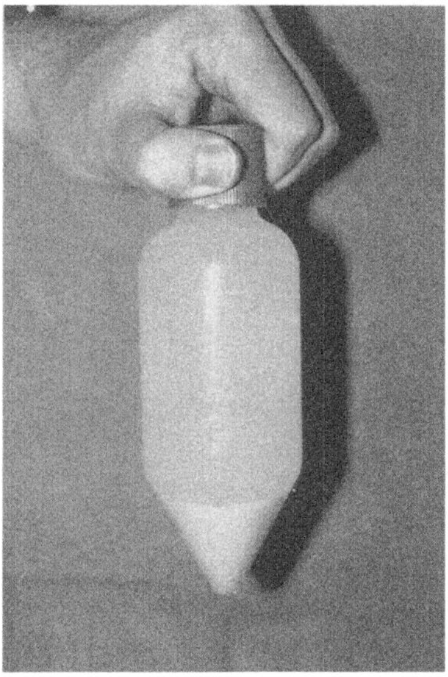

Figure 6. Post-centrifugation Corning tube containing mixed pancreatic material pelleted at the bottom
(see Color Plates, p. xxi)

Purification: For purification [20,21,22,23], solutions with different density gradients have to be used, i.e. Ficoll 1108, 1096 e 1037. The pellet obtained at the end of the previous isolation stage is separated from the HBSS and mixed with Ficoll 1108. The remaining Ficoll gradients are then layered on the solution obtained, using special bags if a Cobe 2991 type cell-separator is used [24], or tubes for normal centrifugation. In both cases, islet purification is obtained after tissue centrifugation of 10-20 minutes. At the end of the purification phase, the islets are located between the layer of Ficoll 1037 and that of 1096 (Fig.7).

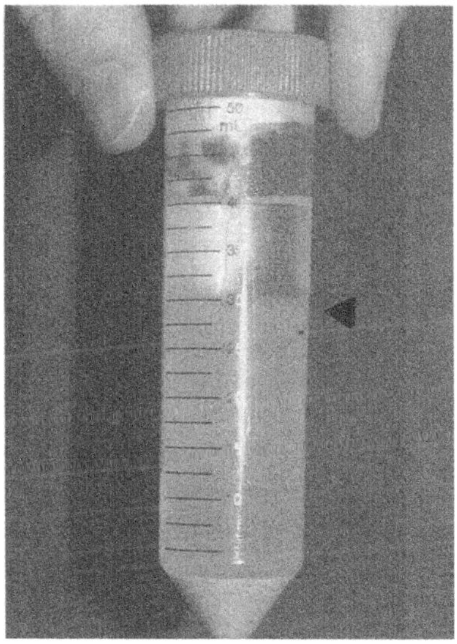

Figure 7. At the end of the purification phase, islets are pelleted at the interface between Ficoll solutions 1096 and 1037. Non- islet material is deposited at the bottom. (see Color Plates, p. xxi)

After 2 or 3 additional washes by centrifugation to completely remove the Ficoll solution, islets are counted and, if the number is sufficient (4/500.000), they are mixed with the transplant media (HBSS, albumin and heparin) and loaded into the transfer bags, to be carried either into the operating theatre or into the x-ray suite for transplantation.

Islet graft

Pancreatic islet cell isolation and purification were not the only obstacles to be overcome by the different authors dealing with the problem of islet transplantation. An additional obstacle concerned the identification of a suitable implant site, which had to be necessarily heterotopic.

Over the years, different heterotopic sites have been experimented with

[25,26,27,28], since transplantation success was found to be heavily dependent on capacity of islet adaptation surrounding tissue. The following sites have been tested: subcutaneous, intramuscular, intrathymic [20,30], under the renal capsule [31], omental [32] and intraperitoneal. However, successful results have only been obtained with the intrahepatic site, which is currently extensively used in all centers where islet cell- transplantation is carried out [33,34].

Intrahepatic transplantation has been attempted ever since the late 70's experience by Lazarow and Sutherland [35] and is currently performed by means of islet embolization in the portal system. Besides offering better engraftment results, the intrahepatic site requires a simple transplantation technique. The procedure can be carried out in two different ways:

1) Open surgery: after performing a medial minilaparotomy, the mesenteric vascularization of an intestinal loop is identified and a tributary vessel to the portal system is isolated. After ligating the distal end of the vessel, cannulation is performed with a medium to large gauge venous catheter which is connected to the transfer bag containing the islet cells embedded in the transplant media. After checking vessel patency, islets are subjected to embolization by gravity for 10-20 minutes. Infusion must be slow in order to avoid hypertension or portal thrombosis and promote better islet dispersion in the hepatic parenchyma (Fig.8).

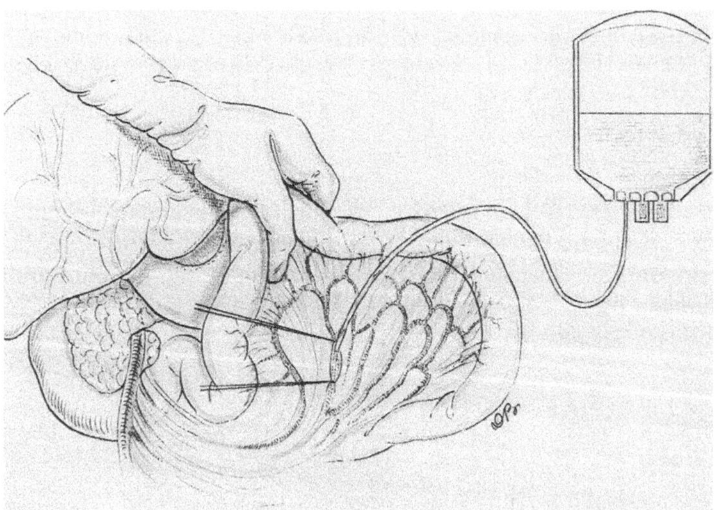

Figure 8. Pancreatic islet transplantation approach with cannulation of a vessel in the mesenteric district (schematic representation).

2) Percutaneous graft: an ultrasound-guided or fluoroscopy-based intraportal injection is administered by transparietohepatic approach [36]. After echo-doppler confirmation of portal patency, the $10^{th}/11^{th}$ intercostal spaces and the medial axillary line are used as landmarks for peripheral portal branches. Under local anaesthesia, a Chiba needle is percutaneously introduced into the liver parenchyma under ultrasound control. If the x-ray-based technique is used, needle placement is monitored by injecting a small amount of fluoroscopy-visible radio-opaque contrast medium. A catheter is passed through the needle until the intrahepatic bifurcation of the portal vein is reached with the distal end of the catheter. The proximal end is connected to the transfer bag and islets are transplanted using a method which is exactly the same as the one used for the previous procedure. (Fig.9).

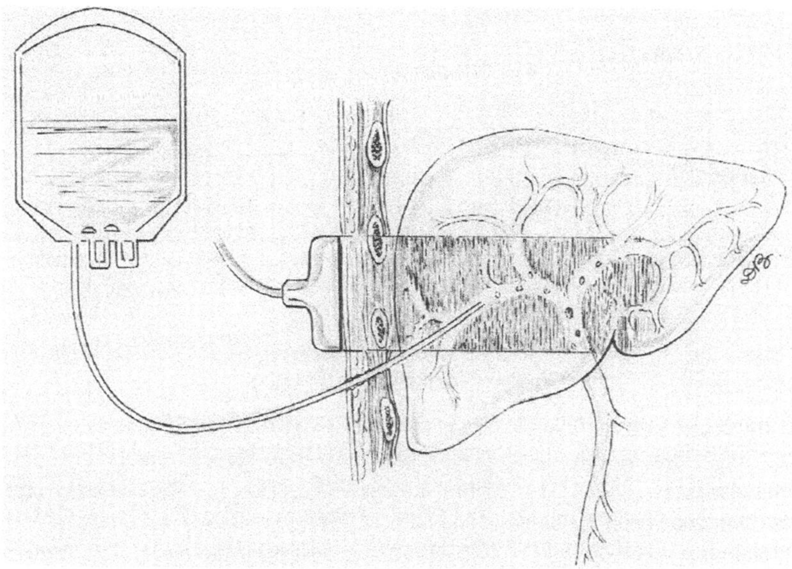

Figure 9. Pancreatic islet transplantation by intraportal injection through the hepatic wall (schematic representation).

International islet transplant registry

The ITR (Islet Transplant Registry) [15] was established in order to collect world-wide data on pancreatic islet transplants in humans, and is co-ordinated by M.Brendel, M.D., from Giessen University (Germany).

The general goals of the Registry are the following:

-Data collection on all islet allo-, auto- and xenotransplants throughout the world.
-Execution of scientific data analysis, group comparisons and research group co-ordination.
-Publication of analysis results in an annual newsletter distributed to all interested institutions.
-Promotion and maintenance of contacts among all institutions dealing with pancreatic islets.

ITR data include all scientifically documented islet transplants up to the end of December '96 , totalling 330 allotransplants (Fig.10) performed in centres throughout the world (Tab.1).

PANCREATIC ISLET TRANSPLANTATION 335 cases

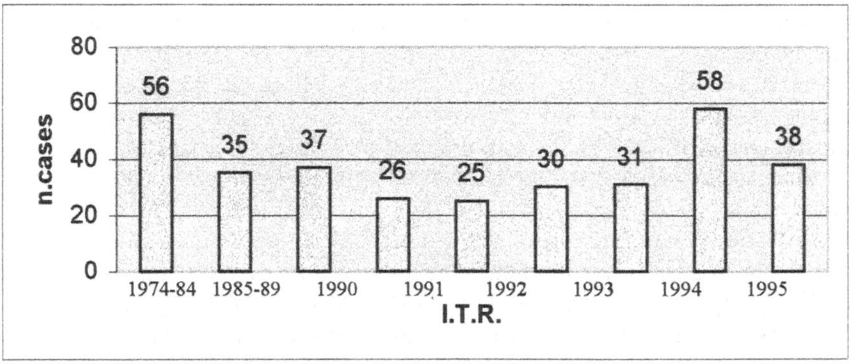

Figure 10. The number of grafts has considerably increased since 1990, after adopting the automated isolation method and improving purification techniques.

The number of very active centres is however extremely limited; in fact, from '94 to date, only 5 institutions have performed more than three transplants (Giessen 28, Minneapolis 15, Miami 14, Milan 8, and Pittsburgh 7). The greatest number of transplants has been executed at the Dept. of Surgery of the University of Minnesota (Minneapolis) directed by Dr Sutherland, i.e. 54 up till the end of '96. Based on the recipient category, we can conclude that simultaneous islet and renal transplantation (37%), and islet transplantation in previous renal transplant recipients (32,5%) account for 69.5% of all transplants performed, while isolated islet transplants have increased to 17,9%. The remaining cases were performed in association with transplants of liver (10,4%) and other organs. Transplant function results, based on recipient category, indicate that the groups "islets after renal transplant" and "islet+kidney" show the best functional results (Fig.11). As regards the graft site, the intrahepatic site is most frequently selected for intraportal embolization and no other site can give satisfactory results.

Moreover, an analysis of the data collected at the different centres shows that insulin-independence can be obtained by complying with four requirements:

1) Cold ischemia time of retrieved pancreas <8 ore.
2) Transplantation of >= 6.000 Islet Equivalents (IEQ) / kg of recipient weight.
3) Intraportal approach to intrahepatic graft site.
4) Induction of immunosuppression with Anti-lymphocytic Globulin (ALG).

If all the above criteria are complied with, insulin-independence is obtained in 46% of all cases, as shown by a study carried out on 75 patients and documented in the International Registry (Tab.2).

Table 2. Islet functional survival one year after transplantation is 46% in all the cases in which the four fundamental criteria described in the paper were respected. Survival drops to 22% if one or more of the above requirements are not complied with.

ISLET FUNCTIONAL SURVIVAL
1 YEAR after TRANSPLANTATION in 75 PATIENTS (1990-94)

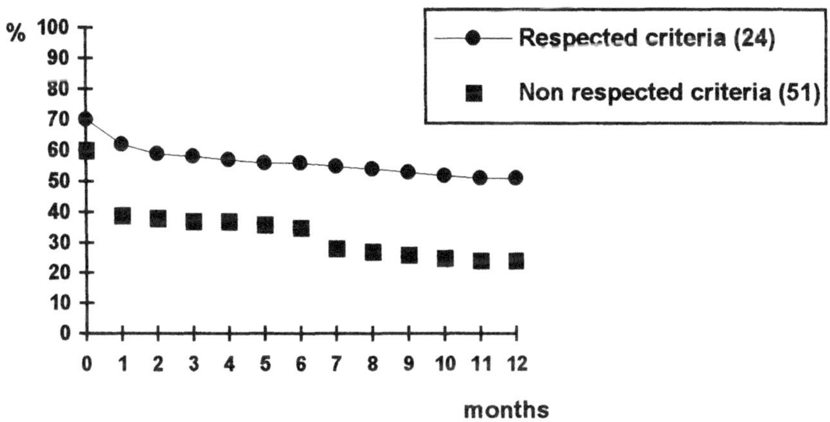

Personal experience

Our school has been dealing for some time with the surgical treatment of insulin-dependent diabetes mellitus (IDDM), by carrying out clinical and experimental activities. Several years ago, experimental studies were started on hybrid artificial pancreas (HAP), using islet tissue retrieved from rat pancreata, introduced by means of a special catheter provided with a millipore membrane. The catheter was then placed into the portal vein of pigs with alloxane-induced diabetes. Results were satisfactory only in the very short term, since insulin release stopped after less than one month. Animals were sacrificed, and retrieved catheters were found to be coated with an exuberant fibrin layer which prevented recirculation and caused insulin secretion discontinuation. Later on, in 1978, after segmental transplantation, with Neoprene intraductal injection, had been introduced into clinical practice (Dubernard e coll.), we performed the first segmental pancreas transplant in a chronic pancreatic patient that had undergone total pancreatectomy. In the following years, additional allografts and a number of segmental allografts were performed, both with and without simultaneous renal transplant.

Following the international guidelines, we are currently interested in pancreatic islet-transplantation, and have carried out a great number of experiments in order to check the reproducibility of Ricordi's automated method, which, alongside with islet-purification,is a key element for success (Fig. 12).

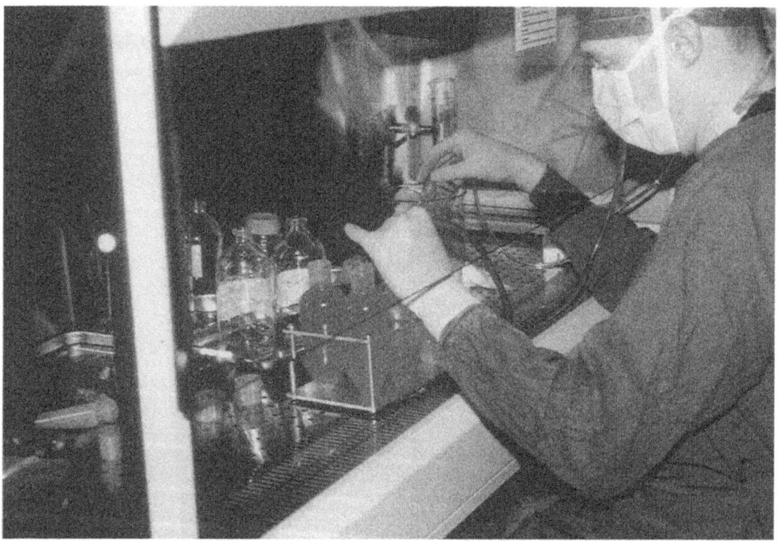

Figure 12. Preparation of the solutions necessary for pancreas digestion in a laminar flow room. (see Color Plates, p. xxi)

We have concluded that the isolation and purification methods enable us to obtain an adequate number of viable pancreatic islets (morphologically intact and functionally active) that can eventually be transplanted [37]. The average number of cells obtained after each successful processing cycle has been 390,000 IEQ. This is an extremely satisfactory result that paves the way for single-donor fresh

islet transplantation, with no need for cryopreserved islets. By transplanting a single and fresh sample, exacerbation of all the immunogenetic reactions triggered off by multiple cryopreserved sample transplants from different donors can be prevented.
The functional aspects have been assessed by means of static function tests and solutions with increasing glucose concentrations, which have confirmed islet capacity to stimulate an insulin secretion which is proportional to the increasing glucose load. Morphological assessments were performed by means of light microscopy studies, using hematoxylin-eosin staining, and then carrying out immunohistochemical investigations in order to identify insulin granules in β-cells (Fig.13a-b).

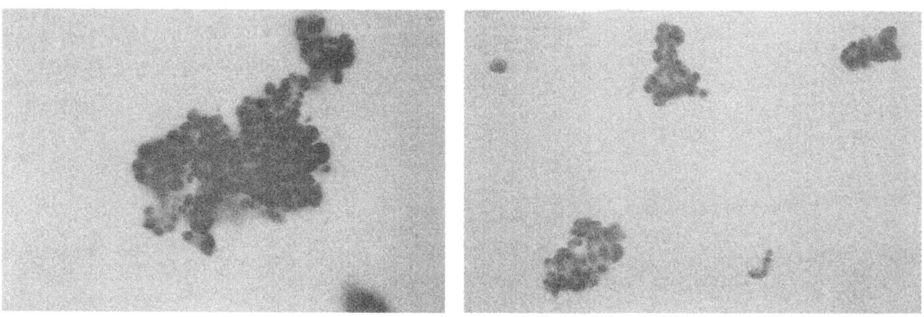

a b

Figure 13 . Identification of intact islets: normal nucleus/cytoplasm ratio, normal nucleus and intercellular contacts. No pyknosis and/or intracellular necrosis and no cytoplasmatic degeneration (40x magnification) (a). By immmunohistochemical analysis with antichromogranin A antibody, islet cells are identified that are rich intracytoplasmic granules (25x magnification) (b).
(see Color Plates, p. xxii)

The same morphological and functional assessment was repeated on cryopreserved pancreatic islet samples, in order to identify and evaluate any possible freezing-induced damage in the islets to be added to the fresh ones for transplantation, and to be able to obtain the best functional results. In the last few cases, we have also performed an electron microscopy study on purified islets, to confirm perfect morphological conditions and functional capacity [38]. Electron microscopy studies have enabled us to observe directly insulin secretion and identify β-cell-stimulated granule exocytosis (Fig. 14 a-b-c-d).

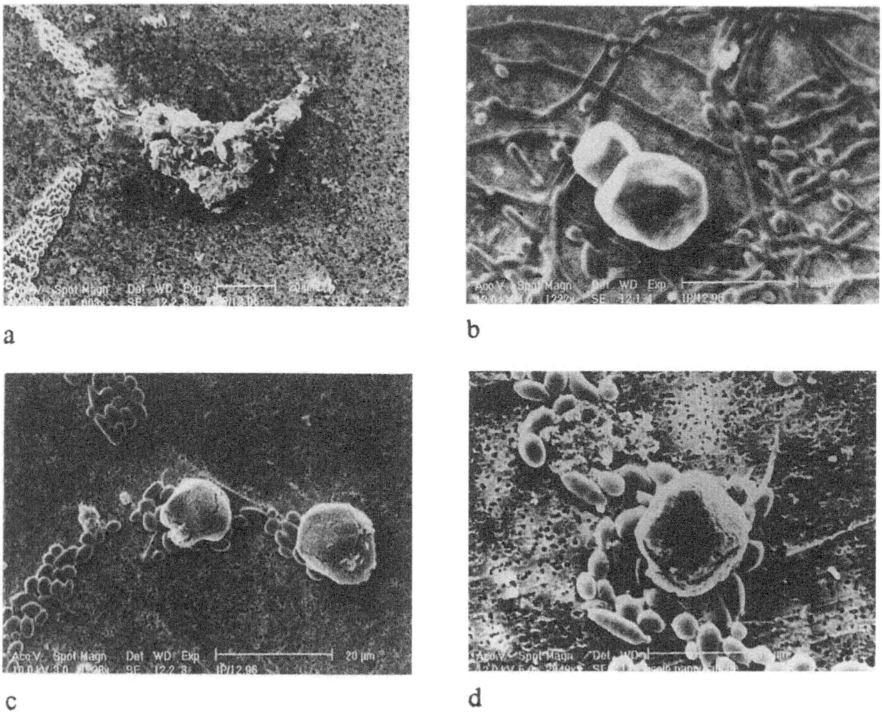

Figure 14. Electron microscopy magnification (=603X) of an intact pancreatic islet in cellular culture (a); Beta-cell magnification (=1222X) embedded in pancreatic islet matrix (b); Magnification (=1228X) of a beta-cell secreting insulin-rich vesicles (c); Magnification (=2456X) of detail of a beta-cell during insulin-rich vesicle exocytosis (d).

Thanks to these SEM studies, actual islet viability has been confirmed.
Based on these experimental results, we believe that Ricordi's automated method can be perfectly and effectively reproduced, as we have been able to confirm that it is possible to obtain an adequate number of morphologically intact and functionally active islets suitable for transplantation.

Table 1. List of pancreatic islet allotransplants (plus one xenotransplant) grouped up by institution and year till December 31, 1996.

Institution (Islet Transplantation/ Islet Isolation)	Year of Transplantation <90	90	91	92	93	94	95	Σ
• Minneapolis	24	1	4	5	5	2	10	51
• Pittsburgh	-	17	6	4	3	4	3	37
• St. Louis	13	3	3	2	4	2	-	27
• Miami	5	4	2	1	1	3	9	25
• Giessen	-	-	-	1	5	5	12	23
• Milan	1	4	3	3	4	4	4	23
• Genoa	13	-	-	-	-	-	-	13
• Berlin (Charité)	8	-	-	-	-	-	-	8
• Zurich	8	-	-	-	-	-	-	8
• Detroit	7	-	-	-	-	-	-	7
• Edmonton	2	2	-	1	-	1	1	7
• Oxford	-	-	1	1	1	1	3	7
• Paris	3	3	1	-	-	-	-	7
• Perugia	3	1	1	-	-	2	-	7
• Madrid	-	-	-	2	1	1	2	6
• Brussels	-	-	-	-	-	1	4	5
• Odense/Milan	-	-	-	-	-	-	5	5
• San Francisco/ LA(UCLA-VA)	-	-	-	-	1	1	3	5
• London (Ontario)/ St. Louis	-	2	1	1	-	-	-	4
• Leicester	-	-	2	1	-	-	-	3
• Los Angeles (UCLA-VA)	-	-	-	3	-	-	-	3
• Padua/Verona	2	-		-	1		-	3
• Los Angeles (St. Vincent)	-	-	-	-	2	1	-	3
• Charlestown	-	-	2	-	-	-	-	2
• Hanover	2	-	-	-	-	-	-	2
• Newcastle -upon-Tyne	2		-	-	-	-	-	2
• Berlin (Moabit)	1	-	-	-	-	-	-	1
• Bristol	1	-	-	-	-	-	-	1

continue

Table 1.(continued)

• Geneva	-	-	-	-	-	1	-	1
• Heidelberg/Giessen	1	-	-	-	-	-	-	1
• Homburg	-	-	-	-	1	-	-	1
• Innsbruch/Milan	-	-	-	-	-	-	2	2
• Leiden	1	-	-	-	-	-	-	1
• London (Ontario)	-	-	-	-	-	1	-	1
• New York	1	-	-	-	-	-	-	1
• Omaha	-	-	-	-	-	1	-	1
• Petah Tiqwah	1	-	-	-	-	-	-	1
• Wuerzburg/Giessen	-	-	-	-	1	-	-	1
Σ	**99**	**37**	**26**	**25**	**30**	**31**	**58**	**306**

References

1. Ricordi C. 1892-1992 one century of transplantation for diabetes. Pancreatic islet cell transplantation. R.G. Landes Company Austin 1992: XV.
2. Warnock G, Ryan EA, Kneteman NM, Rajotte RV. Transplantation of pancreatic islet cells into type I diabetic humans: the University of Alberta experience. In: Ricordi C. Ed. Pancreatic islet cell transplantation. Austin, Texas (USA): R.G. Landes Company, 1992: 400-9.
3. Alejandro R, Strasser S, Esquenazi V, Burke G, Nery J, Miller J, Shapiro ET, Ricordi C, Mintz DH. Long-term survival of intraportal islet allografts in type I diabetes mellitus. In: Ricordi C. Ed. Pancreatic islet cell transplantation. Austin, Texas (USA): R.G. Landes Company, 1992: 410-3.
4. Socci C, Ricordi C, Di Carlo V, Falqui L, Maffi P, Pozza G, Davalli AM, Secchi A. Substitution of the endocrine pancreatic function in IDDM patients. In: Ricordi C. Ed. Pancreatic islet cell transplantation. Austin, Texas (USA): R.G. Landes Company, 1992: 414-22.
5. Gores PF, Najarian JS, Sutherland DER. Clinical islet allotransplantation. The University of Minnesota Experience. In: Ricordi C. Ed. Pancreatic islet cell transplantation. Austin, Texas (USA): R.G. Landes Company, 1992: 423-33.
6. Ricordi C, Alejandro R, Fontes PAC, Starzl TE, Carroll P, Zeng Y, Shapiro R, Tzakis A, Rilo HLR, Fung JJ. Islet transplantation in diabetes: the Pittsburgh experience. In: Ricordi C. Ed. Pancreatic islet cell transplantation. Austin, Texas (USA): R.G. Landes Company, 1992: 448-53.
7. London NJM, Robertson GM, Feehlay J, Bolia A, James RFL, Chadwick D, Burden F, Bell PRF. Human islet transplantation: the Leicester experience. In: Ricordi C. Ed. Pancreatic islet cell transplantation. Austin, Texas (USA): R.G. Landes Company, 1992: 454-61.
8. Federlin KF, Bretzel RG, Hering BJ. Islet transplant registry. In: Ricordi C. Ed. Pancreatic islet cell transplantation. Austin, Texas (USA): R.G. Landes Company, 1992: 462-72.
9. Williams PW. Notes on diabetes treated with extract and by graft of sheep's pancreas. *Br Med J* 1994; 1303.
10. Moskalewski S. Isolation and culture of the islets of Langerhans of the Guinea pig. *Gentile Comp Endocrin* 1965; 5: 342.
11. Lacy PE, Lostianowsky M. Method for the isolation of intact islets of Langerhans from the rat pancreas. *Diabetes* 1967; 16: 35.
12. Ballinger WF, Lacy PE. Transplantation of intact pancreatic islets in rats. *Surgery* 1972; 72: 175.
13. Ricordi C, Lacy PE. Automated method for isolation of human pancreas islets. *Diabetes* 1988; 37: 413.

14. Tzakis AG, Ricordi C, Alejandro R. Pancreatic islet transplantation after upper abdominal exenteration and liver replacement. *Lancet* 1990; 336: 402.

15. International islet transplant registry. Newsletter n. 7 - Vol. 6 (n. 1, december 1996).

16. Ricordi C. Pancreatic islet cell transplantation. R.G. Landes Company Austin 1992.

17. Lacy PE. Islet transplantation. The future. In: Ricordi C. Ed. Pancreatic islet cell transplantation. Austin, Texas (USA): R.G. Landes Company, 1992: 394-9.

18. Kneteman NM, Lakey JRT, Warnock GL, Rajotte RV. Pancreas procurement and preservation: impact on islet recovery and viability. In: Ricordi C. Ed. Pancreatic islet cell transplantation. Austin, Texas (USA): R.G. Landes Company, 1992: 72-81.

19. Latif ZA, Noel J, Alejandro R. A simple method of staining fresh and cultured islets. *Transplantation* 1988; 45: 827-30.

20. Downing R, Morrisey S, Kiske D, Scharp DW. Does the purity of intraportal islet isografts aspect their endocrine function? *J Surg Res* 1986; 41: 41-6.

21. Gotoh M, Maki T, Satomi S. Immunological characteristics of purified pancreatic islet grafts. *Transplantation* 1986; 42: 387-90.

22. London NJM, Toomey P, Contractor H. The effect of osmolality on the purity of human islet isolated. *Transplant Proc* 1992; 24: 312-6.

23. Olack B, Swanson C, Mc Lear M. Islet purification using euro-ficoll gradients. *Transplant Proc* 1991; 23(1): 774-6.

24. London NJM, James RFL, Bell PRF. Islet purification. In: Ricordi C. Ed. Pancreatic islet cell transplantation. Austin, Texas (USA): R.G. Landes Company, 1992: 113-23.

25. White SA, Dennison AR, Swift SM, Davies JM, Clayton HA, Burden AC. Intraportal and splenic human islet autotransplantation combined with total pancreatectomy. *Transplant Proc* 1998; 30: 312.

26. White SA, Birch JF, Forshaw MJ, Power DM, Dennison AR. Splenic human islet autotransplantation; anatomical variations of splenic venous drainage. *Transplant Proc* 1998; 30: 314.

27. Barbich M, Hyon SH, Vieiro Laucirica M, Mullen J, Sorroche P, Furzi A. Effect of embolization of impure islets on liver histology and biochemical variables. *Transplant Proc* 1998; 30: 415.

28. Altmann JJ, Tessier C. Arteriolar epiploic site for islet transplantation in man. *Diabetologia* 1981; 40: 64A.

29. Di Silvio M, Murase N. Intrathymic transplantation of hepatocytes is facilitated by the addicyion of pancreatic islets. *Transplant Proc* 1992; 24: 2987.

30. Korgsen O, Jansson L, Anderson D. Effects of hyperglicemia on function of isolated mouse pancreatic islets transplanted under kidney capsule. *Diabetes* 1989; 38: 510-5.

31. Sutherland DER, Braymann KL, Farney AC, Matas AJ. Evaluation of intrathymic islet transplantation in the prediabetic period. *Surgery* 1992; 112: 319-26.

32. Ao Z, Matayoshi K, Iwata H. Development of an omental pouch site for islet cell transplantation. *Transplant Proc* 1992; 24: 2789.

33. Alejandro R, Burke G, Mintz DH. Intraportal islet allografts in type I diabetes mellito. *Transplant Proc* 1992; 24: 959-60.

34. Carrol PB, Ricordi C, Tzakis A, Alejandro R, Rilo HRL, Fontes P. Intraepathic human islet transplantation at the University of Pittsburgh: results in 25 consecutive cases. *Transplant Proc* 1992; 24: 3038-9.

35. Sutherland DER, Matas AJ, Goetz FC, Najarian JS. Transplantation of dispersed islet tissue in humans. *Diabetes* 1980, 29(S1): 31-44.

36. Rilo HRL, Brow K, Tzakis A, Fontes P, Carrol P, Shapiro R. Percutaneous approach for human islet transplantation. *Transplant Proc* 1992; 24: 3054-5.

37. Greco VM, Conti A, Colacci AM, Santini D, Casadei R, Capelli M. Il trapianto di isole pancreatiche. Studio morfologico e valutazione funzionale in vitro di isole purificate crioconservate. Atti XIX Congresso Nazionale SIRC, Varese, 10-11 maggio 1996; 159-67.

38. Marrano D, Greco VM, Conti A, Okoro HU, Casadei R, Leone A. Modelli sperimentali per lo studio in vivo e in vitro della vitalità e delle proprietà immunogeniche delle isole pancreatiche. Rapporti ISTISAN 97/19: primo progetto di ricerca, sostituzioni funzionali, organi artificiali e trapianti d'organo 1997; 249-52.

Author Index

Subject Index

GPSR Compliance

The European Union's (EU) General Product Safety Regulation (GPSR) is a set of rules that requires consumer products to be safe and our obligations to ensure this.

If you have any concerns about our products, you can contact us on ProductSafety@springernature.com

In case Publisher is established outside the EU, the EU authorized representative is:

Springer Nature Customer Service Center GmbH
Europaplatz 3
69115 Heidelberg, Germany

Batch number: 10584688

Printed by Printforce, the Netherlands